Small Animal Anesthesia
CANINE AND FELINE PRACTICE

TITLES IN THIS SERIES

SMALL ANIMAL ANESTHESIA
CANINE AND FELINE PRACTICE

Diane McKelvey, D.V.M. and K. Wayne Hollingshead, D.V.M.

SMALL ANIMAL SURGICAL NURSING

Diane L. Tracy, B.A., ED.M.

VETERINARY CLINICAL
LABORATORY PROCEDURES

Margi Sirois, B.S., R.V.T.

SERIES EDITOR

Douglas F. McBride, D.M.V.

Director
Veterinary Technology
LaGuardia Community College
Long Island, New York

Mosby's Fundamentals of Veterinary Technology

Small Animal Anesthesia

CANINE AND FELINE PRACTICE

Diane McKelvey, D.V.M.

Veterinary Technology
Centralia College
Huron Park, Ontario

K. Wayne Hollingshead, D.V.M., M.Sc.

Professor
Small Animal Medicine and Surgery
University College of the Cariboo
Kamloops, British Columbia

*with **71** illustrations*

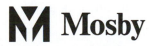

St. Louis Baltimore Berlin Boston Carlsbad Chicago London Madrid
Naples New York Philadelphia Sydney Tokyo Toronto

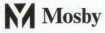
Mosby

Dedicated to Publishing Excellence

Editor: Linda L. Duncan
Developmental Editor: Jo Salway
Project Manager: Karen Edwards
Production Editor: Gail Brower
Design Coordinator: Elizabeth Fett

Printed in the United States of America
Composition by BI-COMP Incorporated
Printing/Binding by Maple-Vail Book Mfg. Group

Mosby–Year Book, Inc.
11830 Westline Industrial Drive
St. Louis, Missouri 63146

Library of Congress Cataloging in Publication Data

McKelvey, Diane.
    Small animal anesthesia : canine and feline practice / Diane
McKelvey, K. Wayne Hollingshead.
        p.   cm.—(Mosby's fundamentals of veterinary technology)
    Includes Index.
    ISBN 0-8016-7961-3 (hardcover)
    1. Dogs—Surgery. 2. Cats—Surgery. 3. Veterinary anesthesia.
I. Hollingshead, K. Wayne. II. Title. III. Series.
SF991.M27   1994
636.7'089796—dc20   94-1541
                                                                              CIP

94 95 96 97 98 / 9 8 7 6 5 4 3 2 1

TO OUR FAMILIES

Preface

Of all the disciplines taught to veterinary technician students, none is more challenging than veterinary anesthesia. It takes only a few minutes to teach someone the rudiments of how to run an anesthetic machine or how to check an animal's capillary refill time, but this by no means qualifies that person to be a veterinary anesthetist. Competent anesthesia, in its best sense, demands the following:

- A detailed knowledge of the actions, advantages, and possible side effects of injectable and inhalation agents used in veterinary anesthesia
- A thorough understanding of physiologic functions such as respiration, heart rate, and blood pressure, not only in the awake animal but also in the anesthetized patient
- The ability to accurately monitor an animal's vital signs and depth of anesthesia during the preanesthesia phase, the anesthesia period itself, and the recovery phase
- The ability to respond to an emergency with competence and assurance
- Complete familiarity with the anesthetic equipment used in small animal practice, particularly the various anesthetic machines
- Knowledge of specialized techniques, such as local analgesia, postoperative analgesia, and the use of muscle-paralyzing agents and ventilators

Although an anesthesia textbook or course can impart this knowledge, many hours of hands-on experience with animals is necessary in order to develop the skills and judgment of a competent anesthetist. Such experience leads the anesthetist to develop a healthy respect for the individual variations among patients and the numerous ways in which animals encountered in practice can differ from those described in textbooks.

Even more important than knowledge and experience, however, are the attitudes the anesthetist must develop and maintain in order to practice anesthesia with safety and a high level of patient care. Compassion, vigilance, and caution are as important as technical skill and knowledge. In fact, the anesthetist's attitude is probably as important as his or her knowledge in determining the safety of anesthesia for each patient. In the case of a trained veterinary technician, more mistakes are likely to be made because of inattention, fatigue, boredom, and laziness, than because the anesthetist had insufficient knowledge, judgment, or skill.

The anesthetist cannot afford to make many mistakes, since there is no other area of veterinary practice assigned to technicians in which poor quality of care can have such dire consequences. As anesthetist, the technician takes on the responsibility of maintaining the animal's well-being during a period in which the animal is under the influence of powerful drugs, some of which have the potential to seriously harm or kill the animal. This is a great responsibility, one which technicians have worked hard for many years (and are still working hard) to achieve. It is also a legitimate source of pride for many technicians that they have learned and mastered the techniques of anesthesia and have thereby earned the privilege of becoming veterinary anesthetists.

The question of the veterinary technician's role in anesthesia is still being debated within the veterinary community. In most jurisdictions, the legislation governing veterinary medicine gives the veterinarian the authority to delegate the responsibility for patient care, including anesthesia, to a qualified and competent staff member. Some veterinarians believe that certain procedures, such as intubation, should be reserved for veterinarians alone. Others accept that a well-trained technician can induce anesthesia, intubate and monitor patients, and perform other demanding tasks with assurance and skill. As authors, we have taken the latter view and have attempted to describe the full range of duties that can be legally delegated to technicians. It is our belief that as veterinarians accord status and recognition to veterinary technicians, they enhance the status of veterinary medicine as a whole.

Anesthesia, by its nature, is an inexact science, and many statements made in this book are subject to debate. Rather than presenting every opinion on every subject, we have elected to present views that currently reflect well-accepted opinion within veterinary anesthesiology circles. That is not to say that every statement made in this book is unfailingly accurate; no doubt time will reveal that the present understanding of anesthesia is incorrect or incomplete in some respects. We trust that the graduate veterinary technician will actively seek continuing education opportunities in anesthesia, as in all other disciplines, to maintain a high level of professionalism and knowledge.

Diane McKelvey

K. Wayne Hollingshead

Acknowledgments

We acknowledge the contributions of the following persons: Dr. Doris Dyson, who reviewed the manuscript and gave many valuable suggestions; Dr. Samuel Longiaru, who prepared the tables; and Jeanne Robertson, who drafted many of the figures. We would also like to thank Dr. Roger Warren, whose book "Small Animal Anesthesia" was the precursor of this present volume and also the source of many of the illustrations.

Contents

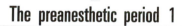

The preanesthetic period 1

2

General anesthesia 55

3

Anesthetic agents and techniques 119

4

Anesthetic equipment 163

5

Workplace safety 214

6

Anesthetic problems and emergencies 235

7

Special techniques 283

The preanesthetic period

1

Define the term *preanesthetic period.*

Understand the reasons for patient evaluation.

Understand the need for obtaining a proper history, know how to take a complete history, and know what pitfalls may be encountered when taking a history.

List the information that makes up the minimum data base for a patient.

Understand the rationale for obtaining the owner's consent for anesthesia.

State the parameters of a proper physical examination.

Understand the importance of species, breed, weight, and obesity as they relate to the use and choice of anesthetic drugs.

State the five physical classifications for patients as specified by the American Society of Anesthesiologists.

Describe the various aspects of preanesthetic preparation including choice of protocol, fasting, rationale for IV catheterization, and types of IV solutions that can be used and why they might be chosen.

State which preanesthetic agents are commonly used, the rationale for their use, their mode of action and effects on the body, and the associated adverse side effects.

Preanesthesia is a term that describes the period immediately preceding the induction of anesthesia. Throughout the preanesthetic period and the anesthetic period that follows, the goal of the technician is to work with the veterinarian to achieve efficient, safe, and effective anesthesia with minimal stress to the patient. This chapter describes the responsibilities of the technician during the preanesthetic period.

One of the most important duties of the technician is to help obtain patient information through history, physical examination, and diagnostic tests. This information is useful not only to the technician/anesthetist but also to the veterinarian, who must determine the patient's physical condition and select the anesthetic protocol. The technician also may be responsible for preanesthetic care of the patient including fasting, intravenous catheterization, and other procedures ordered by the veterinarian. To prepare for anesthesia, the technician must also ensure that the necessary equipment and supplies are available and in good working order (this will be further described in Chapter 4). Finally, the technician is usually responsible for administering preanesthetic drugs to the patient, as requested by the veterinarian, and must have a thorough knowledge of the actions and adverse side effects associated with these drugs.

PATIENT EVALUATION

Technicians working as anesthetists in small animal practice soon become accustomed to the wide variety of patients presented to the clinic. Animals vary in age, temperament, and physical appearance; some are healthy, and some are critically ill or injured; some are presented for minor procedures, whereas others are to undergo lengthy, more complicated surgery. Given this diversity, it is unrealistic to assume that the same anesthetic techniques should be used for all patients. Furthermore, it would be dangerous to expect all patients to react to a given anesthetic agent in the same way. It is therefore vital that the veterinarian and technician gather as much information as possible on each patient before initiating anesthesia to discover any factor that might lead to anesthetic complications. Accordingly, it is recommended that a *minimum patient data base* be obtained for each patient. If the information obtained on a given animal reveals a potential problem, the veterinarian may choose to alter the planned anesthetic procedure or postpone (or even cancel) the anesthesia.

The minimum patient data base should include the following, at the discretion of the veterinarian:
1. A patient history
2. The nature of the procedure to be performed with the patient under anesthesia
3. A complete physical examination
4. Diagnostic tests requested by the supervising veterinarian, including radiography, electrocardiography, urinalysis, hematology, and clinical chemistry

5. In consultation with the veterinarian, determination of the patient's physical status and anesthetic risk

Patient history

No examination of an animal is complete without an adequate history. Obtaining a good history requires skill and care and, like all arts, must be continually practiced and refined. If the technician asks questions that require only a "yes or no" answer, the history may be incomplete or misleading. Thus to ask, "Does your dog drink much water?" would not encourage the client to provide specific information. Asking, "How much water does your dog drink?" would require the client to describe the *amount* of water consumed but not judge whether he or she believes the amount to be abnormal. If the client replied, for example, "About 4 liters," the questioner then would be able to evaluate the information and may decide that 4 liters of water per day is excessive for a 2-kg Chihuahua, despite the owner's possible belief that this is normal.

Another common error is to ask leading questions of the owner. With reference to the previous example, asking the question "Your dog doesn't drink much water, does she?" would suggest to the owner that the appropriate response should be "No, I guess not." A technician asking such a question would fail to obtain an accurate patient history.

To obtain a complete history for any patient requiring anesthesia, the technician should ask the owner the following questions:
1. What is the procedure to be performed on the animal (e.g., surgery, dentistry, diagnostic procedure)?
2. How old is the pet?
3. Has the animal had any previous illnesses, and if so, what was the medical or surgical treatment? Obviously, the patient's record may supplement the owner's information. A history that includes diseases of the heart and circulatory system, respiratory system, kidneys, liver, blood, nervous system, endocrine organs, or gastrointestinal tract may be of significance to the anesthetist and surgeon and should be brought to the attention of the veterinarian.
4. Has the animal exhibited any signs of illness in the past 24 hours, including lack of appetite, coughing, sneezing, vomiting, diarrhea, or any other condition that is of concern to the owner? When was the animal last sick or ill, and has the animal recovered from this disease as far as the owner knows? Any reports of recent illness should alert the veterinarian or technician to focus particular attention on the physical examination of that organ system. Animals suffering from disease may be at increased risk of anesthetic complications because of dehydration, fever, or electrolyte abnormalities. Sick animals also may introduce pathogens into the hospital, posing a risk to other patients unless they are placed in isolation.

5. How well does the animal tolerate exercise? The owner may be able to describe the amount and type of daily exercise or play that is normal for the animal. Dyspnea or fatigue following mild exercise such as walking up a flight of stairs may indicate the presence of cardiovascular or respiratory disease, both of which should be of concern to the anesthetist.

6. Has the animal undergone recent treatment with drugs or insecticides? Many medications, including corticosteroids, insulin, anticonvulsants, antibiotics, and flea control products, may alter the effect of anesthetics.

7. Is there any history of allergies or drug reactions? The owner may be able to recall the animal's reaction to anesthetic agents used in the past. This information is particularly important if the animal has experienced prolonged recovery or personality changes following a previous anesthesia. In addition, if the animal has exhibited signs of an anaphylactic or other allergic reaction to any medication, this should be noted on the record and the information conveyed to the veterinarian.

8. When was the animal last vaccinated, and against which diseases was it vaccinated? Many veterinary clinics require current vaccinations for all healthy patients entering the clinic to prevent the spread of contagious diseases between patients.

9. What is the reproductive status of the animal? Has the animal been spayed or castrated? In the case of an intact female, has the owner observed any recent estrous cycle activity? Is it possible that the animal is pregnant? These questions are of particular importance if the animal is presented for an ovariohysterectomy, as the animal's reproductive status may affect the length and difficulty of the surgery. Animals in heat also may have increased blood clotting times, because of the effect of estrogen on the clotting cascade. This may result in excessive bleeding during surgery.

10. Has the owner observed any of the following: abnormal bleeding or bruising? fainting? seizures? difficulty in passing stool or urine? If the owner answers "yes" to any of these questions, the veterinarian should be consulted, since a serious illness may be present.

At the same time the patient history is obtained, it is customary to obtain a signed release authorizing anesthesia and surgery. It is illegal in many jurisdictions to undertake surgery or anesthesia on an animal without the owner's written consent. Such consent must be "informed," meaning that the owner is warned before anesthesia of any unusual risks associated with the anesthesia or surgery. Standard consent forms are available from practice management consultants and from state and provincial veterinary associations. Owners should be asked to provide a telephone number at which they may be reached during the day, if an emergency or unforeseen complication should arise. It is also advisable that a written estimate of fees be presented to the owner before initiating the procedure.

Obviously, a great deal of information must be obtained for each patient before initiating anesthesia. Ideally, the history is obtained in person by the veterinarian or technician. A trained receptionist may be able to assist, particularly when a young, healthy animal is presented for an elective surgery such as castration or ovariohysterectomy. It is important to ensure that any hospital employee who admits a patient and speaks to the owner not only obtains a history but also relays that information to the anesthetist by means of a written record or oral report.

In some cases it may be difficult to obtain the history in person. Some clinics prefer to have the owner fill out a prepared history form, particularly if the clinic has a high volume of patients. In any practice, difficulties may arise when an animal's owner is in a hurry and reluctant to stop and answer questions; however, it is usually possible to obtain a telephone number and call for more information at a prearranged time. Occasionally the person bringing the animal into the clinic is not the owner and is unfamiliar with the pet. In this case, every effort should be made to contact the owner by telephone to obtain a more complete history.

In a busy practice, it is often difficult to set aside adequate time to obtain a good history, and the technician may be tempted to shortcut or omit one or more questions. The importance of obtaining a complete history on each animal cannot be overemphasized. The experienced anesthetist knows that a thorough history will help avoid unpleasant surprises during anesthesia and surgery. A dog that has been coughing regularly and tires easily when chasing a ball may well have a cardiac problem unknown to the owner. If this problem is not described in the animal's history, the technician may be surprised to find herself dealing with an anesthetized patient suffering from pulmonary edema, circulatory failure, and ultimately, cardiac arrest.

Physical examination

A complete physical examination should be conducted on every animal presented for anesthesia. Although the examination is usually carried out by a veterinarian, the technician should be familiar with the procedure. In some jurisdictions, veterinary technicians are certified to perform basic physical examinations provided they are acting under the direct supervision of a licensed veterinarian.

The physical examination is important because it may reveal the following:
1. The presence of respiratory or cardiovascular disease, which can increase the risk of anesthetic complications and possibly death.
2. The presence of a disorder such as an enlarged liver or abnormally small kidneys, either of which may indicate a reduced ability to detoxify or excrete anesthetic agents.
3. Conditions requiring veterinary attention. Some of the more common disorders that are easily detected by physical examination include ear mite infestation,

otitis externa, dental disease, overgrown nails, the presence of fleas, and anal sac impaction. Often the owner is unaware that these disorders are present and, once informed, will authorize the veterinarian to treat the disorder while the animal is anesthetized.

4. Physical factors that may affect the procedure to be performed with the patient under anesthesia. One surprisingly common example is the discovery that a cat brought in for an ovariohysterectomy is actually a male. It is far better to discover this mistake before undertaking anesthesia than to become aware of the problem during surgery! Another common example is the presentation of a cryptorchid animal for castration: the owner should be informed that the animal is a cryptorchid and that an increased fee may be charged for the surgery.

It is often helpful to have the owner present during the physical examination to give pertinent history regarding any physical abnormalities that are found. Any unusual findings should be brought to the attention of the veterinarian for confirmation. It is the veterinarian's responsibility to formulate an appropriate treatment plan and advise the technician accordingly.

Some veterinary clinics routinely recommend that animals that are to undergo elective surgeries be brought into the clinic for an appointment before the day of surgery. Procedures that can be done at this time include obtaining a complete history, performing a physical examination in the presence of the owner, administering necessary vaccinations, undertaking routine preanesthetic screening such as heartworm tests, giving information on preanesthetic fasting of the animal, obtaining signed consent forms, and giving the owner an estimate of surgery and anesthesia fees. By scheduling such an appointment several days before the planned surgery date, time is available for unforeseen problems to be discovered and addressed well in advance of surgery.

The complete physical examination should include the signalment, disposition, and activity level of the animal and an examination of the organ systems.

Signalment

The signalment includes the species, breed, weight, age, sex, and whether the patient is neutered. Some of this information is best obtained from the animal's history, but as previously mentioned, it is wise to double-check the owner's opinion on issues such as the animal's gender and age.

Species and breed. First, identify the patient's species. Each species has a characteristic response to specific drugs. A cat may metabolize drugs differently than a dog. The technician or veterinarian may occasionally encounter an unfamiliar species, such as a rabbit, iguana, or parrot, and should consult specialty references and the veterinarian before undertaking the anesthetic procedures.

The differences in anatomy and physiology among the various breeds also may affect the response to an anesthetic agent or procedure. For example, endotracheal intubation is often difficult in a brachycephalic dog such as a bulldog. Brachycephalic dogs also are more likely to have breathing difficulties during anesthetic recovery because of airway obstruction caused by excess soft tissue in the oropharyngeal area. Sighthounds such as the greyhound or saluki may experience a prolonged recovery from thiobarbiturate anesthesia because of the relative absence of body fat and slow metabolism of barbiturates compared to other breeds of dogs.

Weight. It is important to weigh each animal accurately before anesthesia, since anesthetic dosages and intravenous fluid drip rates are calculated according to body weight. Simply estimating an animal's weight may lead to incorrect dosages, particularly in smaller patients. Animals lighter than 15 kg should be weighed on a pediatric scale to reduce the error that occurs when larger scales are used. The patient's weight should be compared to previous weights (as noted on the patient record) to determine whether weight gain or loss has occurred. Changes in weight may reflect changes in the patient's nutritional intake or overall state of health.

Age. The age of the patient can be an important consideration when deciding the anesthetic protocol or types of drugs used. The neonate (up to 2 weeks of age) or pediatric animal (2 to 8 weeks) is much less capable of metabolizing any injectable drug than is an adult animal, since the necessary liver metabolic pathways are not fully developed. At the other end of the scale, a geriatric animal may be unable to tolerate normal doses of some drugs because of poor hepatic or renal function. The net result in either case may be a slow recovery from anesthesia, particularly when injectable agents are used.

Disposition and activity level

Before initiating anesthesia, the veterinary technician should observe the animal's temperament and activity level, both of which will affect the selection of the anesthetic agents and their route of administration. For example, an animal that is anxious or aggressive may not become adequately sedated if a phenothiazine tranquilizer is used. In such cases, combining a phenothiazine tranquilizer with an opioid or using a neuroleptanalgesic agent may be preferable. On the other hand, animals that are calm and easily handled may be adequately sedated with phenothiazine tranquilizers alone, or the veterinarian may elect to omit sedation.

Aggressive animals are occasionally presented for anesthesia and surgery. Special handling techniques such as anesthetic chamber inductions or the oral administration of ketamine, xylazine, or Innovar-Vet may be necessary to restrain such patients without endangering hospital staff.

Examination of organ systems

There are probably as many ways to perform a thorough physical examination as there are veterinarians and technicians. The main criterion is that the examination be done in a systematic manner (e.g., from head to tail) and, ideally, should include all of the following:

1. *Notation of overall body condition* (e.g., dehydrated, emaciated, obese, weak, pregnant). Obesity is commonly observed in companion animals presented for anesthesia and poses some difficulties to the anesthetist. Obese animals often have reduced exercise tolerance and may show signs of dyspnea at rest, indicating inadequate cardiovascular and respiratory function. Venipuncture and auscultation may be difficult in these animals. When anesthetizing obese animals, drug dosages should be calculated based on the animal's *ideal* weight (however difficult this is to imagine) rather than the actual weight. The animal's size is indeed increased by the deposition of fat stores; however, the size of the target organ of anesthesia (the brain) is unaffected.

   Excessive thinness is also of concern to the anesthetist, since it may indicate the presence of an underlying disorder, such as renal failure or chronic parasitism. Animals with little body fat also may be unusually sensitive to the effect of some anesthetics and are prone to hypothermia.

   Pregnant animals present unique challenges to the anesthetist. Patients presented in early gestation or mid-gestation are at risk when given drugs such as xylazine that may cause abortion. Animals brought in for cesarean surgery also merit special consideration: the patient must be sufficiently anesthetized to allow the procedure to be performed humanely, yet the anesthetics may adversely affect the newborn puppies or kittens.

2. *Notation of body temperature*. The normal temperature range in the cat is 37.8 to 39.2° C (100.0-102.5° F). The normal range in the dog is 37.5 to 39.2° C (99.5-102.5° F). The veterinarian should be informed if the patient's temperature is outside the normal range.

3. *Examination of the head, including eyes, oral cavity, pharynx, ears, and nose.* The technician should examine the animal for wheezing or stertor (snoring) to determine whether an airway obstruction is present. Any disorder that could impede endotracheal intubation, such as the presence of redundant tissue in the oropharynx or difficulty in opening the mouth, should be noted. The gingivae should be observed for mucous membrane color and capillary refill time (CRT), which indicates whether cardiovascular function is adequate. If the gingivae are pigmented, mucous membrane color and CRT may be observed at other sites, such as the conjunctiva of the lower eyelid, the entrance to the vulva, or the tip of the prepuce.

4. *Observation of the pupillary light reflex and consensual light reflex* (Fig. 1-1). The pupillary light reflex is elicited by shining a beam of light (usually from a penlight or other portable light source) into one eye and noting whether the pupil of that eye constricts in response to light (direct reflex). At the same time, constriction of the pupil of the other eye should also be noted (consensual

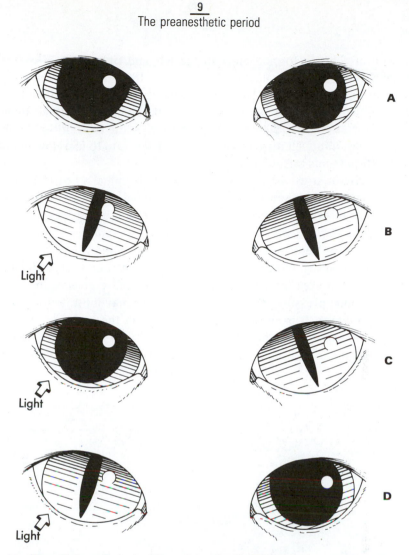

Fig. 1-1. Pupillary light reflex. **A,** Normal pupils. **B,** Direct and consensual light reflex (normal). **C,** Consensual but no direct light reflex (abnormal). **D,** Direct but no consensual light reflex (abnormal).

reflex). Normal animals have both a direct and a consensual light reflex when light is shined in each eye in turn, although this reflex may be altered by the use of some preanesthetic and anesthetic drugs.

5. *Auscultation of heart and lungs.* Auscultation of the chest is performed to determine heart rate and rhythm and to check for the presence of abnormal heart or lung sounds. Auscultation of the lungs is best performed by listening to at least four different areas of the chest, including the right and left anteroventral lung fields and the right and left dorsal lung fields. Auscultation of the heart

should also be performed on both the left and right sides of the chest. The normal range of heart rates for dogs is 70 to 180 beats per minute (bpm), with smaller breeds tending to have more rapid rates than larger breeds. The heart rate in giant breeds should be less than 100 bpm. The normal range of heart rates for cats is 110 to 200 bpm. In both species, the rhythm should be reasonably regular, although it is common for the heart rate to increase slightly during inspiration (sinus arrhythmia).

Exercise or stress of handling may cause an animal's heart rate to increase. Heart rate should be measured on a calm animal and, if possible, not immediately after inserting a thermometer or collecting a blood sample.

6. *Palpation of pulse and comparison of pulse rate and heart rate.* For the dog and cat, the pulse is most easily palpated at the femoral artery, on the medial side of the rear leg. Other sites that may be palpated include the metatarsal and metacarpal arteries (Fig. 1-2). Palpation of the pulse gives some indication of systolic blood pressure: a weak or absent pulse may indicate hypotension (low blood pressure). It is also important to compare the heart rate with the pulse rate: if the two are not the same (usually, the heart rate exceeds pulse rate), a pulse deficit exists, which may indicate the presence of cardiovascular disease.

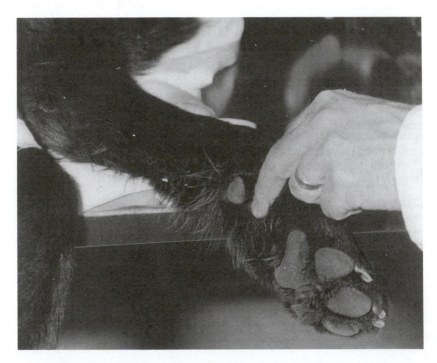

Fig. 1-2. Palpation of the metatarsal/metacarpal artery.

7. *Determination of respiratory rate and observation for dyspnea.* The normal respiratory rate for dogs is 10 to 30 breaths per minute and for cats is 25 to 40 breaths per minute. Animals experiencing *dyspnea* (difficult, labored breathing) may exhibit signs such as mouth breathing, flared nostrils, exaggerated chest or abdominal movements on inspiration, wheezing, and reluctance to lie down. In extreme cases, an animal with breathing difficulty may exhibit *cyanosis* (mucous membranes appear purple or blue). Any animal showing signs of dyspnea should be brought to the veterinarian's attention immediately. Dyspnea must be differentiated from rapid but normal breathing and from panting.

8. *Examination of the thorax, abdomen, and limbs to note any cutaneous lesions, condition of hair coat, and presence of parasites.* Although examination of the skin is seldom relevant to the anesthesia itself, it may indicate the presence of a disorder requiring treatment.

9. *Observation for lameness or localized pain in the extremities.*

10. *Palpation of superficial lymph nodes.* Enlarged lymph nodes may indicate the presence of a local or systemic infection, allergy, or neoplastic disease (cancer), all of which would be of concern to the anesthetist and surgeon.

11. *Abdominal palpation for pain, organ size and location, and the presence of fluid, gas, fetuses, or feces.*

12. *Observation of mammary glands for signs of lactation (in the case of intact females), particularly if the animal is pregnant or postpartum.* The vulva should also be observed for indications of estrus activity or the presence of a discharge.

Diagnostic tests

In a small animal practice, it is normally the responsibility of the veterinarian to decide which diagnostic tests are recommended for any given patient. The technician's responsibilities usually include obtaining blood and urine samples and either performing the tests or forwarding the samples to a diagnostic laboratory. All test results should be reviewed by the veterinarian.

There are no universally recognized guidelines for preanesthetic diagnostic tests. Depending on the clinic policy, certain tests may be routinely performed on every animal presented for anesthesia. Additional tests may be requested by the veterinarian, based on the patient's age, history, and the results of the physical examination. Economic considerations may limit, in some cases, the number and type of tests approved by the client.

The diagnostic tests and procedures that provide information of particular interest to the anesthetist and supervising veterinarian include the complete blood count, urinalysis, blood chemistries, blood clotting tests, blood gases, electrocardiogram, and radiographs.

Complete blood count

The most commonly requested preanesthetic test is a complete blood count (CBC), which includes the determination of packed cell volume (PCV), hemoglobin (Hb), total plasma protein (TPP), and evaluation of a blood smear for white blood cell, red blood cell, and platelet abnormalities. Normal values for these parameters in the dog and cat are given in Table 1-1 (some variation may be expected depending on age, breed, and geographic location).

The information obtained from the PCV and Hb indicates the ability of the blood to deliver oxygen to the tissues. A PCV above normal limits suggests that the relative amount of red blood cells is increased. This is due most often to fluid loss leading to dehydration. A PCV that is elevated is of concern to the anesthetist, since hemoconcentration and increased blood viscosity will be present, which will, in turn, lead to poor tissue perfusion and a reduction in cardiac output. On the other hand, a PCV below the normal range may indicate anemia caused by blood loss, hemolysis, or failure to produce adequate numbers of red blood cells. The net result in each case is decreased capacity to supply oxygen to the tissues.

The total plasma protein value is also of interest to the anesthetist. An increase in TPP, similar to an increase in PCV, may indicate dehydration. A decreased TPP usually indicates hypoproteinemia, which may be due to renal, hepatic, or gastrointestinal disease. Alterations in TPP are particularly significant to the anesthetist

TABLE 1-1

Normal values for selected parameters in dogs and cats

Parameter	Canine	Feline
Heart rate (bpm)	70-180	110-200
Temperature	99.5-102.5° F 37.5-39.2° C	100.0-102.5° F 37.8-39.2° C
Respiratory rate (breaths/min)	10-30	25-40
Hb (g/dl)	14-18	9-16
TPP (g/dl)	5.7-7.8	6.3-8.3
PCV (%)	35-54	25-45
Total leucocyte count ($\times 10^9$/L)	6.0-18	6.0-20
Pao_2 (mm Hg)	91-97	91-115
$Paco_2$ (mm Hg)	30-43	28-43
Arterial pH	7.36-7.46	7.34-7.43

Modified from Muir WW, III, Hubbell JAE: *Handbook of veterinary anesthesia*, St Louis, 1989, Mosby.

because the patient's response to anesthetic drugs may be altered. Many anesthetic agents are distributed within the blood, such that a portion circulates freely and a portion is bound to plasma proteins. Only the portion of the drug that is free and unbound to plasma proteins may affect the drug receptors. In the hypoproteinemic patient, a decreased proportion of drug is bound to plasma proteins, resulting in an increase in the proportion of unbound drug and, consequently, an increased drug potency for that particular patient.

A CBC should also include a differential count and an examination of white blood cells, which may indicate whether the animal is undergoing severe infection or stress. Such conditions may be exacerbated by anesthesia and surgery and may also increase anesthetic risk.

Urinalysis

The results of a urinalysis, particularly the urine specific gravity, provide information on the ability of the kidneys to excrete many anesthetic agents. Any animal with a urine specific gravity within the isosthenuric range (1.007-1.015) should be brought to the veterinarian's attention, as further tests may be needed to assess renal and endocrine function. Urine dipstick results are also useful, allowing rapid screening for conditions such as diabetes mellitus, liver disease, and urinary tract infection. The interpretation of urinalysis results may be aided by microscopic examination of urine and by blood chemistry results such as blood urea nitrogen (BUN).

Blood chemistry

Some patients presented for anesthesia may be known or suspected to suffer from renal, hepatic, endocrine, or other disease. In many cases the degree of organ dysfunction can be determined through appropriate biochemical tests, the most common of which include alanine aminotransferase (ALT), alkaline phosphatase (AP), BUN, creatinine, blood glucose, and serum electrolytes such as sodium and potassium. Normal values for these parameters vary with the instrumentation used and should be obtained from the laboratory doing the tests. Interpretation of test results requires specialized knowledge of disease and is therefore the responsibility of the veterinarian.

Blood clotting tests

Blood clotting tests usually are performed only on animals with suspected coagulation disorders or animals of breeds known to be commonly affected by von Willebrand's disease, such as the Doberman pinscher and Scottish terrier. A toenail cuticle or buccal bleeding time gives a rough estimate of blood clotting ability and can be easily performed on any anesthetized animal. To perform a toenail cuticle bleeding time, the nail is cut slightly short using a pair of nail trimmers, such that the quick is entered and a small amount of bleeding results. The nail is allowed to bleed without any effort to wipe away accumulated blood. In a normal animal, bleeding should stop within 4 minutes. The buccal bleeding time is performed by nicking the tissue on the inside of the cheek using a small lancet. As with the toenail bleeding time, bleeding should stop within 4 minutes. More precise evaluation of hemostasis can be obtained through the use of more sophisticated tests such as partial prothrombin time (PPT) and platelet counts. A patient with reduced ability to clot blood will require special handling by the anesthetist and the surgeon, because hemorrhage during surgery may result in prolonged recovery, shock, or death.

Blood gases

Determination of the partial pressure of arterial blood carbon dioxide ($Paco_2$), arterial blood oxygen (Pao_2), and blood pH is not routinely done in general practice. Sample collection must be done with care: blood intended for Pao_2 analysis must be obtained from an artery (as opposed to CBC and blood chemistry samples, which are taken from a vein). Once obtained, the sample must be stored on ice, and the values should be measured within 2 hours. Many veterinary biochemistry laboratories are equipped to perform these tests, and in areas where a veterinary laboratory is not readily available, a human hospital laboratory may be willing to accept samples from nonhuman patients.

Although sometimes difficult to obtain, blood gas values are one of the few accurate assessments of respiratory function available to an anesthetist in practice. Blood gas results indicate whether the patient is obtaining oxygen and delivering it to the tissues and how efficiently the lungs are eliminating carbon dioxide. The anesthetist must ensure that the oxygen level stays high enough to support cellular metabolism and, at the same time, must avoid accumulation of CO_2 in the blood (hypercapnia). If the $Paco_2$ is increased, it is likely that the patient is not breathing often enough or deeply enough. Normal $Paco_2$ is approximately 40 mm Hg. Values greater than 45 mm Hg are suggestive of respiratory depression, and even higher values (over 60 mm Hg) indicate a serious problem and the need to assist ventilation by means of bagging or the use of a ventilator (see Chapter 7).

The Pao_2, on the other hand, measures the oxygenating capacity of the lungs. Normal Pao_2 in an unanesthetized patient is approximately 90 to 100 mm Hg. Values below 80 mm Hg indicate hypoxia, and animals with a Pao_2 below 60 mm Hg require oxygen supplementation and possibly ventilation assistance to maintain minimal oxygen delivery to the tissues. These values are based on the assumption that the animal is breathing room air, which is approximately 21% oxygen. If the animal is breathing 100% oxygen from an anesthetic machine, the expected Pao_2 in the healthy patient is up to 5 times greater.

Blood pH measurement, often performed at the same time blood gas determinations are made, helps the anesthetist determine the acid-base status of the body. From the anesthetist's standpoint, the pH of the blood is particularly important, since it will affect the potency of a barbiturate given to an animal. Animals with medical conditions such as urinary tract obstructions, renal failure, or shock may be acidotic and, as such, require less barbiturate than do animals with a normal blood pH.

Electrocardiogram

The electrocardiogram (ECG) monitors the electrical activity of the heart muscle, allowing the veterinarian to assess the pattern and rhythm of the myocardial contractions. Abnormalities in the size, duration, shape, and regularity of the ECG tracing are a useful source of information on cardiac function. An ECG is not routinely done on every patient before anesthesia but is usually reserved for those patients with known or suspected heart disease, chest trauma, or electrolyte disturbances, such as hyperkalemia (abnormally high potassium concentration in the blood). The ECG also can be used to screen for cardiac disease before anesthesia of higher risk animals, such as geriatrics. The results of an ECG may allow the veterinarian to determine the type of cardiac dysfunction present, if any, and to evaluate the risk of anesthesia for a particular patient.

Radiography

Because of economic considerations, chest radiographs are not routinely obtained for every patient that is to receive a general anesthetic. Radiography may be warranted in animals that show signs of dyspnea or those in which abnormal heart or lung sounds are detected on the physical examination. It is also advisable that animals that have undergone major trauma (such as being hit by a car) undergo chest radiographs before any surgery, including fracture repair. This will alert the veterinarian to the presence of pneumothorax, pleural effusion, or pulmonary trauma before making the decision to anesthetize the patient.

Patients must not be stressed during radiography procedures, particularly if dyspnea is present. In some cases the patient should stand for the chest radiograph, instead of being placed in lateral or dorsal recumbency, to minimize patient discomfort and anxiety.

Oxygen delivery by mask or nasal cannula will often reduce dyspnea and increase safety during radiography and other procedures.

Miscellaneous tests

Depending on the geographic location of the practice, other diagnostic tests may be routinely performed before anesthesia. For example, veterinary practices in some areas of the United States require a heartworm test be performed before anesthesia in all canine patients.

Classification of patient status

The patient's minimum data base (physical examination, history, and results of diagnostic tests) should be evaluated by a veterinarian, and a status should be assigned to the patient before the anesthetic protocol is chosen and the anesthesia is initiated. Several classification systems have been proposed, the most widely accepted of which is that proposed by the American Society of Anesthesiologists, given in Table 1-2. Classification of risk is subject to personal interpretation, and

TABLE 1-2
Classification of patient physical status

Category	Physical condition	Examples of clinical situations
Class I Minimal risk	Normal healthy animals No underlying disease	Ovariohysterectomy; castration; declaw; hip dysplasia radiograph
Class II Slight risk	Animals with slight to mild systemic disturbances Animals able to compensate No clinical signs of disease	Neonate or geriatric animals; obesity; fracture without shock; mild diabetes; low-grade heartworm infestation
Class III Moderate risk	Animals with moderate systemic disease or disturbances Mild clinical signs	Anemia; anorexia; moderate dehydration; low-grade kidney disease; low-grade heart murmur or cardiac disease; moderate fever
Class IV High risk	Animals with preexisting systemic disease or disturbances of a severe nature	Severe dehydration; shock; anemia; uremia or toxemia; high fever; uncompensated heart disease
Class V Grave risk	Surgery often performed in desperation on animals with life-threatening systemic disease or disturbances not often correctable by an operation; includes all moribund animals not expected to survive 24 hours	Advanced cases of heart, kidney, liver, lung, or endocrine disease; profound shock; major head injury; severe trauma; pulmonary embolus

From Warren RG: *Small animal anesthesia,* St Louis, 1983, Mosby.

two anesthetists might disagree, for example, on whether a particular animal should be assigned to class II (slight risk) or class III (moderate risk). Whatever the preoperative status assigned to an animal, it should be recorded in the animal's hospital record and in the anesthetic logbook.

The technician acting as anesthetist should not hesitate to discuss abnormal findings from the minimum data base with the veterinarian, since such information may lead to changes in the planned anesthetic protocol. The presence of organ dysfunction in an animal does not necessarily require that anesthesia be postponed or cancelled, although this may be necessary in some situations. Often anesthesia may be successfully achieved by selecting the agents that are least likely to have adverse effects on the animal. For example, if the physical examination and diagnostic tests suggest that heart disease is present in a 13-year-old dog presented for surgery, the veterinarian may choose to use isoflurane instead of halothane, because halothane may induce potentially dangerous cardiac dysrhythmias. If the patient is severely ill, the veterinarian may decide that the animal's condition must be stabilized before an anesthetic is administered. Patients that are severely dehydrated, acidotic, anemic, or suffering from a serious systemic disease or electrolyte imbalance are poor anesthetic risks, and every attempt should be made to correct the condition before anesthesia, if time allows. If the planned procedure is not immediately necessary to save the patient's life and the patient's condition may be improved by nursing care, it is likely that anesthesia can be safely postponed.

SELECTION OF THE ANESTHETIC PROTOCOL

Factors that influence selection

In all jurisdictions in the United States and Canada, it is the veterinarian, rather than the veterinary technician, who chooses (prescribes) the anesthetic drugs for a given patient, as well as the dose and the route of administration of each agent. In most hospitals the veterinarian establishes one or two standard anesthetic protocols to be used for routine surgeries on healthy patients. However, the standard protocol must be evaluated for its suitability for any individual patient, and changes should be made to the protocol when necessary for the safety of the patient. The technician who has a good understanding of anesthetic principles and demonstrates sincere interest in patient care and monitoring can communicate valuable observations and suggestions to the veterinarian. Nevertheless, the supervising veterinarian has the ultimate responsibility for the patient's safety and must make the final decision regarding the anesthetic protocol.

The patient's physical status is not the only factor that determines the anesthetic protocol to be used. Other factors that affect the veterinarian's decision are described below.

Availability of facilities and equipment

Some anesthetic techniques require the use of specialized equipment. For example, halothane or isoflurane anesthesia requires the use of a precision vaporizer designed for use with a volatile liquid anesthetic.

Familiarity with the agent

In all procedures, familiarity and skill with the chosen anesthetic and preanesthetic agent are desirable. For most patients, any one of several anesthetic procedures is likely to result in successful and safe anesthesia, and it is reasonable to use the method with which the anesthetist is most familiar, provided patient safety is assured. It is seldom beneficial to anesthetize a critically ill patient with a new combination of drugs that the anesthetist may have heard or read about but has never tried before.

Nature of the procedure requiring anesthesia

Procedures vary in their anticipated duration and the amount of analgesia and restraint required. For example, local analgesia may be suitable for short procedures in which the patient requires only minimal restraint. On the other hand, patients that are to undergo thoracic or abdominal surgery usually require general anesthesia.

Special patient circumstances

Anesthetics that may be appropriate for animals undergoing a routine surgery, such as ovariohysterectomy or castration, may not be the first choice for every surgical procedure. For example, the choice of anesthetic for a cesarean section is partially determined by the need to avoid agents that may cause respiratory depression in the newborn puppy or kitten.

Cost

Anesthetic agents vary in cost, and in a situation in which two agents are of equal value from the standpoint of patient safety, the less expensive may be preferable.

Speed

Critically injured animals may require rapid induction of anesthesia to initiate emergency therapy. For example, a patient that has an obvious hypovolemia because of blood loss cannot wait for a premedication that may be given intramuscularly and takes 15 to 20 minutes to take effect. Rapid induction using a combination of preanesthetic and induction agents given intravenously may be preferable in this case.

PREANESTHETIC PATIENT CARE

During the preanesthetic period the technician should ensure that the patient receives appropriate nursing care, including fasting, intravenous catheterization, and any other procedures requested by the veterinarian. The technician also must ensure that each patient is clearly identified, usually by means of a card attached to its cage or an identification band placed around the animal's neck.

Withholding food before anesthesia

Animals that are anesthetized without prior fasting may vomit or regurgitate stomach contents during anesthesia or in the early recovery period. As anesthetized animals lack the ability to swallow, vomitus in the airway may be aspirated into the trachea, bronchi, and lung alveoli. If the vomitus blocks the airways, immediate respiratory arrest may result. An animal that survives the episode ultimately may develop aspiration pneumonia several days after the incident.

To prevent vomiting during the anesthetic period, it is generally accepted that food should be withheld from adult dogs and cats for 12 hours before anesthesia and that water should be withheld for 2 hours before anesthesia. These times are based on research that indicates that complete emptying of food from the stomach requires an average of 10 hours in the dog. Birds, "pocket pets" such as hamsters and guinea pigs, and dogs and cats younger than 3 months of age should be fasted for a shorter period or not at all because of their tendency to develop hypoglycemia. The technician must ensure that animals that are dehydrated or suffering from renal disease receive adequate intravenous fluids to prevent further dehydration when water is withheld.

Despite the owner's insistence that the animal was fasted, animals may vomit during the preanesthetic, anesthetic, or recovery periods. Fortunately, when it happens, the animal is most often well into the recovery period; the swallowing reflex is present then and aspiration is unlikely. Possible explanations for vomiting in a supposedly fasted animal are individual patient variation and owner noncompliance.

Some protection against vomiting may be offered by the use of preanesthetic drugs with antiemetic properties (e.g., acetylpromazine). Also, the use of cuffed endotracheal tubes helps prevent aspiration of regurgitated or vomited stomach contents, provided the endotracheal tube remains in place until the animal regains the swallowing reflex during recovery. In the case of animals that are known to have ingested food within a few hours of anesthesia, preanesthetics with emetic properties may be given (e.g., xylazine in cats and morphine in dogs) to ensure emptying of the stomach before general anesthesia.

Animals undergoing gastrointestinal procedures may require special feeding and care. This is often necessary to minimize the amount of digestive material within the gastrointestinal tract at the time of surgery. If a surgical procedure involving the stomach or intestine is planned, food is generally withheld for 24 hours and water is withheld for 8 to 12 hours before anesthesia. If surgery of the colon is planned, it may be advisable to administer one or more enemas within 12 hours of the procedure.

The anesthetist should be aware that although preanesthetic fasting is recommended, prolonged fasting may be detrimental to the animal. Many seriously ill animals are anorexic and, in fact, may refuse to eat for several days before and after anesthesia. For example, a dog that has been hit by a car may be presented to the veterinary clinic with a fractured femur and pneumothorax. The veterinarian may elect to postpone fracture repair for several days to allow the pneumothorax to resolve. The animal may be in too much pain, too frightened, or too weak to eat throughout this period. By the time the surgery is performed, the animal may have gone without eating for over 4 days. Lack of nutrition impedes the healing process and prolongs recovery. If necessary, every effort should be made to reestablish caloric intake in the anorexic animal, whether by syringe bolus feeding, the use of feeding tubes, or intravenous nutrition.

Correction of preexisting problems

Animals presented for anesthesia are sometimes found to be suffering from systemic disorders such as dehydration, anemia, respiratory distress, shock, or hypothermia. As already mentioned, these patients are at increased anesthetic risk, and in the interest of patient safety, it may be best to postpone anesthesia to allow time for appropriate nursing care. In some cases, as in a ruptured gastrointestinal tract or uncontrolled internal bleeding, the veterinarian may decide that the risk of delaying surgery outweighs the increased anesthetic risk and will elect to proceed with anesthesia. These patients, perhaps, pose the greatest challenge to the technician's skills as an anesthetist and as an intensive care nurse.

Intravenous catheterization

Reasons for catheterization

Not all animals are catheterized before anesthesia; however, the presence of an intravenous (IV) catheter is of potential benefit to both the patient and the anesthetist. Reasons for catheterization include the following:
1. Intravenous catheters allow the safe use of anesthetic agents that may be irritating if injected perivascularly, such as thiobarbiturates.

2. Intravenous catheters allow simultaneous injection of incompatible drugs such as diazepam and oxymorphone using separate syringes and a catheter adapter (Fig. 1-3).

3. Intravenous catheters allow the rapid administration of emergency drugs, such as epinephrine and prednisone sodium succinate, and for this reason they are particularly recommended for high-risk patients. They are useful not only during the anesthetic period itself, but also during the recovery period, when treatment of complications such as bleeding, respiratory obstruction, or seizures may require intravenous access.

4. Intravenous catheterization allows the administration of balanced electrolyte solutions or saline during surgery. Fluid administration is not mandatory for routine surgeries in healthy animals but is highly recommended for some patients, including the following:
   - Animals that are debilitated or in shock
   - Animals undergoing any surgery that may result in significant blood loss, including cesarean sections
   - Animals that are dehydrated because of renal, gastrointestinal, or other systemic diseases

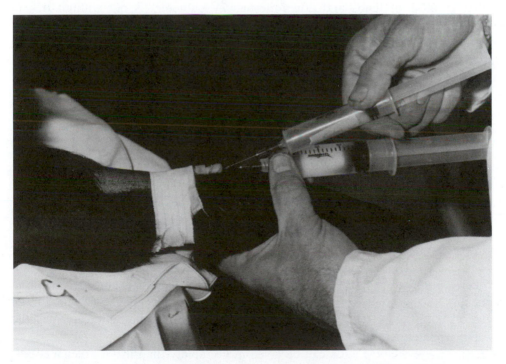

Fig. 1-3.   Simultaneous injection of two drugs through a catheter adapter.

- Animals undergoing lengthy surgery. Many anesthesiologists advise that a secure IV access (by indwelling catheter or butterfly) be established for any animal undergoing a surgical procedure lasting over 1 hour, so fluids or drugs may be given if the need arises. The incidence of cardiovascular compromise is greater in animals undergoing lengthy anesthesia (over 2 hours) than for animals undergoing routine short procedures, and fluid administration is therefore more critical in these patients.

5. Some animals require a constant infusion of electrolytes or drugs such as insulin during anesthesia. These animals are usually catheterized, and the drug is mixed with the IV fluids for convenient administration.

6. Some types of anesthetic agents, particularly propofol and pentobarbital, are given "to effect," such that the drug is given intravenously in small amounts adequate to maintain unconsciousness. In these animals, use of an intravenous catheter is preferable to needle and syringe, as accidental dislodgement of the needle within the vein may lead to perivascular drug administration and the development of a hematoma. Accidental manipulation of the needle and syringe also may lead to inadvertent administration of excessive amounts of drug.

Risks of catheterization

Administration of fluids and drugs through IV catheters is not without risk of complications. The introduction of air should be avoided, although significant air embolism is unlikely if a peripheral vein is used. Accidental overhydration also may occur, with animals weighing under 5 kg being at greatest risk.

Fluid administration rates

The rate of fluid administration varies depending on the patient and the procedure. The following guidelines may be useful:

- *Maintenance fluids:* Daily maintenance fluids are commonly given to hospitalized patients at a rate of 2 ml/kg/hr (large dogs) to 4 ml/kg/hr (small dogs/cats).
- *Fluids given during anesthesia:* A fluid infusion rate of 10 ml/kg/hr is the standard fluid administration rate during routine anesthesia and surgery and is safe for almost all patients. Animals suffering from cardiovascular, respiratory, or renal disease are at increased risk of overhydration and may benefit from a slower infusion rate (5 ml/kg/hr) during surgery. Fluids can be given more rapidly, particularly if bleeding or decreased blood pressure is encountered during a surgery (20 ml/kg in the first 15 minutes is recommended). If excessive blood loss occurs, the anesthetist should ensure that 3 ml of fluids is given for every 1 ml of blood lost. If blood transfusion therapy is used, the amount of blood given should approximately equal the amount of blood lost.
- *Rapid rehydration:* Fluids can be given more rapidly than the maintenance and surgery rates given above. Healthy dogs may tolerate up to 40 ml/kg for 1 hour.

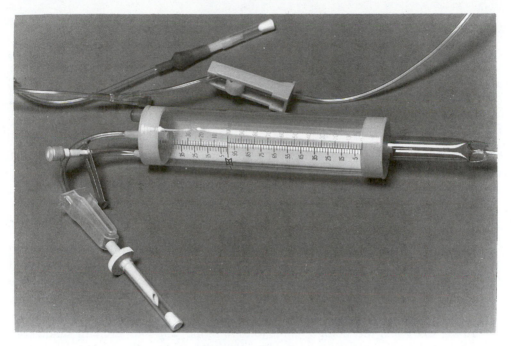

Fig. 1-4. Burette.

Cats are more prone to overhydration than dogs, and for this reason the fluid infusion rate should not exceed 20 ml/kg/hr unless the animal is in shock.

- *Shock therapy:* When treating shock, fluids are given at very rapid flow rates: up to 90 ml/kg/hr for dogs and 50 to 70 ml/kg/hr for cats.

When in doubt, the technician should consult with the veterinarian regarding the optimum fluid administration rate and should carefully monitor the amount of fluids being given to the patient during surgery. The use of a burette (Fig. 1-4) decreases the risk of accidental volume overload by allowing the accurate measurement and administration of small volumes of fluids rather than direct administration from a bag or bottle.

When monitoring any anesthetized patient being given IV fluids, the anesthetist should be alert for signs of overhydration. These include ocular and nasal discharge, chemosis (edema and swelling of the conjunctiva), increased lung sounds, increased respiratory rate, and dyspnea.

Types of IV fluids

The choice of intravenous (IV) fluids is governed by the animal's condition and the veterinarian's preference. Crystalloid solutions, which are water-based, are the most commonly administered type of fluid. There are three types of crystalloid solutions. (See Table 1-3 for composition of fluids.)

TABLE 1-3

Composition of intravenous fluids and plasma

Solution	pH	Carbohydrate content	mEq/L				
			Na⁺	K⁺	Ca⁺²	Mg⁺²	Cl⁻
Plasma	7.5	5.6% dextrose	144	5	5	1.5	107
0.85% NaCl	5.4	None	154	0	0	0	154
5% dextrose	5.0	5% dextrose	0	0	0	0	0
Lactated Ringer's	6.5	Plain, 2.5%, or 5% dextrose	130	4	3	0	109

From Short CE: *Principles and practice of veterinary anesthesia*, Baltimore, 1987, Williams & Wilkins.

1. *Balanced electrolyte solutions.* As the term *balanced electrolyte solution* implies, the solution contains several electrolytes (most often sodium, potassium, chlorine, magnesium, and calcium) in concentrations that reflect the electrolyte composition of blood. Lactated Ringer's solution is one of the most commonly used balanced electrolyte solutions.
2. *Saline solutions.* Physiologic saline (0.85% saline) and half-strength saline contain only sodium and chloride ions in water. These solutions may be preferred over lactated Ringer's for some animals, including patients suffering from hyperkalemia or liver disease. Occasionally, very concentrated (up to 7%) saline solutions, also called hypertonic saline, are administered to patients in shock.
3. *Dextrose solutions.* Solutions of 2.5% or 5% dextrose in water are commonly used in animals suffering from hypoglycemia and in animals receiving insulin. Dextrose solutions are also useful in neonatal animals and debilitated animals, both of which benefit from a ready source of calories during anesthesia.

   The anesthetist must exercise caution when administering drugs and crystalloid fluids concurrently, since undesirable interactions may occur between the drug and the fluid. Diazepam, for example, precipitates in almost any fluid. Sodium bicarbonate and whole blood should not be mixed with fluids containing calcium.

   Some patients require the administration of *colloid* solutions, which are not water based and have a much higher specific gravity than crystalloid solutions. Examples of colloid solutions include the following:

- *Plasma or blood.* Transfusions of plasma or blood are particularly useful in treating animals suffering from acute blood loss or severe anemia. Patients with extensive burns often suffer from severe plasma loss, and a plasma transfusion may be required. Plasma or blood is also useful in hypoproteinemic animals and patients with coagulation disorders.
- *Synthetic colloids.* Patients suffering from shock are sometimes given synthetic colloids such as dextran and pentastarch. Unlike crystalloid solutions, colloid

solutions remain in circulation and help maintain circulating blood volume for a considerable time.

Other preanesthetic patient care

On occasion the technician or another staff member may be directed by the veterinarian to provide specific preoperative care. Some patients require the administration of medication such as insulin injections or heartworm prophylaxis. Antibiotics may be required for animals with existing infections or when the planned surgery involves a contaminated area (such as the gastrointestinal tract). The technician should obtain specific instructions from the veterinarian on the route, dose, and type of medication to be administered to each patient.

PREANESTHETIC AGENTS

Preanesthetic agents are drugs that are administered to an animal before general anesthetics. The most commonly used preanesthetic agents are atropine, acetylpromazine, xylazine, diazepam, and opioid agents. Either a single drug or a combination of drugs may be administered to any given animal. Suggested dosages for the common preanesthetic agents for use in dogs and cats are given in Table 1-4.

Reasons for the use of preanesthetic agents

The potential benefits associated with the use of preanesthetic agents are summarized in Table 1-5. The most important reasons for the administration of preanesthetic agents are the following:

1. To calm or sedate an excited or vicious animal. Sedation not only enhances patient comfort, but also simplifies the task of the anesthetist. However, not every patient requires sedation; in the case of debilitated, injured, or sick animals, even light sedation may cause excessive central nervous system (CNS) depression. Conversely, some vicious animals may be unaffected by even high doses of tranquilizing medications, particularly phenothiazines. In these and all other clinical situations, the anesthetic protocol must be chosen to reflect the needs of the individual patient.
2. To reduce or eliminate possible noxious side effects resulting from the use of general anesthetics. General anesthetics, such as barbiturates, ketamine, and the inhalation anesthetics halothane, isoflurane, and methoxyflurane, may cause undesirable side effects in addition to their anesthetic action. For example, ketamine causes excessive salivation in some patients. Cardiac dysrhythmias and bradycardia sometimes are seen in animals given the inhalation anesthetic halothane. Some opioid drugs (narcotics) may induce bradycardia, vomiting,

TABLE 1-4

Suggested dosage ranges of common preanesthetic medications
for use in healthy dogs and cats (for analgesic dosages, see Table 1-9)

Drug	Canine dosage (mg/kg)	Feline dosage (mg/kg)
Acetylpromazine	0.04-0.2 SC or IM 0.02-0.05 IV Maximum 3 mg	Same Same
Atropine	0.02-0.04 SC, IM, IV	Same
Butorphanol	0.1-0.5 SC or IM 0.05 IV	Same Same
Diazepam	0.2-0.4 IM (not always effective) 0.1-0.5 IV Maximum 10 mg	Same Same
Glycopyrrolate	0.01-0.02 SC or IM	Same
Innovar-Vet	1 ml/7-10 kg IM 1 ml/10-20 kg IV	None None
Meperidine	3-5 IM	5 IM
Morphine	0.25-1.0 SC or IM	0.1-0.3 SC or IM (may produce excitement)
Oxymorphone	0.1-0.3 IM 0.05-0.10 IV Maximum 3 mg	0.1-0.3 IM 0.02 IV Maximum 1 mg
Xylazine	1-2 IM 0.2-0.5 IV	Same Same

Data from Morgan RV: *AAHA formulary,* Denver, 1988, American Animal Hospital Association; Muir WW, III, Hubbell JAE: *Handbook of veterinary anesthesia,* St Louis, 1989, Mosby; Warren RG: *Small animal anesthesia,* St Louis, 1983, Mosby.

diarrhea, and flatulence. Preanesthetic agents, particularly the anticholinergics atropine and glycopyrrolate, are commonly given to prevent these unwanted effects.

3. To reduce the amount of general anesthetic that is required to induce anesthesia. The use of preanesthetic medications, such as tranquilizers and opioids, will result in significant sedation of the animal. Although this level of sedation is insufficient to allow surgery, the animal may require the administration of only a small quantity of general anesthetic to produce true anesthesia. Reduction of the amount of general anesthetic given to the patient allows rapid induction and

TABLE 1-5

Benefits associated with the use of selected preanesthetic agents

Benefit	Preanesthetic agent
Tranquilize or sedate the animal to facilitate catheterization, masking, or injection of an induction agent Reduce patient apprehension Smooth patient recovery	Phenothiazines (acetylpromazine) Thiazines (xylazine) Opioids (meperidine, butorphanol, oxymorphone) Diazepam (debilitated animals only)
Decrease quantity of general anesthetic used	All of the above
Muscle relaxation	Xylazine Diazepam
Induce vomiting in unfasted animal	Xylazine Morphine
Minimize bradycardia that occurs during intubation, handling of viscera, or as side effect of many anesthetics	Atropine Glycopyrrolate
Minimize salivation	Atropine Glycopyrrolate
Decrease GIT motility, thereby preventing vomiting, diarrhea, and flatulence that may occur with some opioids	Atropine Glycopyrrolate
Provide intraoperative or postoperative analgesia	Opioids
Prevent intraoperative or postoperative seizures	Diazepam

earlier recovery and minimizes the adverse side effects of the general anesthetic on the respiratory and cardiovascular systems. This approach to anesthesia, in which doses of several preanesthetic and general anesthetic agents are used in combination to achieve a satisfactory anesthetic state, is termed *balanced anesthesia.*

4. To decrease pain and discomfort in the postoperative period. If the period of anesthesia is brief, drugs given during the preanesthetic period may exert some analgesic effect even during the recovery period. Opioid agents such as butorphanol are particularly effective in this regard.

Preanesthetic agents are chosen from one or more of several classes of drugs, including tranquilizers, opioids (narcotics), and anticholinergics. The type of drug or combination of drugs is chosen by the veterinarian based on the nature of the procedure, the veterinarian's personal preference, and the patient's species, physical status, and temperament. The timing of the administration of the drug will also vary among patients. If time allows, the veterinarian will usually elect to administer a preanesthetic well before the general anesthetic is given to allow ample time for the preanesthetic to gradually exert its effects. Sedatives, such as acetylpromazine and opioids, are most effective if the animal is left undisturbed until the full effect of the drug is evident. It is sometimes necessary, however, to give preanesthetic drugs at the same time as the general anesthetic, in the form of an intravenous or intramuscular injection. Caution should be used when giving *any* preanesthetic or general anesthetic drug by intravenous injection, because the potential for adverse side effects is increased when this route is used.

No preanesthetic agent is entirely free of side effects, and no single agent is safe for every animal. Table 1-6 gives a summary of the precautions and contraindications associated with the commonly used preanesthetic agents. The anesthetist should also be aware that all preanesthetics except glycopyrrolate cross the placental barrier, and adverse side effects may be observed in the newborn animal if the agents are administered shortly before birth. Because of the potential for side effects, the veterinarian may elect to omit one or more preanesthetics from the anesthetic protocol, particularly in neonatal or geriatric animals.

TABLE 1-6
Precautions for the use of selected preanesthetic agents

Anesthetic or preanesthetic	Situations in which to use caution
Atropine	Tachycardia (heart rate over 140 bpm in a dog, 160 bpm in a cat) Constipation or obstruction
Acetylpromazine	Hypotension (shock) Seizure disorders, head trauma Hypothermia
Diazepam	Cesarean section Neonatal patients
Xylazine	Cardiovascular disease or respiratory disease Debilitated animals Neonates or geriatrics Pregnant animals Large dogs prone to bloat
Opioids	Respiratory disease Head trauma or spinal cord injury Chest injury

Anticholinergics (parasympatholytics)

Two anticholinergic agents commonly used in veterinary medicine are atropine and glycopyrrolate (Robinul-V). Atropine is derived from the deadly nightshade plant and glycopyrrolate is a synthetic quaternary ammonium derivative of atropine. Both drugs may be given by the intravenous (IV), intramuscular (IM), or subcutaneous (SC) routes. As is common for anesthetic agents, the SC and IM dosages are considerably greater than the IV dosage. Atropine is available in several concentrations, including 0.5 mg/ml (1/120 grain/ml), 2.2 mg/ml, and 15 mg/ml. Caution must be used to ensure that the atropine drawn into the syringe is the same concentration as that used to calculate the dosage, or the incorrect amount of atropine may be administered. An anesthetist who calculates a dose of 0.5 ml of atropine, 0.5 mg/ml may cause atropine toxicity in a patient if he or she accidentally draws the drug from the wrong bottle and administers 0.5 ml of atropine, 15 mg/ml.

Mode of action

Anticholinergic drugs, such as atropine, exert their effect by blocking the receptors for the neurotransmitter acetylcholine. Acetylcholine is produced by the parasympathetic part of the autonomic nervous system and is the transmitter at both the *nicotinic* and *muscarinic* receptors (Fig. 1-5). Atropine blocks the action of acetylcholine at the muscarinic receptors, which are the final terminals of the parasympa-

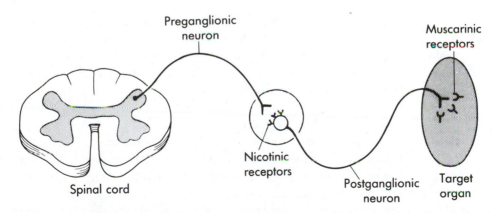

Fig. 1-5. Schematic view of the parasympathetic nervous system. Preganglionic neuron releases acetylcholine at the nicotinic receptors. Postganglionic neuron releases acetylcholine at the muscarinic receptors of the target organ. Atropine affects only the muscarinic receptors.

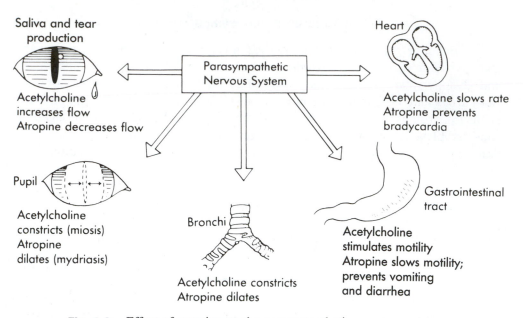

Saliva and tear production

Acetylcholine increases flow
Atropine decreases flow

Heart

Acetylcholine slows rate
Atropine prevents bradycardia

Parasympathetic Nervous System

Pupil

Acetylcholine constricts (miosis)
Atropine dilates (mydriasis)

Bronchi

Acetylcholine constricts
Atropine dilates

Gastrointestinal tract

Acetylcholine stimulates motility
Atropine slows motility; prevents vomiting and diarrhea

Fig. 1-6.   Effect of atropine on the parasympathetic nervous system.

thetic nervous system, and acts to reverse parasympathetic effects. Atropine has no effect on the nicotinic receptors.

The muscarinic receptors are found in the heart, gastrointestinal tract, bronchi, several secretory glands, and the iris of the eye, and it is in these locations that the effect of atropine is readily observed by the anesthetist (Fig. 1-6). When the parasympathetic system is activated (as often occurs during anesthesia), the muscarinic receptors are stimulated by acetylcholine. This is undesirable since it may result in bradycardia, pupil constriction, gastrointestinal stimulation, and salivation; during surgery these effects are all undesirable. By blocking muscarinic receptors, atropine helps to prevent these parasympathetic effects.

Method of use

The onset of atropine action occurs approximately 20 minutes after SC injection, and therefore it is commonly administered 20 to 30 minutes before anesthetic induction. Atropine may be mixed in a syringe and administered intravenously with most other preanesthetic and anesthetic agents including acetylpromazine and ketamine (but not diazepam). Because the onset of action is very rapid following IV administration of atropine, it offers almost immediate protection when given in this way. The duration of effect of atropine is 60 to 90 minutes (less if strong parasympathetic tone is present), and it is common to see bradycardia at the end of a long anesthesia, due in part to the loss of atropine activity.

Effects of atropine

Atropine has many effects that make it a valuable drug in veterinary anesthesia, although its use is not without hazard.

1. Atropine blocks stimulation of the vagus nerve. Several anesthetic procedures and agents may stimulate the vagus nerve, which is an important part of the parasympathetic nervous system. Procedures that stimulate the vagus nerve include endotracheal intubation, handling of the viscera during surgery, and the administration of several commonly used anesthetic agents (including inhalation agents, xylazine, and some opioids). Stimulation of the vagus nerve is undesirable during anesthesia because it causes increased parasympathetic activity, resulting in bradycardia and reduced cardiac output. By blocking the stimulation of the vagus nerve, atropine prevents bradycardia and, in some cases, may cause the heart rate to increase. For this reason, atropine is said to ''protect the heart'' during anesthesia.

2. Atropine reduces salivation (antisialogogic activity). Several anesthetic agents, particularly ketamine, stimulate parasympathetic nerves that promote salivation, which may predispose the animal to aspiration of saliva and possible upper airway blockage. Atropine markedly reduces the production of saliva and, for this reason, is commonly given in conjunction with ketamine.

3. Atropine reduces gastrointestinal activity. Some anesthetic agents (particularly the opioids) increase the peristaltic movement of the gastrointestinal tract, leading to flatulence, vomiting, and diarrhea. Atropine counters these effects by inhibiting intestinal peristalsis. This action also accounts for the inclusion of atropine in several popular antidiarrheal preparations.

4. Atropine causes pupil dilation (mydriasis). This effect is not commonly seen in dogs given usual preanesthetic doses of atropine. In cats, however, mydriasis may occur even at the preanesthetic dosage rates. Mydriasis has been associated with temporary visual disturbances and may also predispose the animal to retinal damage if the eyes are exposed to bright light for a considerable time. The anesthetist should also be aware that animals given atropine may show reduced pupillary light reflex because of the mydriatic effect.

5. Atropine reduces tear secretions. In the awake animal, the cornea of the eye is lubricated by the secretion of tears. Atropine causes a marked reduction in tear production, and the corneas of animals receiving atropine should be protected from dessication by the instillation of ophthalmic ointment. This effect is particularly important when an anesthetic agent such as ketamine is used in addition to atropine. (Animals anesthetized with ketamine do not close their eyelids, resulting in an even greater tendency toward corneal drying.)

6. Atropine promotes bronchodilation. Atropine dilates bronchioles in the lungs, increasing the diameter of these airways. This may be beneficial in some patients; however, an increase in the diameter of the airway results in increased

"dead space" (see Chapter 2). The use of atropine may also be associated with the production of thick mucous secretions within the airways, particularly in cats. This may predispose the animal to airway blockage, and for this reason some veterinarians avoid the use of atropine in cats.

The effects of glycopyrrolate are similar to those of atropine, but the duration of effect may be up to twice as long. Glycopyrrolate may have less tendency to cause tachycardia and cardiac dysrhythmias than atropine. Glycopyrrolate also suppresses salivation more effectively than atropine. For these reasons glycopyrrolate may be preferable to atropine for some procedures in both the cat and the dog, despite its greater expense.

Atropine toxicity

Although it would seem that there are many advantages to using the anticholinergic drugs, they may be contraindicated in certain animals. They should not be given to animals with rapid heart rates (dogs: over 140 bpm; cats: over 160 bpm), as even faster heart rates may result. Because of its tendency to cause tachycardia, atropine should be avoided in animals with clinical signs of congestive heart failure, since the heart is already working to its maximum capacity in these animals. Anticholinergics should also be avoided in animals with constipation or ileus, since these drugs will further reduce peristaltic action of the intestines.

An overdose of atropine may cause drowsiness, dry mucous membranes and thirst, excitability, dilated pupils, or tachycardia. As previously mentioned, atropine toxicity may arise when an incorrect concentration of the drug is administered. Dogs are more susceptible to atropine toxicity than are cats.

Because of the potential for adverse side effects when atropine is administered, some veterinarians omit atropine from their anesthetic protocols. Other veterinarians, however, continue to advocate the routine use of atropine or glycopyrrolate preanesthesia, particularly when ketamine, opioids, or xylazine is to be administered. The use of atropine has also been advocated for brachycephalic dogs to decrease salivation and vagal tone. Atropine may also be used to treat bradycardia or profuse salivation that arises during or after anesthesia.

Tranquilizers and sedatives

This broad group of drugs includes the phenothiazines, benzodiazepines, and thiazine derivatives. In general, agents from each of these classes act on the central nervous system, resulting in a more tranquil or calm animal. These drugs may also cause ataxia and prolapse of the nictitating membrane (also called the third eyelid, Fig. 1-7). Most of these drugs have no analgesic effects. Thus a dog that appears

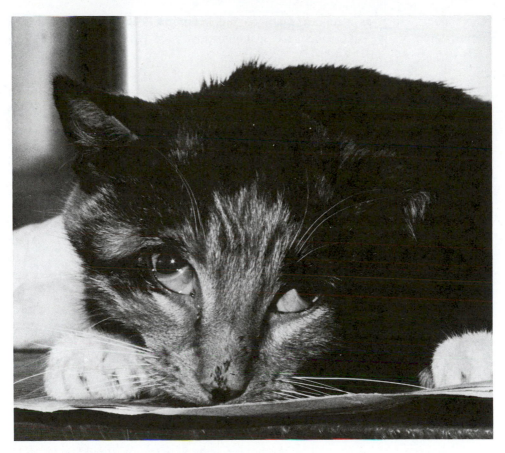

Fig. 1-7. Prolapse of the third eyelid. (From Warren RG: *Small animal anesthesia,* St Louis, 1983, Mosby.)

quiet following sedation may suddenly become alert or aggressive when exposed to a painful stimulus.

Phenothiazines

The phenothiazine group of drugs includes such agents as acetylpromazine (or acepromazine) maleate, chlorpromazine hydrochloride, and triflupromazine hydrochloride. Phenothiazines are probably the most commonly used agents for preanesthetic sedation. Because they do not cause respiratory depression and have minimal adverse effects on the heart, they are considered to have a wide margin of safety. They are effective in many species and may be given in combination with other agents, such as atropine, opioids, and ketamine. Phenothiazines may be administered orally, subcutaneously, intramuscularly, or (with caution) intravenously.

Effects of phenothiazines

The phenothiazines act on the reticular activating center of the brain, with the following clinical effects:

1. *Sedation*. This is the chief reason for the use of phenothiazines as preanesthetic agents.
2. *Antiemetic effect*. Phenothiazines, even at very low doses, help prevent vomiting during the anesthetic period. Sometimes they are used in small animal practice to prevent vomiting caused by gastrointestinal disease or motion sickness.
3. *Antidysrhythmic effect*. Some drugs, including epinephrine and halothane, have a potential to cause cardiac dysrhythmias, which may result in decreased cardiac output. Phenothiazines antagonize this effect and are therefore considered to be antidysrhythmic.
4. *Antihistamine effect*. Histamine is a chemical released by the body as part of the allergic response. Phenothiazines prevent the release of histamine and therefore help reduce allergic reactions. For this reason, phenothiazines should not be used to sedate animals that are to undergo allergy testing.
5. *Peripheral vasodilation*. Phenothiazine agents dilate blood vessels, particularly when given by the IV route. Vasodilation may result in increased heat loss, leading to hypothermia. Even more seriously, vasodilation may lead to a fall in blood pressure (hypotension). Consequently, phenothiazines are not the preanesthetic agents of choice for animals in shock. Animals that experience significant hypotension as a result of phenothiazine administration should be given IV fluid replacement to raise blood pressure. The veterinarian may also prescribe drugs that increase blood pressure by constricting the arteries, including alpha sympathomimetics such as phenylephrine.
6. *Reduction of the threshold for seizures*. Phenothiazines predispose animals to seizure activity. For this reason a veterinarian may elect to omit acetylpromazine when anesthetizing an animal with a history of epilepsy or recent head trauma or in an animal undergoing a procedure such as myelography that may result in postoperative seizures.
7. *Effects on personality*. Occasionally, the administration of a phenothiazine or other tranquilizing agent, such as diazepam or xylazine, may induce excitement rather than sedation. This effect may persist into the postanesthetic period but usually resolves within 48 hours. Owners should be warned that personality changes sometimes occur following the administration of tranquilizing agents, and care should be used when handling patients returning home within 48 hours of anesthesia.

As is evident from the discussion above, the use of phenothiazines is not without risk. Recently it has been suggested that the manufacturer's recommended dose for acetylpromazine is higher than required for preanesthesia and should be reduced by 50% or more to minimize the danger of side effects. High doses of phenothiazine drugs do not cause increased levels of sedation and may induce significant hypotension. The anesthetist should be particularly aware that phenothiazines have increased potency in geriatric animals, neonates, and animals with liver dysfunction, and the dose should be reduced by at least one half in these patients.

Benzodiazepines

The benzodiazepine group includes diazepam (Valium) as well as zolazepam (a component of Telazol), midazolam (Versed), and lorazepam (Ativan). Diazepam, although commonly used in veterinary anesthesia as a preanesthetic or combination induction agent, is not licensed in the United States or Canada for use in animals.

Effects of benzodiazepines

Benzodiazepines probably exert their effects through the release of endogenous GABA, an inhibitory neurotransmitter in the brain. Their usefulness to the anesthetist arises from properties listed below:

1. *Antianxiety and calming effect.* Benzodiazepines, unlike phenothiazines, do not sedate or tranquilize animals. As a result animals given diazepam do not usually appear drowsy; instead, the drug causes the animals to appear less anxious, although still alert. The use of diazepam as the sole premedication agent in healthy young animals is often disappointing because sedation is unreliable. With its normal inhibitions and anxieties removed by the drug, the animal may, in fact, become more difficult to control. The anesthetist should also be aware that like phenothiazines, benzodiazepines have no analgesic effect and will not be effective in calming animals that are experiencing pain.
2. *Skeletal muscle relaxation.* Benzodiazepines induce excellent skeletal muscle relaxation and often are used to counteract the muscle rigidity seen with dissociative agents such as ketamine.
3. *Anticonvulsant activity.* Diazepam is an excellent anticonvulsant drug and commonly is given in combination with agents that have a potential to cause seizures, including ketamine, opioids, and local anesthetics. It is the preanesthetic of choice for animals suffering from seizure disorders. Also, it is used frequently as a preanesthetic for animals that are to undergo a diagnostic or surgical procedure of the spinal cord or brain (such as a cerebrospinal fluid tap or myelography), because it helps prevent postoperative seizures. Diazepam commonly is

given intravenously as a treatment for many types of seizures, including seizures that arise in the postanesthetic period.

4. *Minimal adverse effects*. At therapeutic dosages, benzodiazepines have minimal adverse effects on the cardiovascular and respiratory systems and therefore have a high margin of safety. This property makes them particularly useful for anesthesia of high-risk and geriatric animals.

Benzodiazepines should be used with caution in neonates and animals with known liver dysfunction, because they are poorly metabolized in these patients.

Method of use

Diazepam is most effective and least painful to administer when given by the IV route, rather than IM or SC. When given as a sole agent intravenously, diazepam should be injected slowly, since rapid administration may cause bradycardia.

Unfortunately, diazepam is not water soluble and is not compatible with most other preanesthetic agents. It should not be mixed in a single syringe with atropine, acetylpromazine, barbiturates, or opioids, because a precipitate may result. The only anesthetic agent that is physically compatible with diazepam is ketamine. Ketamine and diazepam can be mixed together in equal volumes and stored up to 1 week.

Because of its tendency to cause excitement and belligerence in healthy animals, diazepam is seldom used as a sole premedicating agent, except in very old or debilitated animals. More commonly, it is used in combination with drugs that induce anesthesia. Although it is very difficult to induce anesthesia in a healthy animal through the use of diazepam alone, diazepam is a very effective inducing agent when supplemented by other agents. In particular, the combination of ketamine and diazepam has gained wide acceptance as a safe and effective IV induction agent in small animals. Diazepam may also be administered concurrently with opioids or ultrashort-acting barbiturates (provided separate syringes are used) to achieve safe, smooth induction of high-risk patients.

The recently introduced benzodiazepine agent midazolam appears to have some advantages over diazepam. It is water soluble and therefore can be mixed with other preanesthetic agents. It is also less irritating to tissues and is more reliably absorbed after IM injection.

Flumazenil (Anexate) recently has been shown to be somewhat effective as a reversing agent for benzodiazepine tranquilizers.

It is interesting to note that benzodiazepine agents are used for a wide variety of purposes in veterinary medicine other than anesthesia. Intravenous diazepam is used as an appetite stimulant in cats, and oral diazepam may be effective in modifying undesirable behavior such as inappropriate urination in cats. Both of these effects may arise from the action of benzodiazepine agents on neurotransmitters within the brain.

Diazepam is classified as a controlled drug in the United States and as a prescription drug in Canada. Some potential for human abuse and theft exists, so the drug should be stored in a secure location.

Thiazine derivatives

Xylazine (Rompun, Anased) is the most commonly used thiazine derivative, having a wide range of applications in veterinary anesthesia. Medetomidine (Domitor) and detomidine (Dormosedan) are other thiazine derivatives used in veterinary anesthesia.

Xylazine is supplied as a 2.0% solution (20 mg/ml) for small animal use and a 10% solution (100 mg/ml) for equine use. The 10% solution can be diluted with sterile water for use in small animals.

Pharmacologically, xylazine is classified as an alpha-2 adrenoreceptor agonist. The site of action is receptors (called *alpha-2 adrenoreceptors*) found on sympathetic nerves within the brain. Xylazine and other alpha-2 adrenoreceptor agonists stimulate these receptors, causing a decrease in the level of the neurotransmitter norepinephrine released within the brain. The result is sedation and analgesia.

Method of use

Xylazine can be used alone or in combination with ketamine, opioids, and many other agents. The required doses of other agents may be reduced when they are given in combination with xylazine, particularly barbiturates (up to 80% reduction) and inhalation agents (up to 50% reduction).

Whether given alone or in combination with other agents, xylazine can be administered intramuscularly or intravenously. Subcutaneous injections have much less effect and are generally avoided. Xylazine can be absorbed through skin abrasions and mucous membranes, and technicians handling xylazine should ensure that any of the drug spilled on human or animal skin is immediately washed off.

Effects of xylazine

Xylazine is a potent sedative, and as with most tranquilizers, it is also a muscle relaxant. Unlike phenothiazine or benzodiazepine agents, xylazine also has some analgesic effect. When combined with other tranquilizers, ketamine, opioid agents, or nitrous oxide, xylazine may provide sufficient analgesia and sedation to allow minor surgical procedures. Analgesia, however, is short-lived (16-20 minutes) and should be supplemented with other agents if a prolonged effect is required.

Xylazine has considerable potential for adverse side effects and is associated with a higher rate of anesthetic complications and death than any other commonly used preanesthetic agent. Adverse side effects are reported most commonly after IV administration and include the following:

1. Xylazine may induce profound cardiovascular changes, particularly when given intravenously or when used without atropine. Bradycardia and second-degree heart block are commonly seen, and hypotension (low blood pressure) also may occur. Xylazine also sensitizes the heart to the dysrhythmogenic effect of epinephrine. Because of these serious effects on the cardiovascular system, the use of xylazine should be avoided in any animal that is debilitated or suffering from cardiac or respiratory disease. Atropine can be given as a premedication or reserved for those animals showing a significant (greater than 33%) drop in heart rate; however, it is not always effective in preventing or treating cardiovascular side effects of xylazine.

2. Respiratory effects of xylazine vary from animal to animal and among species. Following the administration of xylazine, some animals show respiratory depression, whereas others show no ill effects. Severe hypoventilation and cyanosis may occasionally arise from the use of xylazine, particularly in brachycephalic dogs. As a general rule, xylazine should not be administered to animals showing signs of respiratory disease.

3. Xylazine causes vomiting in up to 50% of dogs and 90% of cats. This effect has led to its use as a preanesthetic for animals that have not undergone preanesthetic fasting, although the stomach may not be emptied completely and some risk of vomiting during anesthesia remains. The emetic action of xylazine appears to be unpleasant for the animal but may be somewhat reduced if the animal is premedicated with atropine.

4. Xylazine has been reported to cause abdominal distension resulting from bloating in ruminants and in dogs. For this reason it should not be used as a preanesthetic in breeds of dogs prone to gastric dilation and torsion.

5. Xylazine has been associated with temporary behavior and personality changes in both dogs and cats. This effect also has been reported for other preanesthetic agents, including acetylpromazine, opioids, and diazepam.

6. Xylazine is metabolized in the liver, and its metabolites are excreted in the urine. Adequate hepatic function and renal function are therefore important requirements for any animal receiving this drug.

7. Xylazine may cause profound sleep in some animals.

8. Xylazine reduces the secretion of insulin by the pancreas. Animals sedated with this drug may show transient hyperglycemia, which is not harmful to the animal but may confuse the interpretation of blood samples collected during this period.

Because of the adverse side effects that can occur following xylazine administration, use of a reversing agent is sometimes advisable. Yohimbine (Yobine), given intravenously, is effective in reversing the effects of xylazine, including sedation and bradycardia (see Chapter 3). Tolazoline and 4-aminopyridine have also been used to reverse the effects of xylazine.

Given the adverse effects associated with xylazine use, attention has recently focused on another alpha-2 adrenoreceptor agonist, medetomidine. This agent is more potent than xylazine and may have fewer side effects (including less tendency to cause vomiting). It is not presently licensed for animal use in the United States or Canada. Medetomidine has a specific antagonist, atipamezole (Antisedan).

Opioids

Opioids are a versatile class of drugs that may be used as preanesthetics, induction agents, and analgesics. The name *opioid* is derived from the opium poppy, which is the source of morphine, the first agent of this class to be identified. Opioid agents were formerly known as *narcotics*; however, this term is more properly used to describe only those agents that induce physical dependence (addiction). Several synthetic members of the opioid family, such as butorphanol, have little tendency to induce physical dependence and therefore are not considered to be narcotics.

Mode of action

A great deal of research has been done to determine the site of opioid action within the body. Opioid receptors are found on neurons throughout the body. The natural stimulants of these receptors are chemicals produced by the body, such as endorphins and enkephalins.

The effects of opioids are chiefly the result of their action on receptors located in the brain. Three types of opioid receptors have been found in the brain: mu (μ), kappa (κ), and sigma (σ). Opioid agents differ in their action at each of these sites and therefore in their overall effects within the body. An opioid agent may act as an agonist (stimulating agent) or antagonist (blocking agent) at each type of receptor. Some opioids are considered to be both antagonists and agonists, since they block one type of receptor and stimulate another type (Table 1-7). Morphine, meperidine, fentanyl, and oxymorphone stimulate all three types of receptors and therefore are classified as agonists. Naloxone blocks all three types of receptors and is classified as an antagonist. Butorphanol, which blocks some receptors and stimulates others, is considered to be a mixed agonist-antagonist.

Beneficial effects

Opioid agents have two effects on the nervous system that account for their use in veterinary anesthesia:

1. *Central nervous system (CNS) effects.* Depending on the dose, the particular opioid agent, and the species in which the agent is used, an opioid agent may cause CNS depression or excitement. In dogs the predominant effect is sedation. Cats, however, may react to some opioids by exhibiting bizarre behavior

TABLE 1-7

Effect of opioid drugs on receptors

Receptor	Effects	Agonists	Antagonists or minimal effect
Mu (μ)	Respiratory depression Euphoria Addiction Analgesia Sedation	Morphine Meperidine Fentanyl Oxymorphone	Naloxone Butorphanol
Kappa (κ)	Analgesia Sedation Respiratory depression	Morphine Meperidine Fentanyl Oxymorphone Butorphanol	Naloxone
Sigma (σ)	Hallucinations Euphoria/dysphoria	Morphine Meperidine Fentanyl Oxymorphone	Naloxone Butorphanol

Modified from Orsini J: Butorphanol tartrate: pharmacology and clinical indications, *Compendium* 10:849, Oct, 1988.

patterns, including anxiety, convulsions, or mania, particularly if the drug is given intravenously. For this reason, some opioids (particularly fentanyl) must be avoided in cats, although others are safe at a reduced dosage or when given in combination with tranquilizing agents. Dogs may also show excitement (whining, barking) as a result of opioid administration, particularly if a tranquilizing agent is not used concurrently.

2. *Analgesia.* Opioids have long been considered to be the most effective analgesics known to medicine. The potency varies between members of the class, and fentanyl, butorphanol, and oxymorphone are considered to have a more potent effect than equal doses of morphine or meperidine (Table 1-8). Potency does not imply a stronger analgesic effect, but rather that the same effect is produced with a lower dose. With the routine use of general anesthetics with limited analgesic properties (isoflurane, halothane, ketamine, barbiturates) and the current emphasis on prevention of postoperative pain, the analgesic effect of opioids remains one of the chief reasons for their use in veterinary medicine.

Most animals exhibit a combination of CNS depression and analgesia within 60 seconds of intravenous administration of opioids. Although swallowing may persist, endotracheal intubation is often possible. If high doses are given (particularly to a sick animal), a *hypnotic* state may be produced in which the patient appears

TABLE 1-8

Relative analgesic
potencies of opioids
compared to morphine

Opioid	Potency
Morphine	1.0
Meperidine	0.1
Fentanyl	50-300
Oxymorphone	10
Butorphanol	5-8

profoundly sedated yet can be aroused by sufficient stimulus. Hypnosis is typically more profound than the sedation that is seen with acetylpromazine, xylazine, or diazepam. Recovery is often slow (up to 6 hours in some animals) unless a reversing agent is given.

Adverse effects

Because of associated side effects, opioids must be administered with caution.

1. *Respiratory function.* The most serious side effect is the strong tendency of these drugs to depress respiration, particularly when used with a tranquilizing agent. Opioids cause a decrease in both respiratory rate and tidal volume, resulting in decreased Pao_2 and increased $Paco_2$. Respiratory efforts may become inadequate to lower blood carbon dioxide levels, resulting in significant respiratory acidosis. The respiratory depression seen is dose dependent for most opioid agents, meaning the effect is more pronounced at high doses. Some opioids, however, show a "ceiling effect" in that high doses show no greater depression of respiration than do low doses.

   The tendency of opioids to depress respiration is potentially so severe that high doses of an opioid agent should not be given unless the anesthetist is able to support respiration by manually bagging the animal or by use of a ventilator. If respiratory arrest occurs, it is usually possible to maintain the animal with manual support of respiration until the effect of the opioid has been chemically antagonized or has worn off.

   Interestingly, despite the tendency of opioids to depress respiration, some animals pant after opioid administration. This results from a direct effect of opioids on the temperature-regulating center of the brain, which mistakenly interprets normal body temperature as being elevated.

2. *Gastrointestinal function.* The effect of opioids on the gastrointestinal tract is twofold. The initial effect of many agents is an increase in peristaltic movement, resulting in diarrhea, vomiting, and flatulence. Pretreatment with atropine usually moderates this effect. After the initial stimulation of peristalsis, a prolonged period of gastrointestinal stasis may occur, resulting in constipation.
3. *Physical dependence.* Physical dependence (addiction) is associated with the prolonged use of some opioid agents. Human patients given morphine develop tolerance for its effects in approximately 2 to 3 weeks. Physical dependence is seen after 48 hours of continuous use or 3 weeks of intermittent use. Not all opioids are addictive: those with minimal or antagonistic activity at mu receptors (e.g., butorphanol) have less potential for causing physical dependence.

Other reported effects of opioid agents include:
- Bradycardia (this is less pronounced in animals pretreated with atropine)
- Hypotension resulting from vasodilation
- Cough suppression
- Miosis in dogs and mydriasis in cats
- Increased responsiveness to noise
- Excessive salivation
- Euphoria in human patients

Reversibility

One advantage of the opioid class as a whole is the reversibility of these agents. Several narcotic antagonists (reversing agents) are available, including naloxone hydrochloride (Narcan), levallorphan tartrate, and nalorphine hydrochloride. Technically, levallorphan and nalorphine are classified as agonist-antagonists, whereas naloxone is a pure antagonist. Butorphanol has also been used to reverse pure opioid agonists such as morphine. Of these drugs, naloxone is the preferred reversing agent, because it is the most effective and causes the least respiratory depression.

Narcotic antagonists exert their effect by binding to opioid receptors, acting as blocking agents. By displacing other opioid agents from receptors, they reverse the agonist effect of those agents. Reversal of sedation, respiratory depression, hypotension, bradycardia, and gastrointestinal effects occurs within minutes of IV injection of the antagonist. Unfortunately, reversal of analgesia also occurs. Reversal of analgesia can be avoided by titrating the dose of reversing agent such that respiratory depression is relieved only partially, allowing an acceptable level of analgesia to be maintained. Narcotic antagonists are effective in reversing opioid agents only and are not effective in reversing the effects of phenothiazines, thiazine derivatives, and other nonopioid agents.

Reversal of opioid effects through the use of an antagonist is too expensive for routine anesthesia; however, the technique is extremely useful in emergency overdose situations. Narcotic antagonists are also used for rapid reversal of anesthesia in the compromised or geriatric patient. Narcotic antagonists also are helpful in reviving neonates delivered by a cesarean section performed using opioid agents. One drop of naloxone placed under the tongue of each puppy or kitten is sufficient to reverse the respiratory depression caused by fentanyl or other opioids given to the mother.

The effects of narcotic antagonists are usually observed within 30 seconds of IV injection. The reversing agent may not remove all sedative effects in some animals, and in such cases additional doses are usually ineffective. In fact, repeated doses of some reversing agents may cause CNS and respiratory depression through overload and stimulation of opioid receptors.

Method of use

Opioid agents are used in many ways in veterinary anesthesia. They are commonly found as part of *preanesthetic mixtures* composed of atropine, a tranquilizer such as acetylpromazine, and an opioid (particularly meperidine or butorphanol, see box on p. 44). These preanesthetic "cocktails" are mixed together in advance and given to the patient before anesthetic induction. An opioid is included in these mixtures for its analgesic effects and to potentiate the sedative properties of acetylpromazine. Opioid agents are also commonly used at higher dosages in combination with a tranquilizer, resulting in a type of sedation termed *neuroleptanalgesia*. Animals given these agents exhibit profound sedation and excellent analgesia but can be aroused by sufficient stimulation. Neuroleptanalgesia is discussed further in the following section.

Opioid agents, including butorphanol, oxymorphone, and morphine, are commonly used for the prevention and treatment of *postoperative pain*. (For further discussion see "Use of opioids as analgesics" on p. 45.)

Neuroleptanalgesia

Neuroleptanalgesia is a profound state of sedation and analgesia achieved through the use of an opioid agent in combination with a tranquilizer. The effect of the two agents used together is greater than that of either used alone. Patients under neuroleptanalgesia appear deeply anesthetized but may respond to noise or other stimuli. Random limb movements are also seen.

Neuroleptanalgesia using an opioid-tranquilizer combination is commonly used for procedures that require significant CNS depression. Examples include dentistry, minor surgery such as porcupine quill removal, and diagnostic procedures such as endoscopy or radiography. Neuroleptanalgesics given at low dosages may also be used as preanesthetic agents.

An opioid-tranquilizer combination is available commercially as Innovar-Vet, a combination of fentanyl (a potent opioid analgesic) and droperidol (a tranquilizer).

Formulas for preanesthetic mixtures

Premix

Contains per ml:
   1 mg acetylpromazine
   20 mg meperidine
   0.2 mg atropine

To make up a 10-ml solution, mix together the following:
   Acetylpromazine   1 ml of 10 mg/ml solution = 10 mg
   Atropine   4 ml of 0.5 mg/ml solution = 2 mg
   Meperidine   2 ml of 100 mg/ml solution = 200 mg

   Make the mixture up to 10 ml with sterile water

Preanesthetic dose:
   Dogs: 0.1 ml/kg (Do not exceed 2.5 ml)
   Cats: 0.2 ml/kg

BAA

Contains per milliliter:
   0.25 mg acetylpromazine
   0.2 mg atropine
   2 mg butorphanol

To make up a 20-ml solution, mix together the following:
   Butorphanol   4 ml of 10 mg/ml solution = 40 mg
   Acetylpromazine   0.5 ml of 10 mg/ml solution = 5 mg
   Atropine   8 ml of 0.5 mg/ml solution = 4 mg

   (Atropine may be replaced by 8 ml of glycopyrrolate solution, 0.2 mg/ml)

   Make the mixture up to 20 ml with sterile water

Preanesthetic dose:
   Dogs: 0.05-0.1 ml/kg IM or SC
   Cats: 0.1-0.13 ml/kg IM or SC

Data courtesy of Doris Dyson, Ontario Veterinary College, Guelph, Ontario; Donald C. Sawyer, College of Veterinary Medicine, Michigan State University, East Lansing, Michigan. *BAA,* Butorphanol-Ace-Atropine.

Each milliliter of Innovar-Vet contains 0.4 mg of fentanyl and 20 mg of droperidol. Innovar-Vet is widely used in the dog and is particularly useful for sedating excited or aggressive animals. Because of its potential to cause seizure activity in cats, it is not used in that species. Innovar-Vet is usually given subcutaneously, intramuscularly, or intravenously but also may be given orally at twice the regular dosage. Intramuscular injections may be painful to the animal.

Innovar-Vet has been associated with a high incidence of behavioral changes in the postsurgical period. For example, aggressive behavior has been reported in normally placid animals after the use of this agent. This effect may be caused by the tranquilizer component of the mixture, droperidol (a butyrophenone tranquilizer), which may increase anxiety in some patients. Some veterinarians avoid the use of Innovar-Vet in outpatient animals because of the unpredictable behavior sometimes seen after recovery from this drug. Other reported adverse side effects include hypotension (caused by droperidol) and a persistent head bob or intention tremor after anesthesia, seen most commonly in Doberman pinschers.

Other neuroleptanalgesic combinations may be used in both the cat and dog and can be prepared within the clinic using tranquilizing agents such as acetylpromazine, xylazine, or diazepam and opioids such as morphine, meperidine, oxymorphone, or butorphanol. In some cases the drugs are mixed in the same syringe, or they may be injected separately by the IM or IV route after pretreatment with atropine. Safe use of neuroleptic agents by the IV route requires slow injection over 1 to 2 minutes, because hypotension or CNS stimulation may occur if a large bolus is given.

For all neuroleptanalgesic combinations including Innovar-Vet, the opioid component can be reversed using naloxone or another narcotic antagonist; however, the tranquilizer component cannot be reversed, unless a specific antagonist such as yohimbine is available. The ability to partially reverse neuroleptanalgesia allows its use in geriatric and other higher-risk patients, provided ventilatory support is available in case of severe respiratory depression.

Use of opioids as analgesics

Traditionally, most veterinarians have reserved the use of analgesic agents for patients recovering from orthopedic, thoracic, or other extensive surgery. However, in recent years some veterinarians have advocated the use of analgesics in all patients undergoing major surgery, including ovariohysterectomy. Most general anesthetics (barbiturates, isoflurane, propofol) provide minimal postoperative analgesia, and patients may undergo painful, rapid recoveries when these agents are used. It is logical to assume that animals perceive painful stimuli in the same way humans do, although as in humans there is a wide variation in tolerance to pain. In some cases the presence of pain is not evident because of the stoic nature of the

TABLE 1-9

Suggested dosage ranges of opioid
drugs used for postoperative analgesia

Drug	Species	Dosage	Duration of action
Oxymorphone	Dog and cat	0.03-0.05 mg/kg IM, IV	4-5 hours
Butorphanol	Dog and cat	0.1-0.4 mg/kg IM, SC, IV Maximum 5 mg	1-2 hours (less in cats)
Morphine	Dog Cat	0.1-0.5 mg/kg IM, SC 0.1 mg/kg IM, SC	4-5 hours 4-5 hours
Meperidine	Dog Cat	1-3 mg/kg IM Effectiveness questionable	45 minutes ?
Buprenorphine	Dog and cat	0.01-0.03 mg/kg	8-12 hours

Modified from *Veterinary teaching hospital undergraduate manual*, Guelph, Ontario, Canada, 1992, Ontario Veterinary College.

patients. On the other hand, some animals in pain will show vigorous activity, vocalization, and even frenzy. Still others may appear lethargic and uninterested in their surroundings. Many patients will show increased heart rate, elevated blood pressure, and abnormal respiration patterns. For humane reasons, it is probably best to assume that pain exists after surgery and to provide analgesia. "Pain is the only situation in which if in doubt, go ahead and treat" (Lloyd Davis). Many animal owners are acutely aware of the pain their pets experience after surgery and welcome the use of analgesics in the postoperative period.

It is widely accepted that only the opioid agents (including butorphanol, oxymorphone, and morphine) provide sufficient analgesia to treat acute postoperative pain. These agents vary in their potency and in the side effects associated with their use. Analgesic doses of commonly used opioid agents are given in Table 1-9. Nonopioid agents such as aspirin or acetaminophen and corticosteroids such as prednisone are inferior to opioids in their analgesic properties and are not as suitable as opioids in treating acute postoperative pain.

The timing of the administration of an opioid or other analgesic agent may vary, depending on the surgical procedure and the veterinarian's preference. The convenient times for administration of opioid analgesics in conjunction with anesthesia are:

• Administration during the preanesthetic period
• Administration during the surgery

- Administration just prior to discontinuation of the anesthetic (i.e., just before the anesthetic vaporizer is turned off)
- Administration during the recovery period

The preferred option depends on the nature of the anesthetic agents used and the duration of anesthesia. If the anticipated procedure is short (patient recovery expected within 1 hour of preanesthesia), it is advisable to use an opioid in the preanesthetic period (e.g., using BAA or premix). However, if the procedure is fairly lengthy, an opioid given in the preanesthetic period may no longer be effective in the recovery period. In this case it is advisable to administer additional analgesic toward the end of surgery.

It is not a good practice to wait until an animal shows signs of acute postoperative pain before initiating treatment because:

(a) Many animals will show little or no overt signs, even when experiencing severe pain.
(b) Analgesics usually have a more pronounced effect if given before the perception of pain.

Therefore it is preferable to give the analgesic before the patient wakes up, rather than after. If administration is delayed until the patient is agitated and crying, larger and more frequent doses of analgesic, and possibly concurrent administration of a tranquilizer, may be required.

Regulatory considerations

Most opioid agents are subject to government regulation regarding purchase, handling, and dispensing. The need for detailed record keeping and the potential for abuse or theft of opioid agents is a significant disadvantage of this class of drugs. In the United States, the Controlled Substances Act assigns each opioid to one of five drug schedules according to each drug's potential for abuse. In a similar way, Canadian legislation has classified each opiate as a narcotic, controlled, or prescription drug. Agents classified as narcotics in Canada, or as schedule II substances in the United States, cannot be dispensed or drawn into a syringe except under the direct supervision of a licensed veterinarian. Regulated substances should be kept in a cabinet, safe, or other locked storage place and should not be left on countertops or in other public areas. After withdrawing a dose from a bottle of controlled substance, the bottle should be immediately returned to locked storage. Usage must be accurately recorded in a drug logbook, and inventory must be periodically checked to ensure that no drug is unaccounted for.

Opioid agents commonly used in practice

The opioid agents in common use in veterinary medicine are described below.

1. *Morphine*. The original opioid agent used in human and veterinary medicine, morphine is still occasionally used in veterinary practice as a preanesthetic or

analgesic. Morphine can be used in dogs or cats; however, the canine dosage rate may cause mania in cats, so a lower dosage rate should be used for felines. Morphine has several disadvantages, including gastrointestinal stimulation resulting in vomiting, a strong tendency to cause physical dependence in humans, and a potential to cause severe respiratory depression. It should not be administered IV in an undiluted form because hypotension may result. A constant IV infusion of morphine (0.2 mg/kg/hr) following an initial loading dose of 0.3 mg/kg has been used to provide prolonged analgesia after very painful procedures.

Morphine also may be given by epidural injection (between vertebrae L7 and S1 using a spinal needle) to animals requiring long-term analgesia. (See Chapter 7 for information on epidural technique.) The injection of morphine, 0.1 mg/kg, diluted in saline to a total volume of 1 ml/kg, provides up to 18 hours of postoperative analgesia to the pelvis or rear limbs. When given by epidural injection, side effects such as excitement, gastrointestinal stimulation, and respiratory depression are seldom seen. Preservative-free morphine is recommended for this purpose.

2. *Meperidine* (Demerol, Pethidine). A synthetic opioid, meperidine has been extensively used in the past as a preanesthetic agent. It is commonly used to formulate a preanesthetic cocktail in combination with atropine and low doses of acetylpromazine (see box on p. 44). When administered with a tranquilizer (usually diazepam or acetylpromazine), meperidine also provides safe and effective neuroleptanalgesia in puppies.

Meperidine offers a wide safety margin and causes less respiratory depression and gastrointestinal stimulation than morphine. Unfortunately, its analgesic effect is weak and of very short duration, particularly in cats. For this reason it is not considered to be a good postoperative analgesic. Its use in recent years has been somewhat superseded by other agents, particularly butorphanol.

3. *Butorphanol*. A synthetic opioid with both agonist and antagonist properties, butorphanol was first used as a cough suppressant. Butorphanol is not approved for use in veterinary anesthesia but has found widespread application as a preanesthetic, inducing agent, and postoperative analgesic.

Butorphanol is available in two concentrations, 0.5 mg/ml (Torbutrol), which is approved for use as an antitussive in dogs, and 10 mg/ml (Torbugesic), which is approved for use in horses only. Tablets are also available for long-term administration and may be dispensed for postoperative pain. It is not a scheduled drug in the United States (except in Oklahoma), and record-keeping is unnecessary. In Canada it is classified as a controlled drug, with record keeping requirements.

Butorphanol produces less respiratory depression than most opioids because of the ceiling effect. Panting is sometimes reported, although less frequently than with Innovar-Vet or oxymorphone. Heart rate, blood pressure, and cardiac output may be decreased after the administration of butorphanol; however, the effect is less than that of morphine, and pretreatment with atropine is not required. Butorphanol may be given IV, IM, or SC and is effective and safe for both dogs and cats.

4. *Oxymorphone* (Numorphan). An expensive but useful derivative of morphine, oxymorphone offers potent and long-lasting analgesia without the side effects of many other opioids. Oxymorphone does not stimulate vomiting or diarrhea and causes minimal respiratory depression. Unlike meperidine, it may be given IV, although intravenous administration may cause excitement in the cat. A tranquilizer such as xylazine, acetylpromazine, or diazepam may be used concurrently if additional sedation is required. Oxymorphone mixed with sterile saline and administered by IV drip is a safe induction agent in very sick or debilitated animals. Atropine pretreatment is recommended, as with most opioids. Oxymorphone also has been used effectively as an epidural agent and appears to produce a longer duration of anesthesia than morphine. It also has been used to treat postoperative pain, although it is provided in vials that are inconvenient to use if only a small dose is required. As with butorphanol, oxymorphone has a greater analgesic potency than morphine and a longer duration of analgesia.

5. *Pentazocine* (Talwin). This opioid agent has been used as an analgesic for human patients. Its short duration of action (22 minutes in the dog) makes it unsuitable for postoperative analgesia in veterinary patients.

6. *Buprenorphine*. This opioid agent provides long-term analgesia (8 to 12 hours) in human patients. Information on its use in veterinary patients is scant, and it is presently not approved for use in animals. Although it appears to be a potent analgesic, it may induce significant respiratory depression. Respiratory effects are difficult to reverse with naloxone, although analeptic agents such as doxapram may be effective.

KEY POINTS

1. The technician's duties during the preanesthetic period may include obtaining an adequate patient history, performing a physical examination, and performing diagnostic tests, as requested by the veterinarian.

2. Preanesthetic care of the patient may include fasting and intravenous catheterization. Preparation of equipment and administration of drugs are also the responsibility of the anesthetist.

3. No one anesthetic protocol is ideal for all patients. Rather, the anesthetic techniques and agents used are tailored to the needs of the individual patient. Factors such as previous or concurrent illness, patient age, temperament and species of the patient, nature of the procedure, and preference of the veterinarian are all considered in determining the choice of anesthetic protocol.

4. Diagnostic tests such as the complete blood count (CBC) and urinalysis may provide valuable information regarding the patient's ability to tolerate anesthesia. Procedures such as radiography, electrocardiography, and blood gas determination also may be useful in selected patients but are seldom done on a routine basis.

5. The risk of anesthesia to the patient should be assessed before initiating the procedure. The patient should be assigned to a class based on physical condition, as outlined by the American Society of Anesthesiologists.

6. The patient should be in stable condition, when possible, before being anesthetized; preexisting problems such as dehydration or shock should be corrected.

7. Although intravenous (IV) catheterization offers many advantages in regard to patient safety and convenience for the anesthetist, this procedure is associated with the risk of accidental overhydration. A fluid infusion rate of 10 ml/kg/hr is considered safe for most patients.

8. Preanesthetic agents increase the safety and convenience of anesthesia by reducing the dose of general anesthetic needed, by preventing bradycardia and other parasympathetic effects, and by reducing patient stress and discomfort. All preanesthetic agents, however, have side effects that may be harmful in some patients.

9. Anticholinergics such as atropine and glycopyrrolate help prevent bradycardia, excessive salivation and gastrointestinal activity, and bronchoconstriction. They are particularly recommended for use in animals that are to receive xylazine, opioids, or ketamine. Anticholinergic agents may be harmful when used in animals with preexisting tachycardia, constipation, or ileus.

10. Tranquilizing agents include phenothiazines, benzodiazepines, and thiazine derivatives. Phenothiazines have a wide margin of safety but may cause hypotension in some patients. Benzodiazepines have a calming effect and are excellent

for controling possible seizure activity. Thiazine derivatives are extremely potent and produce excellent muscle relaxation but may cause serious cardiovascular and respiratory complications in some animals.

11. Opioids may be used as preanesthetic agents, as induction agents, as postoperative analgesics, and (in combination with tranquilizers) as neuroleptanalgesics. Their greatest advantage is the profound analgesia they produce in most patients. They have the potential to cause adverse side effects on the cardiovascular, respiratory, and gastrointestinal systems, and prolonged administration may be associated with addiction. Their use is subject to government regulation regarding purchase, handling, and dispensing.

12. The action of some preanesthetic agents may be reversed through the use of specific agents such as yohimbine, flumazenil, and naloxone.

REVIEW QUESTIONS

1. Given the busy nature of a veterinary practice, it is probably best to assume that the same anesthetic protocol should be used on all patients.
   True   False

2. The best question to ask when taking a history would be one that requires a "yes" or "no" answer.
   True   False

3. The following question would be a good example of how to ask a question: "Your dog does not drink much water, does he, Mrs. Jones?"
   Agree   Disagree

4. An owner who volunteers information on the type of medication that his or her pet is receiving is really not giving valued information.
   True   False

5. Different species may have different physiologies in regard to the metabolism of drugs.
   True   False

6. An obese dog will require more anesthetic than a normal weight dog of the same breed.
   True   False

7. The term *isosthenuria* means:
   a. Production of very dilute urine (1.007-1.015 specific gravity)
   b. Urine that contains crystals
   c. Urine that has blood in it
   d. Urine that has bacteria in it

8. Blood tests such as ALT have minimal value for an anesthetist.
   True   False

9. When performing blood gas determinations, it is best that the sample be no older than _____ .
   a. 30 minutes
   b. 1 hour
   c. 2 hours
   d. 12 hours
   e. 24 hours

10. It is always best to withhold food from any patient scheduled to receive a general anesthetic for at least 12 hours before the scheduled procedure.
    True   False

11. Which of the following is *not* a crystalloid solution?
    a. Lactated Ringer's
    b. Normal saline
    c. Dextran
    d. Sterile distilled water

12. Which of the following is not a valid reason for administering a preanesthetic medication?
    a. It reduces the amount of general anesthetic required for induction
    b. It may calm an excited animal
    c. It may reduce possible noxious side effects from the general anesthetic
    d. It increases patient safety by allowing the animal to stay under the general anesthetic for a longer time
    e. It may reduce pain in the postoperative period

13. Most preanesthetics will not cross the placental barrier.
    True   False

14. It is recommended that atropine not be given to an animal that has tachycardia.
    True   False

15. Anticholinergic drugs such as atropine block the release of acetylcholine at the:
    a. Muscarinic receptors of the parasympathetic system
    b. Nicotinic receptors of the parasympathetic system
    c. Muscarinic receptors of the sympathetic system
    d. Nicotinic receptors of the sympathetic system

16. Tranquilizers such as acetylpromazine maleate sedate the animal and give some analgesia.
    True   False

17. In general the opioids can have a significant effect on the cardiovascular and respiratory systems causing bradycardia and respiratory depression.
    True   False

18. A patient that is anemic or moderately dehydrated would be classified as a _____ anesthetic risk.
    a. Class I
    b. Class II
    c. Class III
    d. Class IV
    e. Class V

For the following questions more than one answer may be correct.

19. The suggested minimum data base for any patient may include:

    a. History
    b. Physical examination
    c. Diagnostic tests
    d. Name of the required procedure

20. One should be cautious when using opioids as a premedication for animals suffering from:
    a. Respiratory disease
    b. Head trauma
    c. An inclination to bloat
    d. Chest injury

21. Effects that atropine may have on the body include:
    a. Decreased salivation
    b. Increased vagal tone
    c. Decreased gastrointestinal motility
    d. Mydriasis

22. Clinical signs that are associated with atropine toxicity include:
    a. Excitability
    b. Mydriasis
    c. Tachycardia
    d. Dry mucous membranes

23. Effects that one may see after premedication with the phenothiazine tranquilizers include:
    a. Sedation
    b. Antidysrhythmic effect
    c. Peripheral vasodilation
    d. Reduced salivation
    e. Reduced seizure threshold

24. Characteristic effects of the benzodiazapines include:
    a. Sedation
    b. Muscle relaxation
    c. Significant decrease in respiratory function
    d. Minimal effect on cardiovascular system

25. Physical effects that may be seen following administration of xylazine include:
    a. Hypotension
    b. Mydriasis
    c. Skeletal muscle relaxation
    d. Hypoventilation
    e. Vomiting

26. Effects of opioid administration include the following:
    a. Analgesia
    b. Bradycardia
    c. Panting
    d. Decreased tear production

27. Opioids may be reversed with:
    a. Levallorphan
    b. Naloxone hydrochloride
    c. Atropine
    d. Yohimbine

28. Which of the following drugs will most likely precipitate out when mixed with other drugs or solutions?
   a. Atropine
   b. Acetylpromazine
   c. Diazepam
   d. Butorphanol

29. Drugs that are considered effective in treating for acute postoperative pain in cats include:
   a. Oxymorphone
   b. Butorphanol
   c. Acetylpromazine
   d. Meperidine
   e. Morphine

30. A neuroleptanalgesic is a combination of:
   a. An opioid and an anticholinergic
   b. An anticholinergic and a tranquilizer
   c. An opioid and a tranquilizer
   d. An anticholinergic and a benzodiazepine

ANSWERS FOR CHAPTER 1

1. False   **2.** False   **3.** Disagree   **4.** False   **5.** True   **6.** False   **7.** a   **8.** False
9. c   **10.** False   **11.** c   **12.** d   **13.** False   **14.** True   **15.** a   **16.** False
17. True   **18.** c   **19.** a, b, c, d   **20.** a, b, d   **21.** a, c, d   **22.** a, b, c, d
23. a, b, c, e   **24.** b, d   **25.** a, c, d, e   **26.** a, b, c   **27.** a, b   **28.** c   **29.** a, b, e
30. c

SELECTED READINGS

Haskins SC: *Opinions in small animal anesthesia,* Vet Clin North Am (Small Anim Pract) 22(2), Philadelphia, 1992, WB Saunders.

Johnson JM: The veterinarian's responsibility: assessing and managing acute pain in dogs and cats. I. *Compendium* 13(5):804-807, 1991.

Johnson JM: The veterinarian's responsibility: assessing and managing acute pain in dogs and cats. II. *Compendium* 13(6):911-916, 1991.

Muir WW, III, Hubbell JAE: *Handbook of veterinary anesthesia,* St Louis, 1989, Mosby.

Paddleford RR: *Manual of small animal anesthesia,* New York, 1988, Churchill Livingstone.

Sackman JE: Control of pain in animals, *Compendium* 13(2):181-191, 1991.

Short CE: *Principles and practice of veterinary anesthesia,* Baltimore, 1987, Williams & Wilkins.

Warren RG: *Small animal anesthesia,* St Louis, 1983, Mosby.

General anesthesia

2

PERFORMANCE OBJECTIVES
After completion of this chapter, the reader will be able to:

Define or explain the terms *general anesthesia, tachypnea, induction, hyperventilation, apneustic breathing, hypostatic congestion, reticular activating center, hypertension, hypotension, and central venous pressure.*

Identify or describe the components of general anesthesia, including the various stages and planes.

Understand the techniques, advantages, and disadvantages of IV, IM, and inhalation anesthesia.

Describe the technique of endotracheal intubation and understand the advantages and disadvantages of this procedure.

State the rationale for monitoring an anesthetized patient and know the various parameters that should be monitored.

Describe appropriate ways to position an animal during anesthesia.

State the various tasks or duties that need to be performed during the recovery period.

Understand the concept of safety as it relates to general anesthetics.

T hrough the use of the preanesthetic drugs described in Chapter 1, the anesthetist is able to tranquilize (and in the case of neuroleptanalgesics, profoundly
sedate) a small animal patient. This level of CNS depression is adequate for
minor procedures; however, a state of *general anesthesia* is usually required for
major surgeries. This chapter describes the components of general anesthesia,
including induction, maintenance, and recovery. The classical stages and planes of
general anesthesia and the anesthetic procedures and monitoring associated with
each stage are also described.

DEFINITION OF GENERAL ANESTHESIA

General anesthesia is a state of controlled and reversible unconsciousness characterized by lack of pain sensation (analgesia), lack of memory (amnesia), and relatively depressed reflex responses. Ideally, this state is achieved without significantly affecting the patient's vital systems, particularly respiration and circulation.

In any given patient, general anesthesia may be accomplished through the use
of injectable anesthetics, inhalation anesthetics, or both (Fig. 2-1). *Injectable anesthetics* include barbiturates (thiopental sodium, thiamylal sodium, methohexital,
and pentobarbital sodium), cyclohexamines (ketamine, tiletamine), and propofol.
Injectable neuroleptanalgesic agents, such as Innovar-Vet, also may be used to

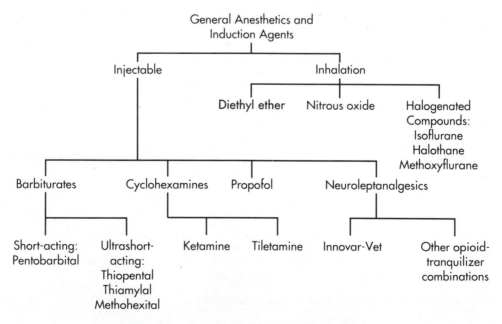

Fig. 2-1. Agents used in general anesthesia.

induce anesthesia, although they are not normally considered to be general anesthetics. *Inhalation anesthetics* used in veterinary medicine include diethyl ether, halothane, methoxyflurane, isoflurane, and nitrous oxide. Patients may be anesthetized with one drug or with several agents used in combination (in a technique called *balanced anesthesia*). The characteristics of general anesthesia are covered in this chapter, and the properties, advantages, and disadvantages of specific agents are discussed in detail in Chapter 3.

COMPONENTS OF GENERAL ANESTHESIA

General anesthesia is brought about through the use of techniques and agents (together called the *anesthetic protocol*) chosen by the veterinarian. The administration of a general anesthetic to any animal varies according to such parameters as temperament of the patient, nature of the procedure to be done, cost and availability of various drugs, and preference of the veterinarian.

Regardless of the anesthetic protocol chosen, any anesthetic procedure may be divided into the following components: preanesthesia, induction, maintenance, and recovery.

Preanesthesia

The preanesthetic period is the time immediately preceding anesthesia, in which patient data are collected, the patient is fasted, and preanesthetic drugs are administered. This period is discussed in Chapter 1.

Induction

The process by which an animal leaves the normal conscious state and enters the anesthetized state is known as *induction*. Usually, the induction process is initiated only after the animal has received premedication drugs, as ordered by the veterinarian, and enough time has lapsed for the drugs to take effect (a minimum of 10 minutes if the drugs are given by the intramuscular [IM] route and 20 minutes if the subcutaneous [SC] route is used). Occasionally, premedications and induction agents may be administered simultaneously, as, for example, when acetylpromazine, atropine, and ketamine are mixed in a syringe and given intravenously to a cat.

The induction agent may be administered to the patient either by injection or inhalation. When injection is used, it is frequently followed by intubation with an endotracheal tube to allow the administration of a volatile inhalation (gas) anesthetic by means of an anesthetic machine. Alternatively, the animal may be directly induced by means of a gas anesthetic delivered by a mask or anesthetic chamber, and no injectable anesthetic is necessary.

Initially, the animal may show signs of incoordination or excitement, followed by progressive relaxation and unconsciousness. The onset of general anesthesia is also characterised by the loss of some protective reflexes, including the ability to swallow or cough.

Maintenance

Following the induction period, the animal enters the *maintenance period,* during which a stable level of anesthetic depth is achieved. Surgery and other procedures are commonly performed during this period. As with induction, a predictable sequence of events occurs during the maintenance period, including the onset of analgesia, skeletal muscle relaxation and cessation of movement, further loss of protective reflexes including the palpebral (eye blink) reflex, and the occurrence of mild respiratory and cardiovascular depression. If anesthetic depth increases, the patient may show more severe respiratory and cardiovascular depression, and in the unusual event of an anesthetic overdose, respiratory and cardiac arrest can occur.

Recovery

The maintenance period ends and recovery begins when the concentration of anesthetic in the brain begins to decrease. The method by which the anesthetic is eliminated from the brain and circulatory system varies, depending on the anesthetic agent.

- Injectable drugs are commonly removed from the blood by the liver and undergo metabolism by liver enzymes. The metabolites are excreted by the urinary system. Some drugs do not undergo metabolism and are excreted unchanged by the kidneys (e.g., ketamine in the cat).
- In the case of short-acting thiobarbiturates, the level of anesthetic in the brain falls as the drug is rapidly absorbed by body fat, and the patient recovers from the anesthetic even though it is still present in the body.
- Inhalation agents are eliminated through the respiratory tract, as anesthetic molecules leave the brain and enter first the blood and then the alveoli of the lung.
- Recovery from either injectable or inhalation anesthesia may be hastened by the action of analeptic agents such as doxapram and reversing agents such as yohimbine discussed further in Chapter 3.

However it is achieved, recovery from anesthesia is in many respects the reverse of the induction process. Reflex activity, muscle tone, and sensitivity to pain are regained as consciousness returns.

SAFETY OF GENERAL ANESTHESIA

General anesthesia is not without risk. The administration of any anesthetic may affect the patient's vital centers, which are the areas of the brain that control cardiovascular and respiratory function and thermoregulation. Death may occur if the activity of these centers is not maintained throughout anesthesia. It is therefore vitally important that the animal be closely monitored during induction, maintenance, and recovery from any general anesthetic. Particular attention should be focused on heart rate, pulse quality, ventilation, mucous membrane color, and capillary refill.

The anesthetist may use several strategies to increase the safety of anesthesia and minimize the adverse effects of general anesthetic agents:

- Preanesthetic drugs, such as atropine or acetylpromazine, may be given to prevent bradycardia and cardiac dysrhythmias during general anesthesia.
- Preanesthetic sedatives such as xylazine, acetylpromazine, and opioids help reduce the dose of general anesthetic required to induce and maintain anesthesia, thus minimizing the adverse side effects of the general anesthetic agent. For example, a patient preanesthetized with acetylpromazine and butorphanol will require significantly less barbiturate to induce unconsciousness than an animal that has not received preanesthetic medication. In some patients, multiple general anesthetic and preanesthetic agents (such as a combination of nitrous oxide, an opioid, and a muscle relaxant) may be used in a balanced anesthesia technique to further minimize the required dose of each agent used.
- All injectable drug dosages should be double-checked before administration to the animal, and the anesthetist should ensure that the concentration of an agent drawn into a syringe is the same as that used for the drug calculations. All syringes containing injectable anesthetic agents should be labeled with the patient's name, type of drug, and drug concentration.
- When inducing an animal or maintaining an animal already under anesthesia, only the *minimum* dose of drug needed to achieve the desired level of anesthesia should be administered. Many injectable agents are given "to effect," which means that only the amount of injectable anesthetic necessary to produce unconsciousness is given, rather than administering the entire dose calculated on a milligram per kilogram basis. This technique is necessary because the amount of drug needed to induce or maintain anesthesia cannot be accurately predicted for a given patient. Most dogs, for example, will achieve a moderately deep state of anesthesia after receiving 15 mg of thiopental sodium per kg body weight. A few dogs will reach a comparable anesthetic depth after receiving only 10 mg/kg thiopental sodium, and others will require 20 mg/kg to reach the same depth. Since the anesthetist can seldom predict the exact dose that a given patient will require, it is safer to give the drug as a series of bolus injections, observing the

animal for signs of anesthesia and discontinuing the administration of anesthetic when the desired depth is reached. This process is known as *titration*.

Factors that may affect the animal's response to a general anesthetic include age, breed, physical condition, preanesthetic drugs given, and the ability of the patient's liver and kidney to metabolize and excrete the drugs. For example, the amount of thiobarbiturate required to induce a quiet, older dog may be one half or less of the dose required to induce an active 2-year-old dog, despite the fact that the dogs may weigh the same. Similarly, a cat with a urinary obstruction may be deeply anesthetized after receiving less than 10 mg of IV ketamine, whereas a healthy cat may require 30 mg of IV ketamine to reach the same depth of anesthesia.

Just as the amount of drug required to *induce* anesthesia varies between patients, the amount of inhalation or injectable agent required to *maintain* anesthesia will also vary. At a given concentration of halothane gas, for example, one patient may show brisk reflexes and appear to be only lightly anesthetized, whereas another may show the absence of all reflexes and a relatively slow heart rate, indicating deep anesthesia. The knowledgeable anesthetist monitors the patient closely and alters the amount of anesthetic given to suit the patient's requirements, rather than relying solely on a calculated dose recommended by a textbook.

• Close observation of a patient during the recovery period is also critical. Various untoward events, such as vomiting, laryngospasm, and convulsions, may occur during the recovery period. Hypothermia is also of concern to the anesthetist, since recovery from anesthesia may be delayed if the animal's temperature has been allowed to fall below the normal range. Problems that may be encountered during the recovery period are described in Chapter 6.

CLASSICAL STAGES AND PLANES OF ANESTHESIA

During the course of general anesthesia, the animal passes through a series of anesthetic stages and planes roughly correlated with changes in anesthetic depth. With the induction of anesthesia, the patient enters stage I, and as anesthetic depth increases, the animal passes through stage II and stage III (the anesthetic depth most appropriate for surgical procedures) and, in some cases, may enter stage IV. These stages and planes are summarized in Table 2-1. Although they were first developed based on work done with the anesthetic agent diethyl ether, the stages may be adapted to describe the effect of other agents, including both injectable and inhalation anesthetics. The signs listed in the table will vary somewhat depending on the agent used and the individual patient's response.

TABLE 2-1

Depth indicators of anesthetic stages and planes

Stage of anesthesia	Behavior	Respiration	Cardiovascular function	Response to surgery	Depth	Eyeball position	Pupil size	Pupil response to light	Muscle tone	Reflex responses
I	Disoriented	Normal, may be panting; respiration rate 20-30 breaths/min	Heart rate unchanged	Struggle	Not anesthetized	Central	Normal	Yes	Good	All present
II "Excitement stage"	Excitement: struggling, vocalization, paddling, chewing, yawning	Irregular, may hold breath or hyperventilate	Heart rate may increase	Struggle	Not anesthetized	Central, may be nystagmus	May be dilated	Yes	Good	All present, may be exaggerated
III, plane 1 Light anesthesia	Anesthetized	Regular; rate 12-20 breaths/min	Pulse strong; heart rate > 90 bpm	May respond with movement	Light	Central or rotated, may be nystagmus	Normal	Yes	Good	Swallowing poor or absent, others present but diminished
III, plane 2 Medium (surgical) anesthesia		Regular (may be shallow); rate 12-16 breaths/min	Heart rate > 90 bpm	Heart and respiration rates may increase	Moderate	Often rotated ventrally	Slightly dilated	Sluggish	Relaxed	Patellar, ear flick, palpebral, and corneal may be present, others absent
III, plane 3 Deep anesthesia		Shallow; rate < 12 breaths/min	Heart rate 60-90 bpm; CRT increased; pulse less strong	None	Deep	Usually central, may rotate ventrally	Moderately dilated	Very sluggish or absent	Greatly reduced	All reflexes diminished or absent
III, plane 4		Jerky	Heart rate < 60 bpm; prolonged CRT; pale mucous membranes	None	Overdose	Central	Widely dilated	Unresponsive	Flaccid	No reflex activity
IV	Moribund	Apnea	Cardiovascular collapse	None	Dying	Central	Widely dilated	Unresponsive	Flaccid	No reflex activity

CRT, capillary refill time; bpm, beats per minute.

Stage I

Immediately after the administration of an inhalation or injectable agent, the animal enters the initial stage of anesthesia, stage I. Animals in this stage are conscious but disoriented and show reduced sensitivity to pain. Respiration and heart rate are normal, and all reflexes are present.

Stage II

Stage II begins with the loss of consciousness. All reflexes are still present and, in fact, may appear exaggerated. The animal is able to chew or swallow, and yawning is common. The pupils are dilated but will constrict in response to intense light.

As the higher centers of the brain release voluntary control of body functions, the animal may exhibit excitement in the form of rapid movement of the limbs, vocalization, and struggling. Breathing may be irregular, and the animal may appear to be holding its breath. Although animals in stage II may appear to be "fighting" the anesthesia, the actions are not under conscious control. Rather, they are thought to occur because the anesthetic selectively depresses neurons in the brain that normally inhibit and control the function of motor neurons.

Throughout stage II, care should be taken to prevent the struggling patient from injuring itself, the restrainer, or the anesthetist. To limit the duration of this "excitement" stage, it is desirable that the patient's depth be increased as quickly as possible by continuing the administration of anesthetic until stage III is reached. Stage II ends when the animal shows signs of muscle relaxation, slower respiration rate, and decreased reflex activity.

Stage III

The third stage is subdivided into four planes, representing increasing anesthetic depth from plane 1 through plane 4. In *plane 1* the respiratory pattern becomes regular, and involuntary limb movements cease. The eyeballs start to rotate ventrally, the pupils may become partially constricted, and the response to bright light is diminished. The gagging and swallowing reflexes are depressed such that an endotracheal tube may be successfully passed, allowing the patient to be connected to a gas anesthetic machine. Other reflexes (such as the palpebral reflex) are present; however, responses are less brisk than in stage II. Although appearing to be unconscious, the patient will not tolerate surgical procedures at this light plane of anesthesia and will move or otherwise react to a painful stimulus.

Animals in *plane 2* of stage III are generally considered to be at medium depth of anesthesia, suitable for most surgical procedures. Surgical stimulation may evoke a response such as increased heart rate or respiration rate, but the patient

usually remains unconscious and immobile. The pupillary light response is sluggish, the eyeballs may be central or rotated, and the pupils are slightly dilated. The respirations are regular but shallow, with a respiratory rate between 12 and 16 breaths per minute in the dog (slightly higher in the cat). Heart rate and blood pressure are mildly decreased. The skeletal muscle tone becomes more relaxed, and many of the normal protective reflexes (pedal, palpebral) are diminished or lost.

In *plane 3* of stage III, the patient appears to be deeply anesthetized. Significant depression of circulation and respiration is often present, and for this reason plane 3 is considered to be excessively deep for most surgical procedures. The respiratory rate is less than 12 breaths per minute, and respirations are shallow. Ventilation assistance in the form of "bagging" with the reservoir bag or assistance from a mechanical ventilator may be desirable in some patients.

Heart rate is also notably reduced in patients at this plane, even in the presence of surgical stimulation. Pulse strength may be reduced because of a fall in blood pressure. The capillary refill time may be increased to 1.5 to 2 seconds. The pupillary light reflex is poor throughout this plane and may be absent. The eyeballs become central, and the pupils are moderately dilated. Reflex activity is often totally absent. Skeletal muscle relaxation is marked, to such a degree that no resistance occurs when the mouth is opened (i.e., jaw tone is slack).

Plane 4 of stage III can be recognized by a "rocking boat" ventilatory pattern. This type of ventilation is characterized by spasmodic, jerky inspirations, caused by a lack of coordination of the intercostal and abdominal muscles and the diaphragm. Plane 4 is also characterized by a fully dilated pupil and the absence of a pupillary light reflex. The eyes may be dry because of the absence of lacrimal secretions. Muscle tone is flaccid. More importantly, there is obvious depression of the cardiovascular system, marked by a dramatic drop in heart rate and blood pressure, accompanied by pale mucous membranes and a prolonged capillary refill time. The patient in this plane is too deeply anesthetized for safety and is in danger of imminent respiratory and cardiac arrest.

Stage IV

If anesthetic depth is increased past stage III, plane 4, the animal enters stage IV of anesthesia. At this stage, there is a cessation of respiration, which is quickly followed by total circulatory collapse and death. Immediate resuscitation is necessary to save the patient's life.

Overview of anesthetic stages and planes

Although these stages and planes would appear easy to differentiate on paper, they are not well defined in every animal. A given patient may show some signs that

indicate stage III, plane 2 anesthesia and other signs indicating stage III, plane 3. The anesthetist must assess as many parameters as possible in order to come to a conclusion regarding the patient's depth of anesthesia.

The appearance of the anesthetic stages and planes also varies somewhat among anesthetic agents. Methoxyflurane, for example, produces greater respiratory depression than halothane. An animal in stage III, plane 3 of methoxyflurane anesthesia may have a respiratory rate of 8 breaths per minute, whereas the same animal at the same plane of anesthesia might have a respiratory rate of 12 breaths per minute when anesthetized with halothane.

What, then, is the "ideal" depth of anesthesia? This question has no easy answer. The anesthetist must ensure that the patient does not perceive a surgical stimulus. At the same time, the anesthetist must avoid excessive anesthetic depth, which may result in depression of the cardiovascular and respiratory systems. The skills involved in achieving successful induction, maintenance, and recovery of anesthetized animals are discussed in the remainder of this chapter.

INDUCTION TECHNIQUES AND AGENTS

Induction using injectable agents

Anesthesia may be induced by either intravenous or intramuscular injection of general anesthetic agents.

Induction by intravenous injection

One of the most common induction methods involves the intravenous (IV) injection of a barbiturate, cyclohexamine, or neuroleptanalgesic agent. Thiopental sodium, ketamine, propofol, and oxymorphone/acetylpromazine are examples of inducing agents that are given intravenously. Typically, a standard dose of the agent is calculated and drawn up into a syringe, then administered as needed to induce unconsciousness and allow endotracheal intubation of the animal without resistance. (For a detailed outline of induction technique, see the box on p. 65.) Once intubated, the animal may be maintained at a moderate or deep level of anesthesia through the administration of an inhalation anesthetic. The use of inhalation anesthetic is not always necessary, however, since it is possible to perform minor surgical and short diagnostic procedures (such as radiography, endoscopy, and quill removal) under injectable anesthesia alone.

The duration of anesthesia varies with the injectable agent used, but is usually less than 20 minutes. If necessary, anesthesia may be prolonged by repeated administration of the intravenous agent. Repeated dosing, however, is generally discouraged because it may lead to the accumulation of large amounts of anesthetic within the body, resulting in a prolonged recovery.

Intravenous induction of anesthesia

The method of administering a drug by IV induction varies depending on the agent used. In most cases the patient is premedicated with a tranquilizer and, if requested by the veterinarian, an anticholinergic. Premedication reduces the dose of anesthetic required and allows smoother induction. *Barbiturates* are usually injected over a 10- to 15-second period by a technique known as *bolus* induction. In this technique, half of the calculated dose is injected IV, such that the patient's anesthetic depth is rapidly increased, resulting in stage III anesthesia with little evidence of stage I or stage II excitement. If the patient is not sufficiently anesthetized to allow intubation 15 to 30 seconds after injection (1 minute if pentobarbital is used), a second dose (one fourth the calculated dose) may be given. This method of administration is continued until the desired depth is reached. In patients with systemic disorders (acidosis, hypoproteinemia, or illness), the amount of barbiturate given in each bolus should be reduced to as little as 5% of the calculated dose. These patients may reach an adequate anesthetic depth at a greatly reduced dosage compared to that given to a healthy patient. During bolus induction with barbiturates, patients may exhibit signs of disorientation and excitement corresponding to stages I and II anesthesia if the barbiturate is given too slowly or if some of the drug is injected perivascularly. For this reason, and to prevent the irritation that occurs when barbiturates are injected outside the vein, an IV catheter is commonly used for the administration of barbiturates (Fig. 2-2).

In contrast to the bolus induction technique used with barbiturates, other agents such as propofol, ketamine-tranquilizer mixtures, and neuroleptanalgesics may be injected much more slowly, over 1 to 2 minutes. Although the animal passes through stage I and stage II in a slow induction of this type, excitement is not usually seen following administration of these agents. Slow inductions have the advantage of minimizing the toxic effect of these anesthetic agents on the cardiovascular and respiratory systems. Bolus injection also may be used for these agents, particularly if rapid induction is desired. One technique for induction using *ketamine-diazepam* is as follows: a bolus of one third the calculated dose is given IV, and a portion of the remainder is injected every 45 seconds until the desired depth is reached. It may be helpful to supplement ketamine or neuroleptanalgesia induction with administration of an inhalation anesthetic by mask, until the animal is well relaxed and intubation is possible.

Propofol also can be used to induce anesthesia by IV administration. A gradual injection technique (25% of the calculated dose given every 30 seconds) has been suggested. More rapid induction is also safe and may be useful in uncooperative patients and in those animals in which the anesthetist wishes to establish rapid intubation and airway control (brachycephalic animals and animals that have not been fasted).

In some animals, even more gradual induction may be achieved by adding a calculated dose of an opioid agent, such as oxymorphone, to a bag of IV fluids. The fluid-opioid mixture is administered to the patient by an IV drip and can be discontinued when the desired anesthetic depth is reached. Alternatively, oxymorphone can be diluted with saline and given slowly by syringe injection until the desired level of anesthesia is achieved. These gradual induction methods provide relatively safe and gentle induction for debilitated or geriatric patients. They are not, however, effective induction methods in healthy patients unless supplemented by some form of inhalation anesthesia.

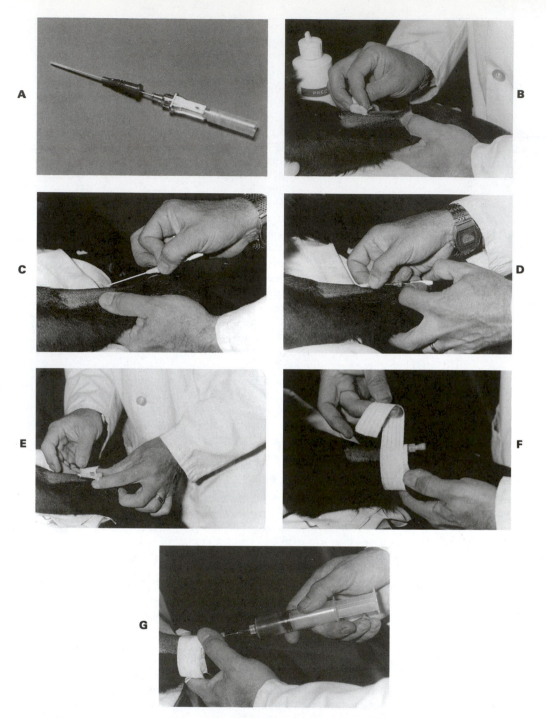

Fig. 2-2. Use of an intravenous catheter for injection of barbiturate. **A,** Intravenous catheter, showing metal stylet used for placement of catheter in vein. **B,** Surgical preparation of cephalic vein. **C,** Insertion of catheter into vein. **D,** Catheter is advanced over stylet. **E** and **F,** Taping of catheter in place. **G,** Injection of drug into catheter cap.

Induction by intramuscular injection

Some induction agents, including ketamine and fentanyl-droperidol (Innovar-Vet) may be administered by intramuscular (IM) injection. This method is useful for uncooperative animals and for animals in which IV injections are difficult, such as ferrets and very young puppies and kittens. (Inhalant inductions also may be used in these animals and are usually preferable.)

Induction by IM injection differs from IV induction in several important respects:

1. For most agents, the dose required for induction of anesthesia by IM injection is 2 to 3 times the IV induction dose.
2. It is difficult to titrate drugs given by the IM route, so usually the entire calculated dose is given.
3. Drugs administered by the IM route require several minutes to reach the brain at a concentration high enough to induce anesthesia. IM induction of anesthesia is therefore characterized by a relatively slow onset of anesthesia. This is in contrast to drugs administered intravenously, which take effect much more quickly, particularly if a bolus induction technique is used.
4. IM administration is characterized by a lengthy recovery period because the animal requires considerable time to metabolize the relatively large dose of drug given by this route.

The characteristics of intramuscular and intravenous anesthesia are illustrated by the use of ketamine, an anesthetic commonly used in cats. When given intravenously at a dose of 5 mg/kg, induction of anesthesia occurs in less than 1 minute. Alternatively, the drug can be given intramuscularly at a dose of 15 mg/kg, inducing anesthesia in 3 to 5 minutes. Recovery from IV ketamine administration is usually rapid, and healthy animals often appear fully recovered within 1 to 2 hours. In contrast, complete recovery from IM ketamine administration may require 8 to 12 hours.

IM administration of induction agents is particularly useful in anesthesia of wild animals and zoo animals. Because it is difficult to approach and handle these animals, the agent is usually administered by means of a blowpipe or tranquilizing gun, or through the use of a squeeze cage. Agents that can be administered by this method include ketamine/xylazine mixtures, neuroleptanalgesics, and opiates (particularly etorphine).

Induction by oral administration

Anesthesia may result when some agents, including ketamine and Innovar-Vet, are given *orally*. This route of administration constitutes extra-label use of these agents. Oral administration is not used routinely, but may be appropriate in some situations. Typically, a single dose of the agent is drawn into a syringe and forcefully squirted into the animal's mouth. Care should be used to avoid aspiration of the material by the patient.

Induction using inhalation agents

Induction of anesthesia may be achieved through the use of rapid-acting inhalation anesthetics, such as halothane or isoflurane. Nitrous oxide is occasionally used to supplement the anesthetic effect of other inhalation agents. The gas anesthetic contained in an anesthetic machine is administered along with oxygen by means of a face mask or anesthetic chamber.

Mask induction

The technique for mask induction is described in the box below. Mask induction is well suited to use with rapid-acting inhalation anesthetics, such as isoflurane, but is more difficult to achieve when a slow-acting anesthetic, such as methoxyflurane, is used. Mask induction is considered to have less risk than induction using injectable agents because the anesthetist can quickly control the animal's depth by adjusting the vaporizer setting. If problems arise, induction can be discontinued immediately.

The main drawback of mask induction is the high level of operating room pollution that can occur. Waste anesthetic gas readily leaks around the mask and is released into the room air.

It is possible to maintain anesthesia by using a mask throughout the surgical procedure; however, most anesthetists prefer to intubate the patient with an endotracheal tube after induction, allowing direct connection to an anesthetic machine.

Technique for mask induction

Either a malleable black rubber mask or a clear plastic mask with a rubber diaphragm may be used for mask induction. The mask should fit tightly on the animal's face to reduce leakage of waste gas and to minimize dead space. The mask is connected to the Y piece of an anesthetic machine and is held in place over the animal's muzzle (Fig. 2-3). To allow the patient to adjust to the mask, 100% oxygen is given for 2 to 3 minutes. The oxygen flow rate should be set at a minimum of 3 to 4 liters per minute (higher flow rates may result in faster induction). The anesthetic vaporizer is then set to deliver 0.5% isoflurane or halothane. The concentration of anesthetic is gradually increased by small increments (e.g., by increasing the vaporizer setting by 0.5% every 30 seconds) until an anesthetic concentration of 3% to 4% is reached.

This method is often well accepted by cats and small dogs, although some struggling may be seen after 2 to 3 minutes, possibly corresponding to stage II excitement. Induction of stage III, plane 1 anesthesia usually requires 5 to 10 minutes, depending on the agent used.

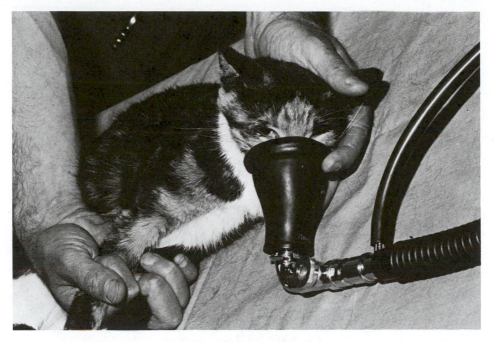

Fig. 2-3. Mask induction of a cat. (From Warren RG: *Small animal anesthesia,* St Louis, 1983, Mosby.)

Anesthetic chamber induction

Induction of anesthesia also can be achieved through the use of an anesthetic chamber (see box on p. 71 and Fig. 2-4). Anesthetic chambers allow the induction of even the most uncooperative animal but are associated with several problems.

- The technique is obviously suited only for use in small patients.
- Some risk of anesthetic complications is present, particularly that of vomiting, and the anesthetist cannot monitor the heart or respiration closely until the animal is removed from the chamber. For this reason, unfasted patients and animals with cardiovascular or respiratory disease should not be anesthetized using this technique.
- There is considerable risk of exposure of hospital personnel to waste anesthetic gas, particularly when removing the patient from the chamber. To avoid waste gas exposure, the chamber must be equipped with a scavenger, and the anesthetic gas should be evacuated before the chamber is opened.
- Both mask and chamber inductions should be avoided in animals for which rapid induction and immediate endotracheal intubation are desired. This category includes all brachycephalic dogs, animals that have not been fasted, and animals

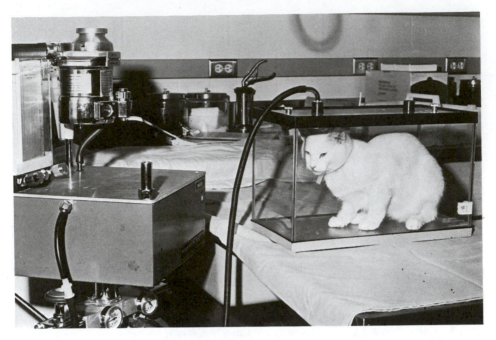

Fig. 2-4. Induction chamber.

with respiratory problems, including those with pleural effusion, diaphragmatic hernia, or pulmonary edema.

Monitoring during the induction period

Regardless of the induction method chosen, monitoring of the patient is of paramount importance throughout the induction period. The heart rate, pulse strength, respiratory rate and depth, mucous membrane color, and capillary refill time should be checked frequently by the anesthetist to ensure patient safety. The animal's reflexes and jaw tone should also be monitored, as they indicate the depth of anesthesia. Endotracheal intubation may be attempted when the patient shows no signs of resistance, gagging, or swallowing when the tongue is grasped and the mouth is opened.

ENDOTRACHEAL INTUBATION

Once anesthesia is induced in the patient, the anesthetist may choose to place a breathing tube (endotracheal tube) in the patient's airway. This tube conducts air

Induction of anesthesia using an anesthetic chamber

To induce anesthesia using an anesthetic chamber, the conscious animal is placed inside the chamber, which contains ordinary room air. The chamber should be large enough for the patient to lie down with its neck extended. Oxygen gas combined with an inhalation anesthetic is delivered to the chamber by means of an air inlet. Typically, a high concentration of anesthetic (4% to 5%) and a high flow rate of oxygen (3 to 5 liters per minute) are used. The anesthetist observes the behavior of the patient and removes the patient from the chamber when the patient loses its ability to stand (loss of righting reflex). This can be tested by rocking the chamber gently.

If the patient is too lightly anesthetized to be intubated immediately after being removed from the chamber, a mask can be used to induce a deeper level of anesthesia.

directly from the oral cavity to the trachea, bypassing the nasal passages and pharynx (Fig. 2-5).

Advantages of endotracheal intubation

Anesthesia with endotracheal intubation offers several advantages over anesthesia in the nonintubated animal.

- If a gas anesthetic machine is to be used, intubation of the patient allows more efficient delivery of the anesthetic gas to the animal than does a mask. Therefore, endotracheal intubation results in reduced exposure of hospital personnel to waste anesthetic gas.
- Intubation improves the overall efficiency of respiration by reducing the amount of dead space within the respiratory passages. *Dead space* is a term that describes those portions of the breathing passages that contain air but in which no gas exchange can occur, namely, the mouth, nasal passages, pharynx, and trachea. By minimizing dead space, the endotracheal tube ensures that a larger proportion of the gas delivered to the patient reaches the exchange surface in the alveoli.
- Intubation allows the anesthetist to deliver oxygen directly to the patient in cases in which respiration must be assisted. Forced delivery of oxygen (with or without an inhalation anesthetic) to a patient by means of a reservoir bag or ventilator is called *intermittent positive pressure ventilation (IPPV)* and is discussed in Chapter 7. This type of ventilation support may be essential in a patient that is having trouble breathing adequately during anesthesia. Positive pressure ventilation

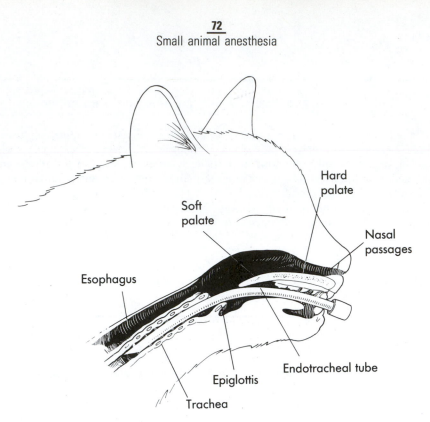

Fig. 2-5. Intubation of a cat, showing anatomy.

through an endotracheal tube is also necessary in animals given neuromuscular blocking agents.

• The presence of an endotracheal tube with an inflated cuff reduces the risk of aspiration of vomitus, blood, saliva, or other material that may be present in the oral cavity or breathing passages. This material may collect during any procedure; however, the risk of aspiration is particularly high during oral surgery or dentistry and in patients that have not been fasted. Because of the usefulness of an endotracheal tube in maintaining a patent airway, it is customary to leave it in place throughout anesthesia and into the recovery period, removing it only when the animal regains the swallowing reflex.

Problems associated with endotracheal intubation

There are several problems and hazards associated with endotracheal intubation.

• As discussed in Chapter 1, intubation may stimulate the activity of the vagus nerve, causing an increase in parasympathetic system tone, particularly in dogs. This, in turn, may cause bradycardia, hypotension (low blood pressure), and cardiac dysrhythmias. Occasionally, cardiac arrest may occur, particularly in an animal with preexisting cardiovascular disease. Atropine given in the preanesthetic period is helpful in preventing parasympathetic stimulation.

- Some species and breeds are difficult to intubate. Brachycephalic dogs, for example, have a large amount of redundant tissue within the oral cavity. This tissue falls over the back of the pharynx when the animal's mouth is opened, obscuring the entrance to the trachea (the glottis). Despite this difficulty, it is important to intubate these animals, because otherwise it may be impossible to maintain an open airway during anesthesia.

- Overzealous efforts to intubate an animal may damage the larynx, pharynx, or soft palate. Particular care should be used when intubating cats, which have a narrow glottis that is easily traumatized. If the tissues of the larynx are irritated during intubation, reflex closure of the laryngeal cartilages may occur. This condition, called *laryngospasm,* may result in blockage of the airway, which must be relieved or asphyxiation will result. To prevent laryngospasm, the anesthetist should avoid trauma to the laryngeal area during intubation. In cats it is also common procedure to spray the larynx with lidocaine and to lubricate the endotracheal tube with lidocaine gel to help desensitize the laryngeal tissues and reduce the risk of laryngospasm. Treatment of laryngospasm is discussed in Chapter 6.

- Certain food animal species and exotic and laboratory animal species are difficult to intubate because the mouth cannot be opened wide enough to allow the anesthetist to see the pharynx or glottis. "Blind" intubation is necessary in these species.

- If the endotracheal tube is inserted too far into the breathing passages, it may enter one bronchus, resulting in the ventilation of only one lung (Fig. 2-6). The tip of the tube should lie midway between the larynx and the thoracic inlet. Palpation of the thoracic inlet while gently moving the tube can assure the anesthetist of correct insertion depth of the tube. Alternatively, the length of the tube can be

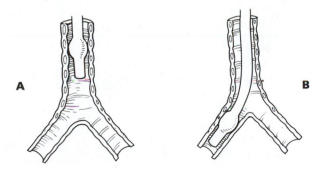

Fig. 2-6. Placement of endotracheal tube in trachea. **A,** Correct placement. **B,** Endobronchial intubation (incorrect).

"premeasured," by determining the distance between the nose and the thoracic inlet of the patient, before anesthesia.

• Many commercially available tubes are designed for human use and are too long for veterinary patients, particularly cats. If an excessively long tube is used, a large portion may extend forward past the animal's incisors, increasing the amount of dead space (Fig. 2-7). The endotracheal tube should be adjusted or trimmed such that the end of the tube is as close as possible to the animal's incisors. When shortening a tube, care must be taken to avoid cutting into the cuff inflation apparatus.

• Pressure necrosis may result if the cuff of the endotracheal tube is inflated excessively. Cats are particularly sensitive to pressure necrosis from endotracheal tubes (possibly the result of the ease of overinflation of the cuffs of small tubes), and in this species it is sometimes recommended that noncuffed tubes or tubes with low pressure cuffs be used. Some anesthetists suggest that if tubes with high pressure cuffs are used, the cuff should be inflated for no longer than 30 minutes before being deflated and moved to a new location in the trachea.

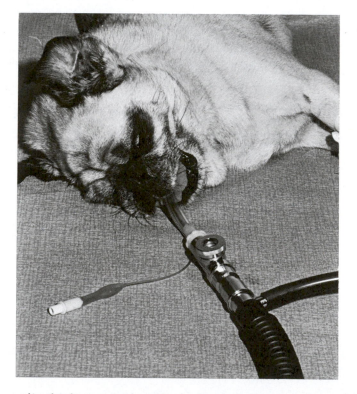

Fig. 2-7. Excessive dead space (endotracheal tube too long or not advanced sufficiently). (From Warren RG: *Small animal anesthesia,* St Louis, 1983, Mosby.)

- Endotracheal tubes may become obstructed by saliva, mucus, blood, or foreign material such as gauze. Obstruction may also occur if the tube is kinked or twisted or the end is occluded by the wall of the trachea. However it arises, obstruction of the endotracheal tube may cause a functional upper airway obstruction in the patient, which is a serious anesthetic emergency.
- Intubated animals require careful monitoring during recovery to ensure that the tube is removed when the animal begins to swallow. If the patient regains consciousness with the tube in place, the tube may be damaged by the patient chewing on it. In fact, patients have been known to chew tubes in half and aspirate the distal portion into the airway. The presence of such a tracheal foreign body obviously would be difficult to explain to the owner.
- Although endotracheal tubes used in human anesthesia are routinely discarded after a single use, it is common in veterinary practice for tubes to be used on several patients. Tubes must therefore be thoroughly disinfected between patients to prevent the spread of infectious diseases such as tracheobronchitis (''kennel cough'').

Because of the hazards associated with the use of endotracheal tubes and for reasons of convenience, not all animals undergo endotracheal intubation during anesthesia. If an endotracheal tube is not used, the inhalation agent is delivered by mask throughout the procedure. Animals lightly anesthetized with intramuscular or intravenous agents for the performance of short procedures also may not require the use of an endotracheal tube if the animal maintains the ability to swallow throughout the anesthesia. Despite these exceptions, intubation is recommended for safety reasons if inhalation anesthetics are used or if a lengthy procedure is performed with the patient under injectable anesthesia.

Endotracheal tubes are further discussed in Chapter 4. Details of the intubation procedure are given in the box below.

Endotracheal intubation procedure

The technique for endotracheal intubation is as follows:
1. All necessary materials should be gathered together before inducing the patient. Several endotracheal tubes of varying sizes should be selected and checked for holes, loose connectors, and excessive wear. The cuff of each tube should be tested to make sure it remains inflated when air is introduced. The amount of air required to inflate the cuff should be recorded.
2. The length of the tube required is determined by measuring the distance from the incisor teeth to the thoracic inlet. The diameter of the tube required can be estimated by palpating the trachea.
3. The tube is lubricated with a sterile lubricant, such as petroleum jelly. In cats,

lubricant containing a local anesthetic, such as Xylocaine, may be used to decrease the incidence of laryngospasm. It is also customary to spray a topical anesthetic on the vocal cords of feline patients before intubation. The intubation should be delayed 1 to 2 minutes to allow the spray to take effect. Commercial laryngeal sprays are available, or 1% lidocaine may be drawn into a tuberculin syringe and aerosolized through a 26-gauge needle. This procedure helps reduce the sensitivity of the laryngeal tissues to intubation trauma and thus helps prevent laryngospasm. Cetacaine was previously used for this purpose, but its use has been largely discontinued because of its tendency to induce methemoglobinemia. Whatever agent is used, only a small amount of topical anesthetic should be administered (0.1 ml), because excessive administration may be toxic.

4. When the animal reaches an appropriate plane of anesthesia, the mouth is opened to allow intubation. An animal showing signs of resistance, such as gagging and swallowing, is too lightly anesthetized to be intubated. The animal is usually restrained in sternal recumbency, although intubation in lateral or dorsal recumbency is preferred by some anesthetists. The neck is extended and the head is raised such that the head and neck are in a straight line, pointing upward (Fig. 2-8). The animal's trunk should be propped upright and not allowed to sag laterally. The upper jaw is held stationary, with the lips pulled dorsally, and the lower jaw is pushed down by pulling the animal's tongue forward and down. The tongue may be held out by either the assistant or the person intubating the animal. The mouth is opened wide enough to allow the anesthetist to clearly see the epiglottis, which normally lies over the entrance to the trachea (Fig. 2-9). The restrainer should not support the animal's ventral neck and head region because this may obscure the laryngeal anatomy, making intubation more difficult.

5. A laryngoscope is often used to assist intubation. This instrument consists of a handle, a smooth blade (which may be curved or straight), and a light source (either a small bulb lamp or a fiberoptic source). Laryngoscopes facilitate intubation by illuminating the pharyngeal area and by moving the epiglottis aside, exposing the glottis and vocal cords. The laryngoscope blade is first used to disengage the soft palate from the epiglottis. It is then placed gently at the back of the tongue, adjacent to the base of the epiglottis (in the case of a curved laryngoscope blade, Fig. 2-9, *inset*) or on the tip of the epiglottis itself (straight laryngoscope blade). This pulls the epiglottis forward and down, allowing the anesthetist to view the entrance to the trachea.

As an alternative to a laryngoscope, some anesthetists use the index finger of one hand to depress the epiglottis and guide the endotracheal tube into the trachea. This method of intubation carries some risk of being bitten by the patient if anesthetic depth is not sufficient. It is also possible to blindly intubate the animal by passing the tube into the mouth with one hand as the other hand holds the mouth open and extends the tongue (Fig. 2-10). In this method, the tube is passed along the roof of the mouth, over the epiglottis, and into the entrance to the trachea. Both blind intubation and digital intubation should be avoided if possible, because significant trauma to pharyngeal and laryngeal tissues is possible with these techniques. Laryngospasm and esophageal intubation also occur more often with these techniques.

6. The endotracheal tube is inserted past the vocal folds and into the trachea. This may be difficult in cats, because the vocal cords are frequently positioned such that they close off the glottis. Intubation in cats is best accomplished by timing the advancement of the tube to coincide with exhalation (when the vocal cords separate and the glottis is open). The endotracheal tube should not be forced past the vocal cords, but gently rotated, if resistance is encountered. The tube should be advanced such that the curve of the tube matches that of the patient's neck.

When advancing a small tube, problems may arise because of bending of the tube during insertion. A thin steel or wooden rod may be inserted into the tube to act as a stylet and prevent bending (Fig. 2-11). The stylet should not protrude beyond the end of the tube, since it may traumatize the laryngeal tissues.

The anesthetist should ensure that the tube enters the trachea and not the esophagus. The entrance to the esophagus lies just dorsal to the entrance to the trachea, and although difficult to see, it easily accommodates an endotracheal tube. Accidental intubation of the esophagus results in delivery of anesthetic and oxygen to the stomach rather than to the lungs, and the patient is unlikely to remain anesthetized if this occurs. Esophageal intubation can usually be avoided if the anesthetist visualizes the entrance to the trachea throughout the intubation procedure and ensures that the tube clearly enters that location.

7. Once the endotracheal tube is in place, its presence within the trachea (rather than the esophagus) should be confirmed. This can be done in one of several ways:
   - If the endotracheal tube is correctly placed, the reservoir bag should expand and contract as the animal breathes in and out. This is one of the most reliable methods for confirming correct location of the tube. Failure of the reservoir bag to inflate or deflate as the animal breathes may indicate esophageal intubation, endotracheal tube obstruction, or inadequate diameter of the endotracheal tube (animal is breathing room air around the tube). Movement of the bag should approximate tidal volume.
   - The mouth can be opened and the entrance to the trachea observed; the tube can be seen to emerge from the glottis if it is in the correct location.
   - In long-nosed breeds, it is possible to palpate the tube with the index finger at the point at which it enters the larynx.
   - A cough may be heard as the tube is inserted. The cough reflex is a normal response to endotracheal intubation, particularly at a light plane of anesthesia; it usually indicates that the tube is entering the correct passageway to the trachea.
   - During expiration, the animal's breath can be felt as it exits the endotracheal tube. If the tube is in the trachea, a tuft of hair placed at the end of the endotracheal tube will also move with the animal's exhalations. Either way, the anesthetist is assured that the tube has been placed in the breathing passages and not in the esophagus.
   - Once the tube is connected to an anesthetic machine, the unidirectional valves should move during inspiration and expiration if the tube is correctly placed. An audible click may be detected as the valves move.
   - The anesthetist may palpate the animal's cervical region, ensuring that only

one firm structure is present, which is the trachea containing the endotracheal tube. Palpation of two firm structures usually indicates that the endotracheal tube is in the esophagus, and the trachea and the tube are being palpated separately. It is often possible to palpate the beveled end of the tube within the trachea, confirming its location.

- Vocalization is impossible if an endotracheal tube is correctly placed. Growling or whining usually indicates that the tube is in the esophagus and must be removed and reinserted in the correct location.

8. The endotracheal tube should be secured in place using a piece of gauze tied around the tube and behind the animal's head or on top of its nose (Fig. 2-12).

9. The cuff of the endotracheal tube should be inflated. The anesthetist should then check for leakage of anesthetic gas around the cuff. This is done by gently squeezing the reservoir bag and listening for a rush of air exiting the oral cavity. If the endotracheal tube size is appropriate and the cuff is inflated adequately, only a small hiss will be evident. If a loud hiss is heard, the anesthetist should inflate the cuff further or obtain a larger tube. If no hiss is heard, the anesthetist should consider deflating the cuff slightly, because it may be exerting excessive pressure on the tracheal mucosa.

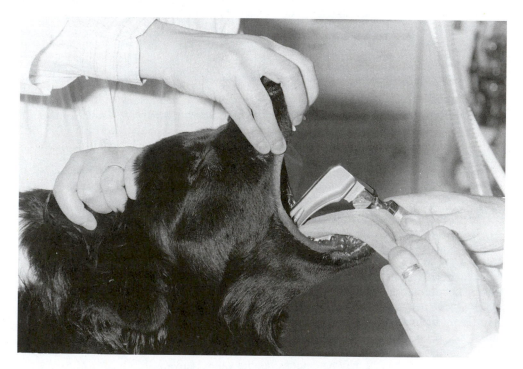

Fig. 2-8. Position of animal for intubation.

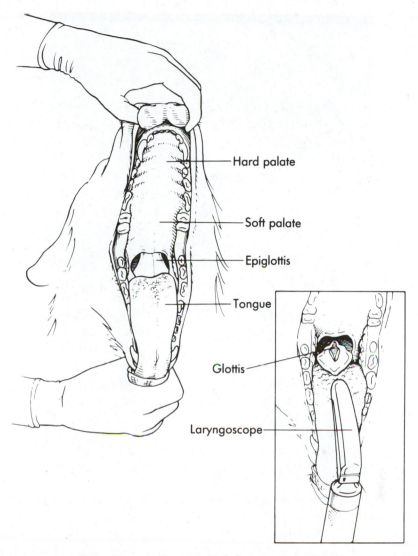

Fig. 2-9. Anatomy of the pharnyx when epiglottis is depressed, glottis is exposed. Endotracheal tube is advanced through glottis.

MAINTENANCE OF ANESTHESIA

Following successful induction of anesthesia, the animal enters a period in which anesthetic depth is adequate for surgical procedures. During this *maintenance period,* the anesthetist has two important tasks. First, he or she must monitor the animal closely, ensuring that the vital signs (particularly heart rate and respiration)

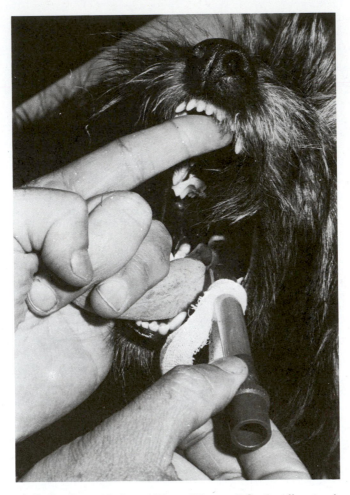

Fig. 2-10. Blind intubation technique. (From Warren RG: *Small animal anesthesia,* St Louis, 1983, Mosby.)

remain within acceptable limits. Second, the anesthetist must maintain the animal at an appropriate anesthetic depth (i.e., one that is neither too light nor too deep). The importance of both of these tasks can hardly be overemphasized. Failure to maintain an adequate depth of anesthesia may result in perception of pain by the animal and premature arousal from anesthesia. On the other hand, maintaining an animal at an excessive depth of anesthesia may lead to a slow recovery or an anesthetic overdose. Attention to vital signs is even more crucial, since failure to monitor and maintain vital signs within acceptable limits may result in death or permanent brain damage.

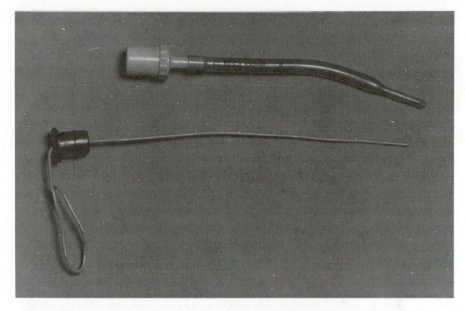

Fig. 2-11. Stylet for endotracheal tube.

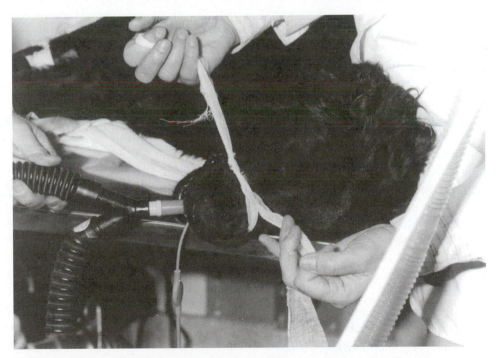

Fig. 2-12. Use of plain gauze to tie endotracheal tube in place.

Parameters to be monitored during anesthesia

Parameters to be assessed at least every 5 minutes throughout anesthesia

√ Respiration rate, depth, and character (assess both reservoir bag movement and chest movements)

√ Mucous membrane color and capillary refill time (CRT)

√ Heart rate

√ Pulse strength

√ Jaw tone, eye position, and palpebral reflex activity

√ Oxygen flow rate and oxygen tank pressure

√ IV catheter placement and fluid administration rate

√ Patient's temperature (may be adequate to palpate paws and ears)

The key to effective and safe anesthesia during the maintenance period is adequate monitoring. The word *monitor* comes from the Latin "monere" meaning "to warn." The anesthetist who monitors the animal under anesthesia closely will usually receive ample warning of problems as they arise. Although continuous monitoring of the anesthetized patient by a veterinary technician is impractical in many veterinary clinics, an attempt should be made to observe and evaluate a healthy anesthetized patient at least once every 3 to 5 minutes. This allows rapid but thorough assessment of depth, cardiovascular and respiratory status, and other parameters (see box). High-risk patients should be checked at more frequent intervals or, if possible, monitored continuously.

Although the anesthetist must observe both vital signs and reflexes, it is important to differentiate between the two. The term *vital sign* refers to those parameters that indicate the response of the animal's homeostatic mechanisms to anesthesia, including heart rate, respiration rate, and capillary refill time. The patient's vital signs indicate to the anesthetist how well the patient is maintaining basic circulatory and respiratory function during anesthesia. The term *reflex* refers to an involuntary response to a stimulus (such as a pinprick or tap). Reflex responses give the anesthetist valuable information on the depth of anesthesia but do not convey information on the patient's homeostatic mechanisms.

Vital signs

Vital signs may be monitored by the anesthetist's senses (touch, hearing, sight) or through the use of electronic devices such as an ECG machine or pulse oximeter. Electronic surveillance, although convenient, should not be relied on to give a complete picture of patient status, as instruments are subject to power failure, interference from artifacts, and loss of contact with the patient. Instrumentation cannot replace the presence of a skilled and conscientious anesthetist.

Vital signs that should be monitored during anesthesia include heart rate and rhythm, blood pressure, central venous pressure, capillary refill time, mucous membrane color, blood loss, respiratory rate and depth, blood gases, and thermoregulation.

Heart rate and rhythm

The minimum acceptable heart rate for anesthetized patients is 70 beats per minute (bpm) in the dog and 100 bpm in the cat. Lower heart rates may indicate excessive anesthetic depth or some other problem and should be brought to the veterinarian's attention immediately. Heart rates of 90 to 120 are common during anesthesia (compared to 70 to 180 bpm in the normal awake dog and 110 to 200 bpm in the normal awake cat). The decreased heart rate normally seen in an anesthetized animal is the result of the depressant effect of most anesthetics on heart rate and myocardial function. However, not all anesthetics reduce the heart rate. Elevated rates may be seen in animals that have received atropine or ketamine.

Cardiac rhythm also may be affected by anesthetic agents, particularly halothane and xylazine. Bradycardia or disturbances in cardiac rhythm should be brought to the attention of the veterinarian for assessment.

Cardiac monitoring may be achieved in several ways, including direct palpation of the chest wall or pulse, auscultation of the chest using a stethoscope, use of an electrocardiogram (ECG), and use of an esophageal stethoscope. Several types of heart monitors are available that detect the patient's ECG and transmit information to the anesthetist by an audible beep, a flash of light, or a digital readout. Display of an ECG on an oscilloscope or paper readout is even more useful, as alterations in heart rhythm and electrical activity may be more easily detected. Some monitors can be adjusted to sound an alarm when the heart rate is above or below limits set by the anesthetist.

Use of an esophageal stethoscope allows auscultation of the heart even if the patient's chest area is covered with surgical drapes and conventional auscultation is difficult. The esophageal stethoscope consists of a thin flexible tube attached to a regular stethoscope. The tube is lubricated with a small amount of water or lubricating jelly and is inserted through the oral cavity into the patient's esophagus and advanced until an audible heartbeat is detected through the earpieces (Fig. 2-13) or through an attached audio monitor. Insertion of the esophageal stethoscope is usually delayed until after an endotracheal tube has been placed to minimize the danger of the stethoscope accidentally entering the trachea.

The presence of a beating heart *does not* necessarily imply that circulation is adequate. Heartbeat must be assessed in conjunction with pulse strength or another measure of blood pressure.

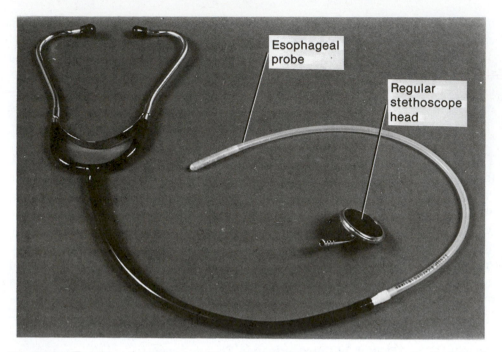

Esophageal
probe

Regular
stethoscope
head

Fig. 2-13. Esophageal stethoscope. (From Warren RG: *Small animal anesthesia,* St Louis, 1983, Mosby.)

Blood pressure

An animal's blood pressure reflects the adequacy of blood circulation throughout the body. Normal systolic blood pressure in the dog or cat is 110 to 160 mm Hg. Normal diastolic blood pressure is 60 to 100 mm Hg. Decreased blood pressure is called *hypotension,* and an increase in blood pressure is termed *hypertension.*

Blood pressure may be influenced by both general anesthetics and preanesthetics. Increasing depth of inhalation anesthesia usually results in a fall in blood pressure, particularly if halothane is used. Certain preanesthetic drugs (i.e., acetylpromazine and xylazine) may also reduce blood pressure by causing the blood vessels to dilate. Animals that are dehydrated or hypotensive (most commonly the result of circulatory shock) before anesthesia are at particular risk of suffering a further drop in blood pressure when given these preanesthetic and anesthetic agents.

Blood pressure may be monitored manually or through the use of instruments. A rough estimate of blood pressure may be obtained manually by determining the strength of the peripheral pulse. The pulse may be detected at any one of several locations, including the femoral, lingual (Fig. 2-14), carotid, and dorsal pedal arter-

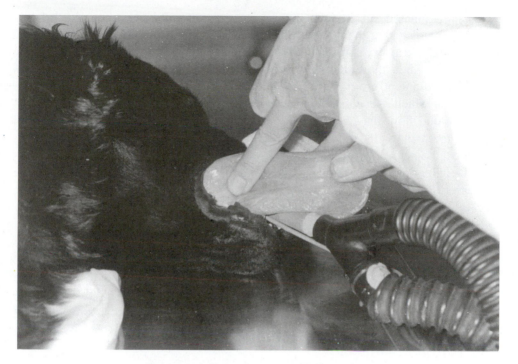

Fig. 2-14. Palpation of the lingual artery.

ies. The pulse should be strong and synchronized with the heartbeat. Difficulty in detecting a palpable pulse may indicate low blood pressure resulting from excessive anesthetic depth or hypovolemia (blood loss). Unfortunately, natural variation in pulse strength among normal animals somewhat limits the usefulness of this method of blood pressure monitoring.

A rough estimate of blood pressure is also given by capillary refill time (CRT), although it is a somewhat insensitive test. CRT is noticeably prolonged when the patient's systolic pressure drops below 70 to 80 mm Hg. Urine production also gives an indication of blood pressure, because it slows or stops when blood pressure falls to subnormal values.

Blood pressure can be monitored most accurately through the use of instruments. External devices may be placed around the patient's leg to detect the strength of a pulse in a peripheral artery. This type of blood pressure monitoring is called *indirect monitoring*. In human medicine, indirect blood pressure monitoring is usually done through the use of a sphygmomanometer and the familiar blood pressure cuff. All indirect blood pressure monitors, whether used on humans or small animals, are based on a simple principle: if a cuff is placed snugly around a limb and is inflated, an artery lying beneath the cuff will be compressed. When a pressure that is higher than the systolic blood pressure is applied by the cuff, blood flow through the artery stops. When the cuff pressure is slowly released, blood flow will resume when the cuff pressure equals the systolic blood pressure. Various types of equipment are used to detect the returning blood flow and indicate the pressure at which it occurs (the systolic blood pressure).

1. The blood flow may be auscultated with a stethoscope (this is the basis of sphygmomanometry in humans but is difficult to do accurately in a dog).
2. An oscillometer may detect the vibration of blood passing through the vessel.
3. A Doppler device may detect an ultrasound echo from blood passing through the vessel (Fig. 2-15).

Regardless of the instrumentation used, systolic blood pressure is normally indicated by a pressure dial (manometer) or by a digital display.

In certain specialized situations, arterial blood pressure may be *directly monitored* through the use of an indwelling catheter in the femoral or dorsal pedal artery. A surgical cutdown or percutaneous insertion technique is used to expose the artery, allowing placement of the catheter. The catheter is connected to a manometer or pressure transducer to display the measured pressure. Because of the difficulty in placing an arterial catheter, direct blood pressure monitoring is common only in research and referral institutions.

Central venous pressure

Just as blood pressure in an artery can be measured, it is possible to measure the pressure of blood flow in a large central vein, such as the anterior vena cava. This value, the *central venous pressure (CVP),* allows the veterinarian to assess how well blood is returning to the heart and the ability of the heart to receive and pump blood. This value is extremely helpful in monitoring animals for right-side heart failure, because it measures the backup of blood in the vena cava that results from this condition. It is also useful in preventing overhydration in animals receiving IV fluids, since CVP values rise as blood volume increases.

CVP can be directly measured by inserting a long catheter percutaneously or by cutdown into the anterior vena cava, in a manner similar to arterial blood pressure. The catheter is inserted into the jugular vein and advanced toward the heart, such that the tip of the catheter lies close to the right atrium. The catheter is connected to a water manometer to obtain a measurement. Normal CVP in dogs and cats is less than 8 cm H_2O pressure. Pressures over 12 to 15 cm H_2O are considered elevated. It is usually more valuable to monitor trends over time, rather than base an assessment on a single reading.

Capillary refill time

The capillary refill time (CRT) is the rate of return of color to a mucous membrane after the application of gentle digital pressure. The CRT reflects the perfusion of the

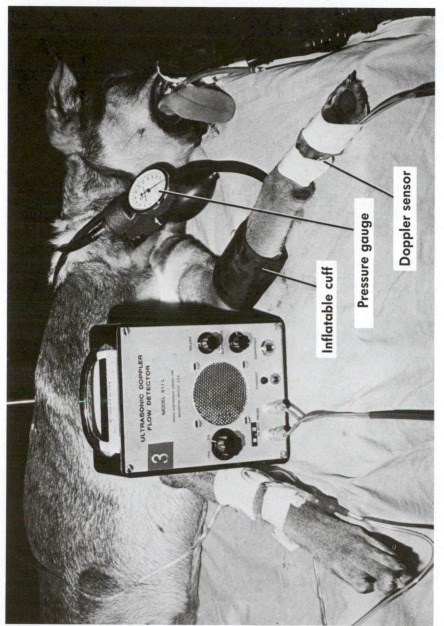

Fig. 2-15. Doppler blood pressure monitor. (From Warren RG: *Small animal anesthesia,* St Louis, 1983, Mosby.)

tissues with blood. Pressure on the mucous membranes compresses the small capillaries and blocks blood perfusion in that area. When the pressure is released, the capillaries rapidly refill with blood, and the color returns, provided the heart is able to generate sufficient blood pressure. However, a short CRT is not an infallible indication that the circulation is adequate; in fact, a normal CRT may be observed shortly after euthanasia in some animals.

A prolonged CRT (more than 2 seconds) may indicate hypotension resulting from excessive anesthetic depth or circulatory shock. CRT is usually prolonged in patients in which the systolic blood pressure is less than 80 mm Hg, and if systolic blood pressure drops below 50 mm Hg, the capillaries may not refill at all. Animals suffering from this degree of hypotension will usually appear cold and have colorless mucous membranes.

Mucous membrane color

The most convenient location for observing mucous membrane color is the gingiva (Fig. 2-16). In the case of dogs with pigmented gingiva, other sites may be used,

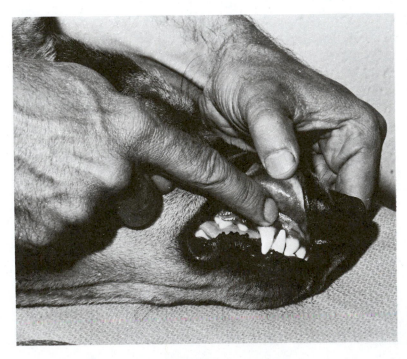

Fig. 2-16. Assessing gingiva for capillary refill time and mucous membrane color. (From Warren RG: *Small animal anesthesia,* St Louis, 1983, Mosby.)

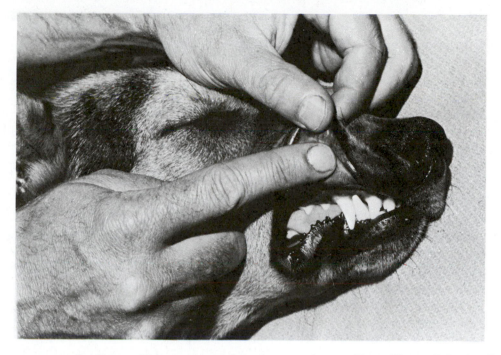

Fig. 2-17. Capillary refill test on buccal mucous membrane. (From Warren RG: *Small animal anesthesia,* St Louis, 1983, Mosby.)

including the tongue, buccal mucous membrane (Fig. 2-17), conjunctiva of the lower eyelid, or the mucous membrane lining the prepuce or vulva (Fig. 2-18). Pale mucous membranes may indicate blood loss or anemia or may result from poor perfusion (as may occur with prolonged anesthesia). Purple or blue mucous membranes indicate cyanosis, a shortage of oxygen in the tissues. Cyanosis during anesthesia is usually the result of respiratory failure or upper airway obstruction and must be addressed immediately.

Blood loss

Blood loss, if excessive, predisposes the patient to shock and anesthetic complications. Blood loss in major surgery may be estimated by counting used sponges. One fully soaked sponge holds 5 to 6 ml of blood. The true amount of blood lost may be up to twice this figure, as it is difficult to measure the amount of blood that has clotted or been retained by surgical drapes or has pooled at the surgery site.

A healthy animal may tolerate a loss of up to 15% of its blood volume without serious circulatory effects. This is approximately 13 ml/kg in dogs and cats.

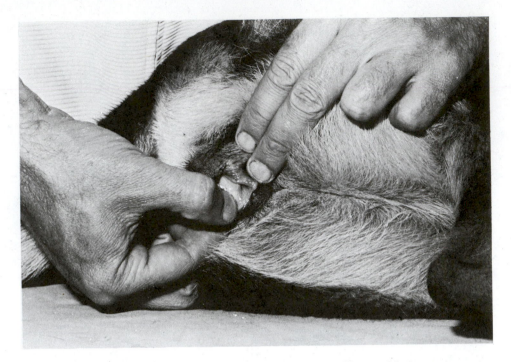

Fig. 2-18. Assessment of mucous membrane color and capillary refill time using vulvar mucous membrane. (From Warren RG: *Small animal anesthesia,* St Louis, 1983, Mosby.)

Respiration rate and depth

The animal's respiration rate may be monitored by observing movement of the reservoir bag or the animal's chest. Normal respiration rate in a conscious animal is 10 to 30 breaths per minute in the dog and 25 to 40 breaths per minute in the cat. At a moderate depth of anesthesia, the normal rate is 8 to 20 breaths per minute, although rates up to 50 may be seen. *During the maintenance period, respiratory rates less than 8 breaths per minute may indicate excessive anesthetic depth and should be reported to the veterinarian.*

The anesthetist must monitor not only the respiratory rate, but also the depth and character of the breathing. With increasing depth of anesthesia, there is normally a decrease not only in the rate, but also in the volume of air taken with each breath (tidal volume). This decrease in respiratory rate and volume is sometimes called *hypoventilation*. Tidal volume decreases by at least 25% in most anesthetized animals, largely because most preanesthetic and general anesthetic drugs decrease the ability of the intercostal muscles to expand the thorax on inspiration. As the animal's breaths become more shallow (i.e., tidal volume decreases), some alveoli in the lung may not receive amounts of air adequate to sustain inflation. As a result, these alveoli partially collapse, leading to a condition called *atelectasis*. In its early stages, atelectasis can be reversed by gentle inflation of the lungs by the anesthetist. In this procedure, called *bagging,* the reservoir bag of the anesthetic machine is carefully squeezed, forcing air into the patient's breathing passages. When bagging a patient, the anesthetist should closely observe the animal's chest to ensure that it rises only slightly, to prevent overinflation of the lungs. Some anesthetists routinely bag every patient under inhalation anesthesia once every 5 minutes. Alternatively, atelectasis may be prevented by mechanical ventilation of the patient through the use of a ventilator (Chapter 7).

In contrast to the hypoventilation that is observed in many anesthetized patients, the anesthetist may occasionally note rapid and deep respirations in some anesthetized patients. An increase in respiratory rate is called *tachypnea,* whereas an increase in depth is termed *hyperventilation.* Tachypnea must be differentiated from panting, in which the breathing is rapid but shallow and air intake is through the open mouth. Panting is a common side effect of opioid drugs, particularly oxymorphone and Innovar-Vet.

True hyperventilation and tachypnea have many possible causes. They are a normal response to increased $Paco_2$ or metabolic acidosis. When an anesthetic machine is used, hyperventilation may indicate that the carbon dioxide (CO_2) is not being adequately removed from the breathing circuit by the CO_2 absorber. Rapid respirations may also indicate an underlying disease, such as pulmonary edema. More commonly, hyperventilation is seen as a response to a mild surgical stimulus. For example, it is often seen when the surgeon pulls on the suspensory ligament of the ovary during an ovariohysterectomy. An elevated respiratory rate may also indicate a progression from moderate to light anesthesia and is one of the first signs of arousal from anesthesia.

Not only the respiratory rate and depth but also the type of respiration may be significant. The anesthetized animal's breathing should be smooth and regular, with both thoracic and diaphragmatic components. Difficult or labored breathing may indicate the presence of an airway obstruction. As previously mentioned, another abnormal breathing pattern, "rocking boat" respiration, is noted in very deep anesthesia.

The time relationship between inspiration and expiration may vary also. Normally, inspiration lasts 1 to $1\frac{1}{2}$ seconds and expiration lasts 2 to 3 seconds. Animals anesthetized with ketamine may exhibit an *apneustic* respiratory pattern, in which inspiration is followed by a prolonged pause before expiration.

Auscultation of the chest may yield useful information not only on cardiac function, but also on respiratory function. Normal respiratory sounds are almost inaudible in the dog and cat: harsh noises, whistles, or squeaks may indicate narrow or obstructed airways or the presence of fluid in the airways or alveoli.

As is evident from this discussion, the rate, depth, and type of respirations must be closely monitored by the anesthetist. Changes in any of these parameters may be the first warning of a change in anesthetic depth or of the onset of an anesthetic problem.

Blood gases

Although observation of respiration is of paramount importance to the veterinary anesthetist, this monitoring may not allow accurate evaluation of the patient's respiratory function. Ventilation may appear normal, yet the animal may be suffering from significant respiratory depression. True assessment of respiratory efficiency requires the use of blood gas analysis ($Paco_2$ and Pao_2) or sophisticated equipment unlikely to be found in a veterinary practice.

Most anesthetized animals show a greatly elevated Pao_2 (up to 500 mm Hg compared to the normal 90 to 115 mm Hg). The Pao_2 is elevated because the patient is breathing 100% oxygen from an anesthetic machine, whereas the unanesthetized animal breathes approximately 21% oxygen in room air. $Paco_2$ is also elevated during anesthesia (45 to 60 mm Hg compared to the normal 28 to 43 mm Hg) because the respiratory depression seen with most anesthetics causes the body to retain CO_2. As a result of the carbon dioxide elevation, hydrogen ions (H^+) are produced according to the equation:

$$H_2O + CO_2 \rightarrow H_2CO_3 \rightarrow H^+ + HCO_3^-$$

The accumulation of hydrogen ions (H^+) results in respiratory acidosis in many anesthetized patients, particularly those showing significant respiratory depression. The blood pH in an anesthetized patient usually reflects the mild respiratory acidosis and is commonly 7.20 to 7.30, compared to the normal animal's blood pH of 7.35 to 7.45.

A rough estimate of respiratory function can be obtained through the use of a pulse oximeter. This device, when attached to the tongue or other hairless area, indicates the percentage of saturated (oxygen-containing) hemoglobin. Low values (less than 95% saturation) indicate a shortage of oxygen in the blood, possibly because of poor ventilation.

Thermoregulation

Throughout anesthesia, the animal's temperature should be maintained as close as possible to the normal range for that species. Although body temperature does not change minute by minute, there is usually an overall drop of temperature with time. Temperature loss is greatest in the first 20 minutes, and the anesthetist should be concerned with preventing temperature loss from the moment of induction. Prolonged general anesthesia may reduce the patient's temperature by 3° C or more. Several factors contribute to this effect:

• Animals are routinely shaved before surgery, and the skin may be washed with antiseptic and alcohol solutions.

- The anesthetized animal cannot generate heat by shivering or muscle activity.
- The metabolic rate of an anesthetized animal is less than that of a conscious animal, resulting in less heat generation.
- During the course of surgery, a body cavity may be opened and the viscera exposed to air at room temperature.
- Several preanesthetic and general anesthetic agents cause vasodilation, resulting in an increased rate of heat loss.

One unfortunate result of hypothermia is prolonged recovery from anesthesia. Hypothermia slows the rate at which liver enzymes metabolize anesthetic drugs, allowing the drugs to remain active in the body for a longer time. In addition, shivering (which is seen in recovering animals) may increase the patient's oxygen demands during the recovery period, leading to hypoxia in some animals.

During anesthesia, rectal temperature should be monitored every 30 minutes. If the rectum is covered by surgery drapes or is otherwise inaccessible to the anesthetist, a rough estimate of body temperature can be obtained by touching the patient's paws or ears. Temperature also may be measured using special thermometers designed for use in the ear canal or esophagus.

Prevention of hypothermia may involve such measures as administering warm IV fluids (rather than fluids at room temperature or refrigerated fluids) and the use of a circulating warm water heating pad (Fig. 2-19), hot water bottles, bubble packing, and foil wraps. It is also important to ensure a comfortable air temperature

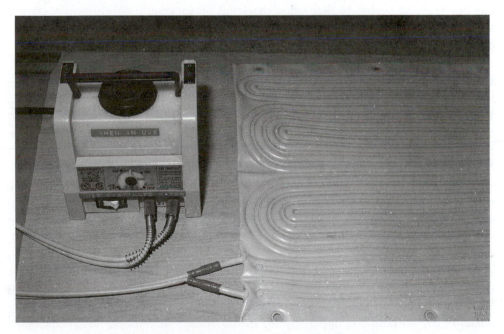

Fig. 2-19. Circulating warm water heating pad..

in the surgery room itself. Patients should not be placed on a stainless steel table or trough unless an insulating layer of newspaper, towels, or a heating pad is provided. Electric heating pads should be avoided, as burns are sometimes associated with their use.

Hyperthermia (increased body temperature) is occasionally seen in anesthetized small animals, particularly in susceptible dogs anesthetized with ketamine, halothane, or succinylcholine. Although rare, this syndrome (called *malignant hyperthermia*) may be fatal if not promptly relieved through the application of cold wet towels and the use of drugs.

Reflexes and other indicators of anesthetic depth

The anesthetist should have at all times an accurate assessment of the patient's depth of anesthesia. Anesthetic depth is a complex balance between the action of the anesthetics and the patient's overall condition. Body temperature, ventilation, blood pH, and blood pressure all have a potent influence on the way in which an anesthetic affects the animal. It is therefore important to monitor the whole animal, assessing the apparent depth in light of the animal's vital signs.

Anesthetic depth is indicated in several ways. Reflex activity, muscle relaxation, heart and respiratory rates, pupil size, and eye rotation are all useful guides in determining how deeply or lightly the patient is anesthetized (Table 2-2). For some anesthetics (particularly cyclohexamine agents, such as ketamine), it may be difficult for the anesthetist to determine the level of anesthetic depth; however, the following guidelines are useful for anesthesia induced by most general anesthetic agents.

Reflex activity

All normal conscious animals demonstrate predictable reflex responses to certain types of stimuli. One example is the cough reflex, in which the animal responds to the presence of foreign material in the trachea by forceful coughing. Reflex responses help protect the animal from injury: in the example above, the cough reflex helps prevent upper airway obstruction and the aspiration of injurious materials into the lung. These protective reflexes are progressively depressed at increasing depths of anesthesia, such that an animal in stage III, plane 3 (or deeper anesthesia) may have few reflex responses or none. The reflexes most commonly monitored in veterinary anesthesia include the palpebral, swallowing, pedal, ear flick, corneal, and laryngeal reflexes.

Palpebral reflex. The palpebral reflex (blink reflex) can be tested by lightly tapping the medial or lateral canthus of the eye and observing whether the animal blinks in response (Fig. 2-20). Some anesthetists prefer to test this reflex by lightly stroking the hairs of the upper eyelid. In the conscious animal, this reflex helps

TABLE 2-2

Indicators of anesthetic depth

Sign	Anesthetic depth		
	Light	**Medium**	**Deep**
Spontaneous movement	Maybe	No	No
Swallowing	Maybe	No	No
Vaporizer setting	Low	Medium (1.1-1.5 MAC)	High
Muscle tone	High	Moderate	None
Palpebral reflex	Active	Moderate	None
Eyeball position	Central	Ventromedial	Central
Pupillary light reflex	Present	May be present	Absent
Shivering	Maybe	No	No
Heart rate	Often elevated	Variable	Often decreased
Respiratory rate	Often elevated	8-30 breaths/min	Often decreased

Modified from Haskins C: General guidelines for judging anesthetic depth, *VCNA* 22(2):432, 1992.
MAC, minimum alveolar concentration.

protect the eye from injury. Most animals retain the palpebral reflex throughout stages I and II and partially through stage III, although individual and species variations exist. The stage at which the palpebral reflex is lost also varies among different anesthetic agents: at a surgical plane of anesthesia, it is usually present in barbiturate anesthesia, occasionally present in methoxyflurane anesthesia, but seldom present in halothane anesthesia. As with most reflexes, loss of the palpebral reflex indicates an increase in anesthetic depth, whereas return of the reflex usually indicates imminent arousal from anesthesia.

Swallowing reflex. The swallowing reflex occurs spontaneously in awake animals; it is usually stimulated by the presence of saliva or food in the esophagus. Lightly anesthetized animals swallow frequently, and this reflex can be readily monitored by observing movement in the patient's ventral neck region. The swallowing reflex is lost at a medium depth of anesthesia and is usually regained just before the patient recovers consciousness. The return of the swallowing reflex during recovery usually indicates that it is safe to remove the endotracheal tube. Animals that vomit after this point usually will swallow rather than aspirate the vomited material, and the endotracheal tube is therefore no longer needed to protect the airway.

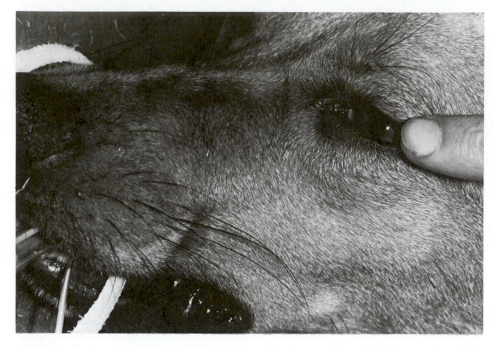

Fig. 2-20. Assessment of the palpebral reflex. (From Warren RG: *Small animal anesthesia,* St Louis, 1983, Mosby.)

Pedal reflex. The pedal reflex is elicited by squeezing or pinching a digit or pad and observing whether the unconscious animal flexes the leg, withdrawing the paw from the examiner (Fig. 2-21). The pedal reflex is a good indicator of anesthetic depth in animals that have been given the general anesthetic pentobarbital. This indicator is not as useful in inhalation anesthesia, because the reflex is normally lost during induction.

Ear flick reflex. The ear flick reflex (pinna reflex) is particularly useful in cats and can be tested by gently touching the hairs on the inner surface of the pinna and observing the resultant twitch of the ear. This reflex may be retained well into stage III, particularly in cats anesthetized with ketamine. This reflex may be difficult to elicit in some animals and may be easily lost if tested too frequently on an individual animal.

Corneal reflex. The corneal reflex can be tested by touching the cornea with a sterile object (a drop of water or artificial tear solution is commonly used) and noting whether the animal blinks and withdraws the eye into the orbital fossa. This reflex is commonly not tested in dogs and cats unless it is necessary to determine if the patient is too deeply anesthetized. This reflex is usually present until stage III, plane 4 anesthesia.

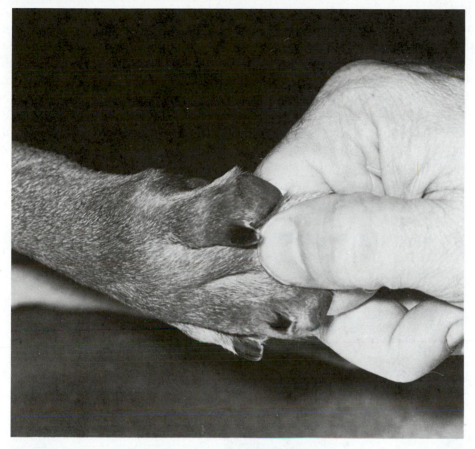

Fig. 2-21. Pedal reflex. (From Warren RG: *Small animal anesthesia*, St Louis, 1983, Mosby.)

Laryngeal reflex. The laryngeal reflex is stimulated when the larynx is touched by an object. The reflex response is an immediate closure of the epiglottis and vocal cords. This reflex normally protects the animal from aspiration of material into the trachea. The laryngeal reflex may be observed during intubation if the animal is not sufficiently anesthetized to allow the tube to be passed. It is easily elicited in cats, in which a sustained laryngeal reflex response is the cause of laryngospasm.

Muscle tone

Muscle tone is also a useful guide to anesthetic depth. With increasing depth, skeletal muscles become more relaxed and offer little resistance to movement. Among the muscles that can be readily assessed are the muscles of mastication, which control jaw tone. Jaw tone is assessed by attempting to open the jaws wide and estimating the amount of passive resistance (Fig. 2-22). Muscle tone also can be assessed by attempting to flex and extend the foreleg at the elbow and carpus. Anal tone also indicates skeletal muscle relaxation and may be assessed by noting the size of the rectal orifice. Some degree of muscle relaxation is desirable for most procedures; however, extreme muscle relaxation resulting in a flaccid jaw tone usually is unnecessary and may indicate excessive anesthetic depth.

The degree of muscle relaxation observed in the patient is dependent not only on anesthetic depth but also on the particular drugs given to the animal, some of which promote relaxation (diazepam, xylazine) and some of which increase muscle tone (ketamine, tiletamine). Specific muscle-paralyzing agents, such as succinyl-

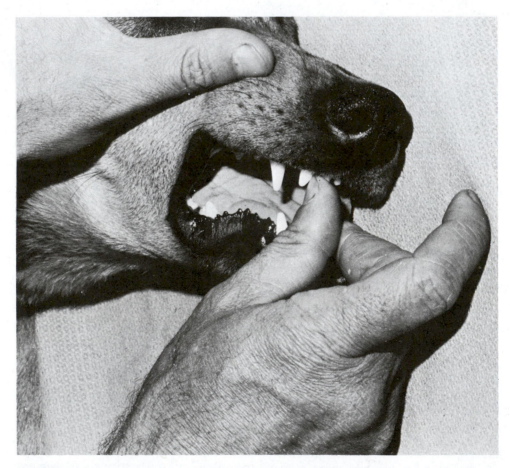

Fig. 2-22. Assessing jaw tone. (From Warren RG: *Small animal anesthesia,* St Louis, 1983, Mosby.)

choline, may be used in combination with general anesthetics to achieve pronounced muscle relaxation for certain procedures (see Chapter 7). This may be advantageous to the surgeon but gives the anesthetist one less parameter with which to monitor anesthetic depth.

Eye position and pupil size

Eye position, pupil size, and the pupillary response to light also may indicate anesthetic depth, although there is considerable variation among individual animals. The eyeball itself is usually central in stage I anesthesia. It becomes eccentric in stage II, making the animal appear to be looking toward its chin (Fig. 2-23). As the animal approaches a surgical plane of anesthesia, the eyeball often becomes more central, and the central position is maintained through increasing depth of anesthesia. Some anesthetics (e.g., ketamine) do not cause eye rotation, even at moderate anesthetic depth.

The size of the pupil also may reflect anesthetic depth: the anesthetized patient normally has dilated pupils (mydriasis) during stage II anesthesia, constricted pupils (miosis) when lightly anesthetized, and more dilated pupils at increasing anesthetic depth. The ability of the pupil to constrict in response to light (pupillary light

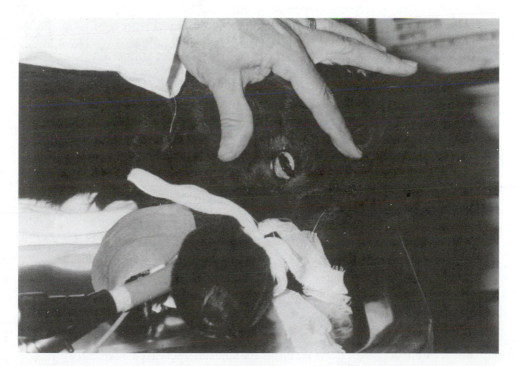

Fig. 2-23. Ventral rotation of the eyeball and prolapse of the third eyelid during anesthesia.

reflex) also diminishes with increasing depth of anesthesia and is usually absent at surgical anesthetic depth. Dilated, central pupils that are nonresponsive to light may indicate a dangerously deep level of anesthesia. The anesthetist should be aware, however, that atropine may cause pupil dilation, particularly in cats. This interaction may confuse the interpretation of pupil size and the pupillary light reflex.

Salivary and lacrimal secretions

The presence or absence of salivary and lacrimal secretions also may give clues regarding anesthetic depth, particularly in an animal that has not received anticholinergics. Production of tears and saliva diminishes with increasing anesthetic depth and is totally absent in deep surgical anesthesia. Because of the relative absence of tears and the subsequent danger of corneal drying, the use of ophthalmic solutions or ointment is advised for all animals undergoing general anesthesia.

Heart and respiratory rates

Heart and respiratory rates may be a valuable guide to anesthetic depth. Both parameters show a tendency to decrease as the animal enters deeper levels of anesthesia and a tendency to increase with lighter anesthesia. Caution should be used, however, in interpreting both heart rate and respiratory rate, because they are subject to many influences in addition to anesthetic depth. For example, an animal's heart rate increases in response to a fall in blood pressure. Heart rate is also elevated by the perception of a painful stimulus. Some preanesthetic and anesthetic drugs (ketamine and atropine) increase heart rate, whereas most other agents decrease heart rate. Heart rate also may be affected by endotracheal intubation, which causes bradycardia. Like heart rates, respiratory rates may reflect anesthetic depth but also vary with the level of oxygen and carbon dioxide in the bloodstream and the anesthetic agent used.

Response to surgical stimulation

One other parameter that may indicate anesthetic depth is the response of the animal to surgical stimulation. As previously mentioned, certain procedures, such as manipulation of viscera or pulling on the suspensory ligament of the ovary, may result in a response that indicates a perception of pain, although the perception is not usually conscious. Animals perceiving surgical stimulation may show an increase in heart rate and blood pressure. Unless the increase in heart rate is considerable, the anesthetist should not necessarily interpret these signs as an indication that the animal's anesthetic depth is inadequate. Minor changes in heart rate during surgery are considered normal, and, in fact, the absence of such a response may indicate an unnecessarily deep level of anesthesia. Increased respiratory rate or signs of voluntary movement by the patient, however, do indicate insufficient anesthetic depth and the perception of pain. Lacrimation, salivation, and sweating (most easily observed on the foot pads) also indicate that the patient may be perceiving a painful stimulus and that depth is inadequate.

Judging anesthetic depth

During the course of anesthesia, the anesthetist should monitor as many parameters as possible and weigh all available evidence before judging the anesthetic depth of the patient. No one piece of information is unfailingly reliable, and it is foolish to determine the anesthetic plane by monitoring only one reflex or vital sign. In addition, each animal is unique and shows an individual response to increasing anesthetic depth. For example, some dogs anesthetized with ketamine maintain the palpebral reflex throughout stage III, whereas others lose this reflex as early as stage III, plane 2. If the palpebral reflex is used as the sole criterion for judging anesthetic depth, the animal that retains that reflex into deep anesthesia may be incorrectly judged to be only lightly anesthetized. Increasing the concentration of anesthetic delivered to such a patient might easily result in dangerously deep anesthesia. Observation of the other indicators of anesthetic depth would likely give the anesthetist a more balanced view of the situation and a more accurate assessment of true anesthetic depth. Examples of the use of judgment in interpreting anesthetic depth are given in the box on p. 102.

Similarly, observation of the amount of anesthetic being delivered to the patient (as for example, by the vaporizer of an anesthetic machine) does not in itself indicate the patient's anesthetic depth. Although high vaporizer settings result in increased delivery of anesthetic to the patient and, subsequently, an increase in patient depth, there is tremendous variation in patient response. One animal may be maintained at stable surgical anesthesia when given a concentration of 1% halothane gas, whereas another animal may require 2% halothane and still another may be satisfactorily maintained at 0.5% halothane. The concentration of anesthetic gas received by the animal also is not necessarily that indicated by the vaporizer setting and may vary with the oxygen flow rate and quality of ventilation received by the patient (see Chapter 4). Nevertheless, a consideration of the vaporizer setting and the length of time that the animal has been anesthetized may help the anesthetist decide if an animal is anesthetized too lightly or too deeply. The basic rule is that if there is doubt about the level of anesthesia in a particular patient, one should decrease the vaporizer setting and monitor the animal until such time as the anesthetic depth can be accurately determined.

Recording information during anesthesia

Complete and accurate medical records are a legal requirement in veterinary practice. Many jurisdictions require some form of anesthetic record be maintained. In many cases, this record must be in the form of a logbook, in which information such

Examples of depth assessment

1. A mature cat has been anesthetized with thiamylal given intravenously. The anesthetist notes that the cat appears unconscious and relaxed. The pulse is strong, and the heart rate is 144 bpm. The respirations are regular, and the rate is 20 breaths/minute. The pupils are centrally positioned. The palpebral reflex is brisk, but there is no pedal or ear flick reflex. The anesthetist wishes to intubate the animal. At this depth of anesthesia, is it possible? What other tests could the anesthetist perform to determine anesthetic depth?

   Answer: The cat appears to be in stage III, plane 1 anesthesia and may be deep enough to intubate. The anesthetist should assess the jaw tone and observe whether there is any resistance when the tongue is gently pulled before assuming that intubation is possible.

2. A 13-year-old dog has been anesthetized by mask induction with isoflurane; after intubation, it is maintained on 2% isoflurane. The anesthetist wishes to ensure that the dog is sufficiently anesthetized to allow removal of a large skin tumor. The dog's respirations are shallow, with a rate of 8 breaths/minute. The heart rate is 90 bpm. There is no response to surgery, and all reflexes are absent. The pupils are central; the jaw tone is slack. Is the animal adequately anesthetized for this procedure?

   Answer: The animal is indeed adequately anesthetized and, in fact, may be at an excessive anesthetic depth. Respiration rate is slow and tidal volume is low. The absence of all reflexes, the central pupils, and the slack jaw tone all indicate that the animal may be in stage III, plane 3 anesthesia. At this point, the anesthetist should consider reducing the isoflurane setting to 1.5% and monitor the animal for signs of decreased depth. After doing this, the anesthetist should carefully monitor the animal for signs of pain perception (increased respiratory rate, movement, lacrimation, sweat on the foot pads) to ensure that the vaporizer setting is high enough for adequate analgesia. Ideally, heart rate and respiratory rate will increase slightly but not enough to indicate imminent arousal (in any case, arousal is unlikely if the animal is receiving 1.5% isoflurane).

3. An 8-year-old dog has been anesthetized with atropine, ketamine, and diazepam, given intravenously, and is now under halothane anesthesia. The dog's heart rate is 100 bpm and the respirations are 8 breaths/minute. The jaw tone appears moderate, but the pupils are central and show no response to light. No reflexes are present. Is the anesthetic depth appropriate?

   Answer: The anesthetist cannot be sure whether the anesthetic depth is appropriate or too deep, since some parameters indicate stage III, plane 2 (heart rate, jaw tone) but others indicate stage III, plane 3 (respiratory rate, reflexes, pupil position and response to light). The patient has been given atropine and ketamine, which may have elevated the heart rate. At this point, the anesthetist should assume that the patient is excessively deep and should reduce the concentration of halothane. At the same time, he or she should monitor the patient for signs of arousal.

as the date, client and patient identification, preoperative physical status, nature of the procedure performed with the patient under anesthesia, and the anesthetic protocol is listed. A brief description of the anesthetic protocol and the animal's response to anesthesia should also be given. Records of this type allow the veterinarian to review the total number of anesthetic procedures that have been carried out in a given time period, as well as review the number of deaths related to anesthesia or the number of animals that developed anesthetic complications. This information may be helpful in assessing the anesthetic protocols and procedures used by a practice.

Information regarding the anesthetic procedure also must be recorded in the patient's record. This allows the veterinarian to quickly review the animal's anesthetic history and may be helpful in determining the best anesthetic protocol to use for future procedures. For example, if the record indicates that the animal has undergone anesthesia with a barbiturate agent and experienced a lengthy recovery, the veterinarian may elect to anesthetize the dog with an alternative agent in the future. On the other hand, if a geriatric dog with congestive heart failure has been recently anesthetized without incident using a particular agent, the veterinarian would be justified in using the same agent for the next anesthesia.

In some situations, an anesthesia form such as that given in Figs. 2-24 or 2-25 is used to record a detailed description of an anesthetic procedure. Forms such as these contain information on the patient's preoperative status (temperature, pulse, and respiration and results of diagnostic tests), the anesthetic protocol used (including fluids administered, amounts and concentrations of drugs given), and the patient's vital signs throughout anesthesia (pulse, respiration, blood pressure, temperature, lab results). The time at which anesthesia commenced and was terminated, the beginning and end of surgery, and the time required for recovery should also be indicated. Typically, the information is recorded chronologically to allow an overview of the patient's responses at every point throughout the procedure. Detailed records of this type are not commonly used in veterinary practice; however, they are very useful in a teaching or research institution.

PATIENT POSITIONING AND COMFORT DURING ANESTHESIA

In addition to monitoring the patient's vital signs and reflexes as described, the anesthetist should ensure that the patient is not compromised by rough handling or careless positioning during the procedure. Examples of appropriate patient care during anesthesia include the following:

• During induction, the animal should be supported as it loses consciousness. Particular care should be taken to avoid striking the animal's head on the table during induction and when the animal is transferred to surgery.

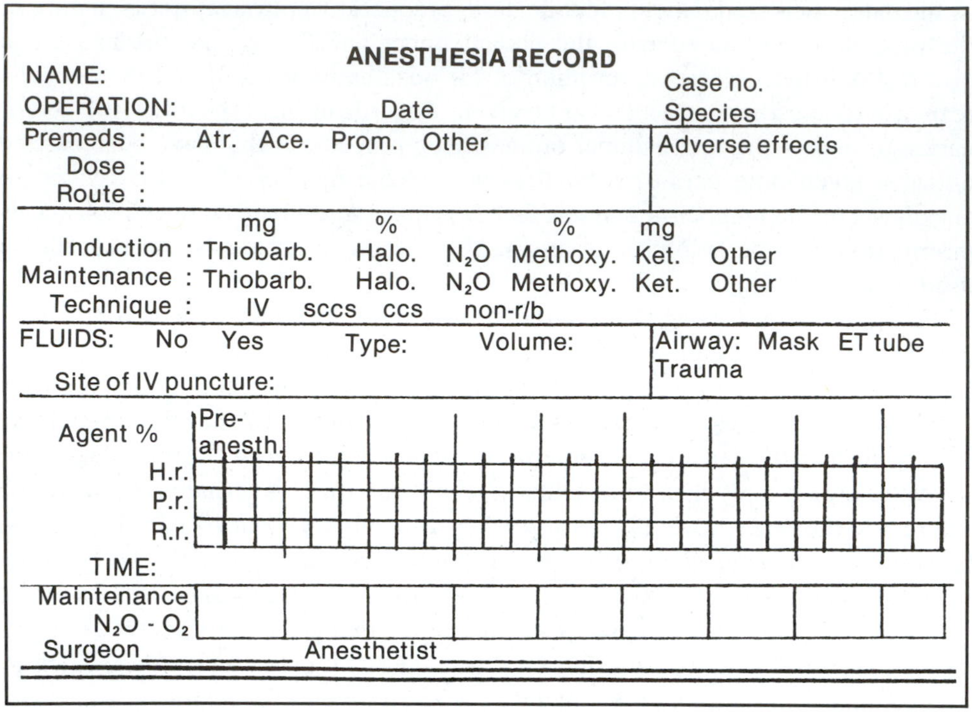

ANESTHESIA RECORD

NAME:		Case no.
OPERATION:	Date	Species

Premeds :   Atr. Ace. Prom.   Other | Adverse effects
Dose :
Route :

	mg	%	%	mg	
Induction :	Thiobarb.	Halo.	N$_2$O	Methoxy.	Ket.	Other
Maintenance :	Thiobarb.	Halo.	N$_2$O	Methoxy.	Ket.	Other
Technique :	IV	sccs	ccs	non-r/b		

FLUIDS: No   Yes   Type: Volume: | Airway: Mask ET tube
Site of IV puncture: | Trauma

Agent %   Pre-anesth.

H.r.
P.r.
R.r.

TIME:

Maintenance
N$_2$O - O$_2$

Surgeon_____ Anesthetist_____

Fig. 2-24. Anesthetic record (short form). (From Warren RG: *Small animal anesthesia,* St Louis, 1983, Mosby.)

- If an intubated patient is to be turned over, the endotracheal tube should be temporarily disconnected from the anesthetic machine. Rolling or twisting the animal while still connected to the machine may cause the endotracheal tube to twist and collapse, resulting in an airway obstruction.
- Before the surgery preparation begins, the anesthetist must ensure that the patient's endotracheal tube is correctly placed (i.e., not in the esophagus) and large enough to prevent significant leakage of waste gas around the tube. Once the surgical preparation starts, it is difficult to position the animal to allow reintubation without compromising aseptic technique.
- The hoses of the anesthetic machine should be supported such that there is no drag on the endotracheal tube, which could result in tracheal trauma by the tube or inadvertent removal of the tube. Care should be used to avoid positions that kink or bend the endotracheal tube (Fig. 2-26), and the position of the hoses and endotracheal tube should be checked during patient transfer and after repositioning. The reservoir bag should be placed such that it is clearly visible at all times.
- When positioning the animal on the surgery table, the anesthetist should ensure

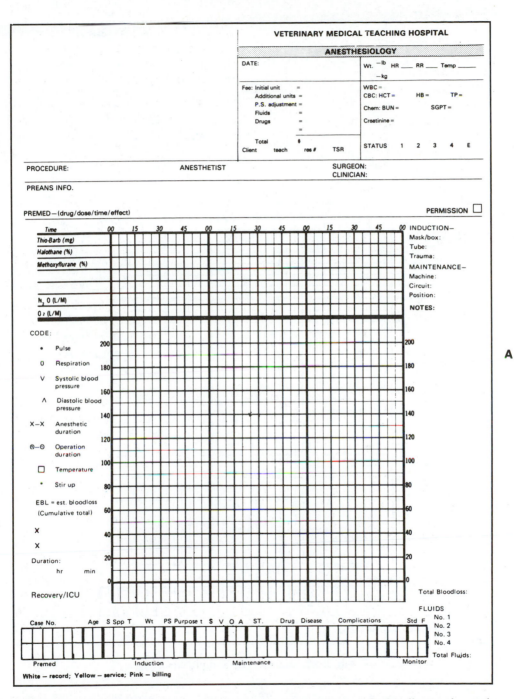

A

Fig. 2-25. **A,** Comprehensive anesthetic record. (From Warren RG: *Small animal anesthesia,* St Louis, 1983, Mosby.)

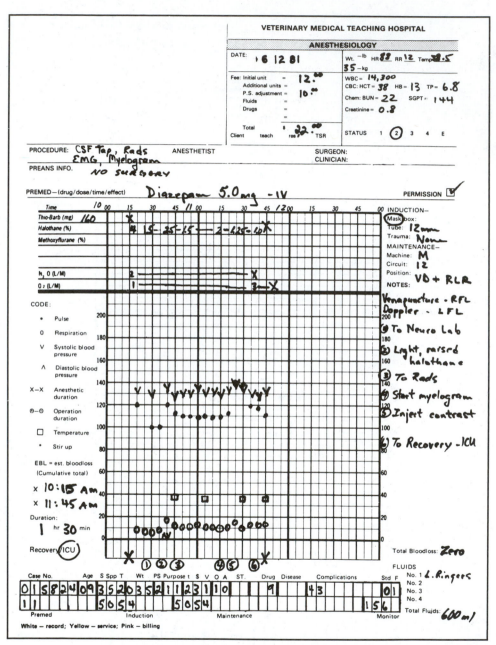

Fig. 2-25, cont'd.   B, Sample case.

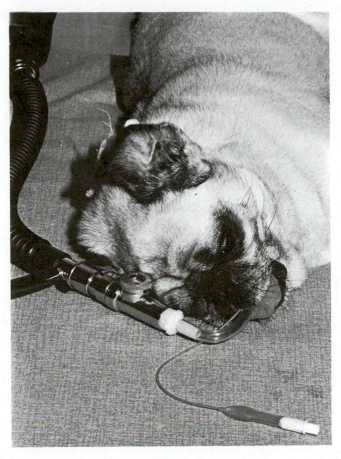

Fig. 2-26.   Kinked endotracheal tube in a dog. (From Warren RG: *Small animal anesthesia,* St Louis, 1983, Mosby.)

that the animal assumes as normal a posture as possible. In particular, overextension or hyperflexion of the neck and limbs should be avoided, because permanent neurologic injury may result. Hyperflexion of the neck also may lead to endotracheal tube obstruction.
- Care should be taken when attaching restraining devices such as ropes or gauze ties to the patient. These devices must not be excessively tight, or blood circulation to the limbs may be compromised.
- Heavy drapes or instruments must not compress the chest of small patients, as they may interfere with respiration.
- The practice of tilting the surgery table allows the surgeon easier access to some abdominal organs, particularly the uterus and ovaries. However, the anesthetist

should be aware that tilting the table more than 15 degrees may cause the abdominal organs to significantly compress the diaphragm, which may, in turn, compromise heart and lung function.

RECOVERY FROM GENERAL ANESTHESIA

The recovery period may be defined as the period between discontinuation of anesthetic administration (whether injectable or inhalation) and the time the animal is again able to maintain sternal recumbency without support. The length of the recovery period depends on many factors, including the following:

1. The length of the anesthesia. As a general rule, the longer the period of anesthetic administration, the longer the expected recovery period.
2. The condition of the patient. Lengthy recoveries are seen in animals suffering from hypothermia or almost any debilitating disease (particularly liver and kidney disease).
3. The type of anesthetic given and the route of administration. Animals given inhalation agents typically show shorter recovery periods than do animals given injectable agents. Lengthy recoveries are particularly common if the injectable agent is given IM rather than IV.
4. The patient's temperature. Hypothermic patients are slow to metabolize and excrete anesthetic drugs.

Stages of recovery

Generally speaking, an animal recovering from general anesthesia gradually progresses back through the same anesthetic stages that were experienced during induction. As the animal moves from deep to moderate to light anesthesia, vital signs and reflexes change in predictable ways. Heart rate, respiratory rate, and respiratory volume increase. The pupil, which had been rotated ventrally, moves back to its normal central position (although it may rotate ventrally again and return to a central position before arousal). Reflex responses, including the palpebral, pedal, and ear flick, become stronger. The animal may shiver. The animal may swallow, chew, or attempt to lick.

Shortly after swallowing, the animal will normally show signs of consciousness, including voluntary movement of the head or limbs, opening the eyelids, and vocalization.

Anesthetist's role in the recovery period

The recovery period is by no means a time of relaxation for the anesthetist. Anesthetic complications and death may occur during this period, even in animals that appear to have no problems during induction or maintenance. Ideally, recovery should occur in an area in which the animal can be watched on a continual basis. An emergency kit, monitoring equipment (stethoscope and thermometer), and oxygen should be readily available.

The duties of the anesthetist during the recovery period include the following.

Monitoring

Vital signs should be evaluated every 5 minutes during the recovery period. Particular attention should be given to mucous membrane color, capillary refill, and respirations. Periodic thorough evaluation is necessary; observation from across the room is not adequate. For example, a recovering animal may have significant bradycardia and respiratory depression, yet show no signs that are evident to the casual observer.

Animals exhibiting abnormal vital signs or a delayed return to consciousness should be examined by the veterinarian. Conditions such as shock, hemorrhage, hypoglycemia, and hypothermia may be present and must be treated as soon as possible. It is also important that the recovering patient be closely monitored for problems such as vomiting, seizures, laryngospasm, and dyspnea, discussed in detail in Chapter 6.

When monitoring recovery from anesthesia, particularly in brachycephalic patients, the anesthetist must take care to ensure that the airway remains open and the tissues receive adequate oxygen. Brachycephalic and other relatively high-risk patients should be observed continuously until fully conscious.

It is advisable that IV catheters or butterflies, if present, should be removed only when the patient appears fully recovered. These catheters allow easy administration of fluids or drugs, in case the patient's condition requires them.

Administration of oxygen

If possible, oxygen should be provided for several minutes after the discontinuation of the anesthetic agent. If an anesthetic machine has been used for the procedure, it is customary to continue oxygen administration at a high flow rate (200 ml/kg/ minute) for 5 minutes or until the animal swallows (at which time the patient must be disconnected from the machine and the endotracheal tube must be removed). This helps flush anesthetic out of the animal's system, allowing faster recovery. It also allows expired waste gas to be evacuated by the scavenger, rather than breathed into the room air. Periodic bagging with the pure oxygen is advisable for as long as the recovering patient is connected to the machine because it helps reinflate collapsed alveoli and increases the rate of anesthetic gas removal. Once the animal has been disconnected from the anesthetic machine, oxygen may be delivered by face mask, nasal cannula, or oxygen cage if the patient requires it. Once extubated, all animals should be placed in sternal recumbency with the neck extended; this position helps maintain a patent airway. Occasionally, fluid or mucus may accumulate in the pharynx or trachea and should be removed by sponges or a suction tube.

Extubation

The endotracheal tube must be removed when the patient shows signs of imminent arousal. In dogs the appearance of the swallowing reflex (signaled by swallowing movements observed in the throat region) is most often cited as the appropriate time to remove the tube, since the returning swallowing reflex will help protect the animal from aspiration if vomiting occurs. Animals that show voluntary limb or head movement or spastic movement of the tongue or animals that attempt to chew the endotracheal tube are close to consciousness and should be extubated even if swallowing has not been observed. One exception to this general rule is brachycephalic dogs: many anesthetists prefer to delay extubation in brachycephalic dogs until the dog is able to lift its head unassisted, because early extubation may lead to significant respiratory distress in these animals. It is wise to prepare for possible respiratory distress in a brachycephalic dog by setting out a laryngoscope, an endotracheal tube, and the appropriate dose of thiopental or another inducing agent near the recovery cage of the animal in case intubation becomes necessary.

In cats the endotracheal tube may be removed when signs of impending arousal are observed, including voluntary limb, tail, or head movements; swallowing; or a very active palpebral reflex. Delaying extubation is inadvisable in cats because it may predispose the patient to laryngospasm.

In all patients, it is necessary to deflate the endotracheal tube cuff and untie any restraining gauze before removal of the tube. Some anesthetists prefer to deflate the cuff and untie the gauze before signs of arousal are seen, so the tube can be quickly removed when swallowing occurs. When removing an endotracheal tube after a dental surgery or prophylaxis or any procedure in which blood or other fluid is present in the oral cavity, the cuff should be left partially inflated to prevent these fluids from entering the air passages.

Stimulation of the patient

In some cases patient recovery may be hastened by gentle stimulation. This may include talking to the patient, pinching the toes, opening the mouth, gently moving the limbs, or rubbing the chest. Stimulation of this type increases the flow of information to the reticular activation center (RAC) of the brain, which is the area responsible for maintaining consciousness in the awake animal. A lack of stimulation to the RAC may cause drowsiness in the conscious animal, and it is therefore speculated that stimulation of this area may help the animal to awaken. It is also advisable to turn the patient every 10 to 15 minutes to prevent pooling of blood in the dependent parts of the body, including the lungs. This condition is called *hypostatic congestion.*

Deep-chested animals are at some risk of gastric torsion when turned, and it is advisable to turn all animals sternally (i.e., the feet are moved under the dog as it turns rather than rolling the patient onto its back).

Reassuring the patient

During the recovery period, the anesthetist should take every possible step to comfort and reassure the awakening patient. The anesthetist should bear in mind that the animal has no means of understanding the events that have led to its present disoriented state. Quiet, calm handling and reassurance are therefore essential.

The anesthetist can take several steps to minimize patient discomfort during recovery. All ties restraining the animal to the surgery table should be removed before the animal regains consciousness. The anesthetist should ensure that all accessory procedures, such as bandaging, chest tube placement, and urinary catheterization, have been completed and the esophageal stethoscope, ECG leads, and thermometer are removed before the patient returns to consciousness. As previously mentioned, it is advisable to leave venous access (indwelling catheter or butterfly) in place until the endotracheal tube has been removed and patient recovery is seen to be uneventful.

Postoperative analgesics should be administered as requested by the veterinarian, preferably before the animal experiences postoperative pain (see section on opioids in Chapter 1). If the animal has received appropriate analgesic administration, it should be able to sleep comfortably and demonstrate minimal signs of pain after the surgery. A change in analgesic dose or frequency or a switch to another analgesic may be necessary if postoperative pain is apparent despite the administration of medication.

Nursing care

Nursing care of the recovering animal should include the application of warm towels, hot water bottles, infrared heat lamps, hot air dryers, or circulating warm water heating pads to all hypothermic animals. The patient often is unable to move voluntarily at this point, and the anesthetist must ensure that the patient is not burned by prolonged contact with an external heat source. Gradual rewarming is preferred to rapid rewarming, since the latter may cause dilation of cutaneous vessels, leading to hypotension.

The patient should be provided with ample bedding or padding material to prevent heat loss and increase patient comfort.

Anesthetized or recovering animals must never be left alone on a table or in a cage with the door open because of the danger of falling. Food and water should not be left in the animal's cage during recovery because it is not unknown for recovering animals to drown in water bowls or suffocate in food bowls. Some patients may be able to drink soon after standing; however, most have little appetite for food for several hours after recovery. Vomiting during the recovery period is common, possibly due to postanesthetic nausea.

Preventing patient self-injury

Some animals may pass through a period of excitement (similar to stage II anesthesia) before regaining consciousness, particularly if pentobarbital was used as part of the anesthetic protocol. As in induction, stage II recovery is characterized by vocalization, delerium, hyperventilation, head thrashing, and rapid paddling movements of the front legs. Occasionally an animal may appear to hallucinate or suffer from disorientation during anesthetic recovery, and patients (particularly those recovering from ketamine anesthesia) may chew at their paws or claw their faces. Animals showing these or similar signs of a "stormy recovery" usually return to normal within a short time, but close observation is necessary to prevent self-trauma and hyperthermia. Any animal that is thrashing or making ineffectual attempts to right itself may disrupt the surgical repair and seriously injure itself.

Summary

The importance of nursing care during the recovery period cannot be overemphasized. Postoperative problems such as hemorrhage, removal of sutures by the animal, vomiting and subsequent inhalation pneumonia, and burns from electric heating pads may be prevented if the animal is closely monitored. The anesthetist's duty toward the patient does not end until the patient is awake and standing, fully recovered from the anesthesia.

KEY POINTS

1. General anesthesia is a state of controlled and reversible unconsciousness accompanied by analgesia, amnesia, and depressed reflex responses. Ideally, respiration and circulation are not affected; however, in practice they may be impaired to a greater or lesser extent.

2. General anesthetic agents may be administered by injection or inhalation. Inhalation anesthesia is generally considered to have a greater margin of safety than injectable anesthesia.

3. The anesthetic period can be broken down into preanesthesia, induction, maintenance, and recovery. Traditionally, anesthetic depth has been described in terms of stages and planes of anesthesia, with stage III, plane 2 being suitable for most surgical procedures.

4. Anesthetic safety is improved through the use of preanesthetic agents, use of the minimum effective dosages, and close monitoring of the patient.

5. Induction of anesthesia may be achieved by intravenous or intramuscular administration of an injectable agent or by mask or chamber administration of an inhalation agent. Regardless of method used, the patient is often intubated immediately after induction and maintained on an inhalation agent.

6. Intubation improves the safety and efficiency of anesthesia; however, it may be associated with problems such as vagal nerve stimulation, laryngospasm, airway obstruction, and pressure necrosis of the trachea.

7. During the maintenance period, the anesthetist must monitor the animal closely to ensure that vital signs remain within acceptable limits. The anesthetist also must monitor reflex activity and other parameters to ensure that the anesthetic depth is appropriate.

8. Vital signs that should be monitored include heart rate and rhythm, blood pressure, capillary refill time, mucous membrane color, respiration rate and depth, blood gas levels, and temperature.

9. Indicators of anesthetic depth include reflexes (particularly the palpebral reflex), muscle tone, eye position, pupil size, and response to surgical stimulation. Heart rate and respiratory rate also may change as anesthetic depth is altered. The anesthetist should assess depth after considering several parameters, since no single indicator is unfailingly accurate.

10. The anesthetist must keep accurate medical records, the nature of which will vary depending on the clinical situation.

11. Patient comfort must be ensured throughout the procedure. This is accomplished by the use of correct positioning and gentle handling procedures.

12. The length of the recovery period depends on many factors, including the anesthetic protocol and the patient's condition. Return to consciousness is accompa-

nied by increasing heart and respiratory rates, increased reflex responses, and voluntary movement.

13. During the recovery period, the anesthetist must continue to monitor the patient's vital signs, particularly temperature. It is often helpful to administer oxygen for several minutes after the anesthetic has been discontinued.

14. In dogs extubation should occur when the swallowing reflex returns; in cats extubation should occur when the patient shows signs of impending arousal, such as voluntary movements or very active reflexes.

15. Other recovery duties may include stimulation of the patient, administration of postoperative analgesics, and general nursing care.

REVIEW QUESTIONS

1. As one increases the depth of anesthesia, there will be a continued depression of the vital centers of the body.
   True   False
2. There are _____ classic stages of anesthesia that an animal may pass through.
   a. 1
   b. 2
   c. 3
   d. 4
   e. 5
3. The surgical plane of anesthesia is generally considered to be:
   a. Stage III, plane 1
   b. Stage III, plane 2
   c. Stage III, plane 3
   d. Stage III, plane 4
   e. Stage IV
4. Breath holding, vocalization, and movement of the limbs are most likely an indication that the animal is in what stage/plane of anesthesia?
   a. Stage III, plane 1
   b. Stage I
   c. Stage II
   d. Stage IV
5. Rocking boat respiration is usually seen in:
   a. Stage II
   b. Stage III, plane 1
   c. Stage III, plane 4
   d. Stage IV
6. Anatomic dead space is considered to be the:
   a. Air within the circuit
   b. Air within the mouth and nose
   c. Air within the mouth, nose, and all airways except the alveoli
   d. Air within the alveoli

7. The process of intubation is quite safe and cannot result in any serious problems.
   True   False
8. The minimum acceptable heart rate for an anesthetized dog is _____ beats per minute.
   a. 60
   b. 70
   c. 80
   d. 90
   e. 100
9. A heart rate that is audibly beating is a good indicator that there is also a strong pulse.
   True   False
10. In general a respiratory rate of less than _____ breaths per minute for an anesthetized patient should be reported to the veterinarian.
    a. 4
    b. 8
    c. 12
    d. 16
11. Tachypnea is:
    a. An increase in respiratory depth (tidal volume)
    b. An increase in respiratory rate
    c. A decrease in respiratory depth (tidal volume)
    d. A decrease in respiratory rate
12. The term *atelectasis* refers to:
    a. Increased fluid in the alveoli
    b. Hyperinflation of the alveoli
    c. A collapsing of alveoli
    d. A decrease in the perfusion of blood around the alveoli
13. A patient that has been anesthetized usually will have a:
    a. Mild metabolic acidosis
    b. Mild metabolic alkalosis
    c. Mild respiratory acidosis
    d. Mild respiratory alkalosis
14. An animal that is in a surgical plane of anesthesia should not respond in any way to any procedure that is being done to it (e.g., pulling on viscera should not change heart rate).
    True   False
15. A 15-year-old dog has been anesthetized by mask induction with isoflurane and after intubation is maintained on 2% isoflurane with a flow rate of 2 liters of oxygen per minute. The heart rate is 80 bpm, respiratory rate is 8 breaths per minute and shallow, the jaw tone is very relaxed, and all reflexes are absent. This animal is in what stage of anesthesia?
    a. Stage III, plane 1
    b. Stage III, plane 2
    c. Stage III, plane 3
    d. Stage III, plane 4
    e. Stage IV

16. After an anesthetic procedure, when is it best to extubate a dog?
    a. Right after you turn off the vaporizer
    b. About 10 minutes after turning off the vaporizer
    c. When the animal begins to swallow
    d. Any time that is convenient

17. The _____ breed of dog is considered to be more likely to vomit after anesthesia or experience airway obstruction, and thus it is often preferable to leave the endotracheal tube in much longer than it would be in other breeds of animals.
    a. Sighthound
    b. Brachycephalic
    c. Shepherd
    d. Spaniel

18. The area of the brain responsible for maintaining consciousness is the:
    a. Reticular activating center
    b. Otic center
    c. Ophthalmic center
    d. Hypothalamus

19. *Hypostatic congestion* may be present at the end of the anesthetic protocol. This term refers to the:
    a. Accumulation of mucus in the trachea
    b. Pooling of blood in the lungs
    c. Buildup of bile in the biliary tract
    d. Pooling of ingesta in one area of the gastrointestinal tract

20. Capillary refill time will be prolonged when the blood pressure drops below:
    a. 110 to 120
    b. 100 to 110
    c. 90 to 100
    d. 80 to 90
    e. 70 to 80

More than one answer may be correct for the following questions.

21. Pale mucous membranes may be an indication of:
    a. Blood loss
    b. Anemia
    c. Decreased perfusion
    d. Hypertension

22. An animal that is hyperventilating may:
    a. Have an increased Pa_{CO_2}
    b. Be in a state of metabolic acidosis
    c. Be responding to a surgical stimulus
    d. Be receiving excess oxygen

23. An endotracheal tube is used to:
    a. Decrease dead space
    b. Allow for a patent airway
    c. Protect the patient from aspiration of vomitus
    d. Allow the anesthetist to ventilate the patient

24. Vital signs that should be monitored during anesthesia include:
    a. Heart rate
    b. Pulse quality

   c. Capillary refill

   d. Respiratory rate

   e. Pulse strength

25. Possible complications of endotracheal intubation include:

   a. Decreased dead space

   b. Pressure necrosis of the tracheal mucosa

   c. Intubation of a bronchus

   d. Obstruction of the endotracheal tube

   e. Spread of infectious disease

26. Which of the following premedication drugs can cause decreased blood pressure?

   a. Acetylpromazine

   b. Atropine

   c. Xylazine

   d. Diazepam

27. An animal under stage III, plane 2 anesthesia would exhibit which of the following signs?

   a. Very brisk palpebral reflex

   b. Regular respiration

   c. Relaxed skeletal muscle tone

   d. Very dilated pupils

28. As you intubate an endotracheal tube into an animal, what clinical signs will indicate to you that the endotracheal tube is in the trachea?

   a. The animal may cough as you insert the tube down the trachea.

   b. You can feel only one tube in the neck region.

   c. The reservoir bag of the anesthetic machine moves as the patient breathes.

   d. When you compress the reservoir bag, the stomach rises.

29. When an animal is under anesthesia, which of the following systems will be depressed?

   a. Respiratory

   b. Cardiovascular

   c. Thermoregulation

   d. Salivary

30. The degree of muscle relaxation exhibited by an animal under anesthesia will be directly correlated to the:

   a. Stage of anesthesia

   b. Type of general anesthetic used

   c. Type of premedication used

   d. Blood pressure

ANSWERS FOR CHAPTER 2

1. True   **2.** d   **3.** b   **4.** c   **5.** c   **6.** c   **7.** False   **8.** b   **9.** False   **10.** b

11. b   **12.** c   **13.** c   **14.** False   **15.** c   **16.** c   **17.** b   **18.** a   **19.** b

20. e   **21.** a, b, c   **22.** a, b, c   **23.** a, b, c, d   **24.** a, b, c, d, e   **25.** b, c, d, e

26. a, c   **27.** b, c   **28.** a, b, c   **29.** a, b, c   **30.** a, b, c

SELECTED READINGS

Haskins SC: General guidelines for judging anesthetic depth, *Vet Clin North Am (Small Anim Pract)* 22:432-434, 1992.

Haskins SC: *Opinions in small animal anesthesia*, Philadelphia, 1992, Vet Clin North Am (Small Anim Pract) 22(2), WB Saunders.

Lee L: Recovery complications in small animal anesthesia, *Vet Tech* 13(5):327-335, 1992.

Muir WW, III, Hubbell JAE: *Handbook of veterinary anesthesia,* St Louis, 1989, Mosby.

Paddleford RR: *Manual of small animal anesthesia,* New York, 1988, Churchill Livingstone.

Short CE: *Principles and practice of veterinary anesthesia,* Baltimore, 1987, Williams & Wilkins.

Warren RG: *Small animal anesthesia,* St Louis, 1983, Mosby.

Anesthetic agents and techniques

3

PERFORMANCE OBJECTIVES
After completion of this chapter, the reader will be able to:

Describe the advantages and disadvantages associated with the use of injectable anesthetic agents.

Describe the advantages and disadvantages associated with the use of inhalation anesthetic agents.

List the barbiturate and dissociative anesthetic drugs that may be used as general anesthetics and be familiar with the following information regarding each agent: mode of action, effect on body systems, factors that may promote their uptake by the brain, route of elimination from the body, and adverse side effects.

List the various inhalation anesthetic agents that are available for use and the advantages and disadvantages of each agent.

Describe the pharmacologic properties of halothane, isoflurane, methoxyflurane, enflurane, and nitrous oxide.

Explain the concepts of uptake, distribution, and elimination of the commonly used inhalation anesthetic agents.

Define and explain the significance of minimum alveolar concentration, vapor pressure, solubility (partition) coefficient, and rubber solubility.

Describe the use of reversal agents and the situations in which their use is indicated.

Explain the proper use of nitrous oxide and the potential dangers associated with nitrous oxide anesthesia.

As described in Chapter 2, general anesthesia may be achieved through the administration of one (or more) potent anesthetic agents. These agents can be divided into two broad classes: injectable drugs (including barbiturates, cyclohexamines, neuroleptanalgesics, and propofol) and inhalation agents (including halothane, isoflurane, methoxyflurane, and nitrous oxide) (see Fig. 2-1). The pharmacology and physiologic effects of general anesthetics is one of the most fascinating areas in the field of anesthesiology and is described in detail in this chapter.

COMPARISON OF INHALATION AND INJECTABLE ANESTHESIA

Although both inhalation and injectable agents are commonly used in veterinary practice, inhalation anesthesia is considered to have a greater margin of safety. The advantages of inhalation anesthesia include the following:

- When an inhalation agent is used, the depth of anesthesia can be readily altered by the anesthetist. Inhalation agents continuously enter and leave the body via the respiratory system, which allows the concentration of anesthetic in the blood or brain to be changed very rapidly. If the patient appears too awake, the concentration of anesthetic delivered by the anesthetic machine to the animal can be increased, resulting in a deeper level of anesthesia. If the anesthetist wishes to bring the patient to a lighter depth of anesthesia or to initiate recovery, the administration of the inhalation agent can be discontinued by turning off the anesthetic vaporizer. In contrast, the depth of the anesthetic state of an injectable agent cannot be readily altered except by injection of additional drug to increase anesthetic depth.

- The elimination of injectable agents is achieved by means of redistribution within the body, liver metabolism, and renal excretion. This is in contrast to the elimination of inhalation agents, which occurs mainly through the lungs. Patient recovery from an injectable agent more dependent on patient metabolism or hepatic and renal function than it is with an inhalation anesthetic. These factors are not always significant in a young, healthy patient; however, they are often of concern to the veterinarian choosing an anesthetic protocol for a patient with preexisting problems. A geriatric cat with chronic renal failure is likely to be anesthetized more safely with an inhalation agent, such as isoflurane, than with an injectable agent, such as ketamine or a barbiturate.

- Inhalation anesthesia allows the constant delivery of high concentrations of oxygen (close to 100%) to the patient. Animals under injectable anesthesia breathe room air containing approximately 20% oxygen.

• Most patients under inhalation anesthesia are intubated, and mechanical ventilation using the anesthetic machine is relatively easy. This increases the safety of the anesthetic procedure, as the anesthetist can respond promptly in case of hypoventilation or respiratory arrest.

The disadvantages of inhalation anesthesia compared to injectable anesthesia are the following:

• Inhalation anesthesia requires an anesthetic machine for delivery of anesthetic and oxygen to the patient. Injectable anesthetics do not require the use of this equipment and, in the short run, may be more economical to use. However, once the equipment has been purchased, the cost of using an inhalation agent is comparable to that of most injectable agents. The cost of each procedure varies with locality and dosage used. The approximate cost (not including equipment) of induction of a 20-kg dog is currently $2.20 for thiopental, $1.17 for ketamine/diazepam, $6.00 for propofol, $.23 for halothane, and $2.07 for isoflurane.

• Inhalation anesthesia has the potential for the escape of waste anesthetic gas into room air. Waste gas exhaled by the patient or leaked from anesthetic equipment results in operating room pollution. Personnel inhaling high levels of waste gas may be at increased risk for reproductive disorders and other health problems (see Chapter 5).

Many years of experience in veterinary anesthesia have shown that both injectable and inhalation anesthetics are effective and can be used with a wide margin of safety. It should be reiterated, however, that both injectable and inhalation agents have an overall depressant effect on the cardiovascular, respiratory, and thermoregulatory systems. Constant vigilance on the part of the anesthetist is necessary to prevent and respond to anesthetic complications that may arise from the use of *any* agent.

INJECTABLE ANESTHETICS

The following injectable anesthetics are used in small animal anesthesia:
1. Barbiturates (including thiopental sodium, thiamylal sodium, methohexital, and pentobarbital)
2. Cyclohexamines (including ketamine and tiletamine)
3. Neuroleptanalgesic agents (a combination of an opioid, such as morphine, meperidine, butorphanol, fentanyl, or oxymorphone, with a tranquilizing agent)
4. Propofol

Recommended dosages for these agents are given in Table 3-1. Dosages are approximate and should be adjusted according to the patient's age, physical status, and veterinarian's recommendations.

TABLE 3-1
Suggested dosage ranges of injectable anesthetic agents

Drug	Purpose	Dose (canine and feline)
Thiopental sodium	Intravenous induction 2% solution (20 mg/ml)	Dog: 10-12.5 mg/kg with premedication; 15-20 mg/kg without premedication; cat: 5-10 mg/kg
Thiamylal sodium	Intravenous induction	8-10 mg/kg with premedication; 15-20 mg/kg without premedication
Methohexital	Intravenous induction 1% solution (10 mg/ml)	5-9 mg/kg with premedication
Pentobarbital	Intravenous anesthesia	15-20 mg/kg with premedication; 22-33 mg/kg without premedication
Ketamine/diazepam (50-50 mixture of 5 mg/ml diazepam and 100 mg/ml ketamine)	Intravenous induction	0.1-0.14 ml/kg
Ketamine (cats only)	Intramuscular (minor procedures) Intramuscular (major procedures) Intravenous induction	11-33 mg/kg 33-44 mg/kg 2-5 mg/kg
Propofol	Intravenous induction Maintenance of anesthesia	3-8 mg/kg 0.5-1 mg/kg every 3-5 minutes or continuous infusion 0.3-0.5 mg/kg/ min
Tiletamine/zolazepam (Telazol)	Intravenous anesthesia Intramuscular (sedation and minor procedures)	Cat and Dog: 2-4 mg/kg Cat: 10-15 mg/kg; dog 4-12 mg/kg

Modified from *Veterinary teaching hospital undergraduate manual*, Guelph, 1992, Ontario Veterinary College.

Barbiturates

Classes of barbiturates

All barbiturates in clinical use are derivatives of barbituric acid. Three classes of barbiturates are used in veterinary anesthesia: oxybarbiturates, thiobarbiturates, and methylated oxybarbiturates. Other classes of barbiturates, including long-acting barbiturates such as phenobarbital, are used as anticonvulsants but not as anesthetics.

Barbiturate drugs vary in their lipid solubility, distribution within the body, rapidity of action, and length of effect.

- **Oxybarbiturates** (also called short-acting barbiturates). One member of this class of drugs that is occasionally still used for anesthesia is pentobarbital (Nembutal, Somnotol). Oxybarbiturates have low lipid solubility and are relatively slow to take effect. The length of anesthesia and the recovery time are greater than with other barbiturate agents. Oxybarbiturates rely on liver metabolism for the termination of their effects.
- **Thiobarbiturates** (also called ultrashort-acting barbiturates). These include thiopental (Pentothal) and thiamylal (Surital, Bio-Tal).
- **Methylated oxybarbiturates**. Methohexital (Brevital) is the only methylated oxybarbiturate commonly used in small animal practice. Both the thiobarbiturates and methylated oxybarbiturates have a rapid effect and short duration of action, and recovery time is relatively brief. These agents are highly lipid soluble, and the termination of their effects is achieved by redistribution of the drug from the brain to muscle and fat.

Mechanism of action

After intravenous administration, barbiturates are quickly delivered to the brain. The speed of absorption into the brain depends on the lipid solubility of the agent, because lipid-soluble agents are absorbed more rapidly than agents with a low lipid solubility. All barbiturate agents produce their effects by depressing the reticular activating center of the brain, causing a loss of consciousness. Their effect is terminated when the agent leaves the brain and is either redistributed elsewhere in the body or metabolized by the liver.

Use in practice

The relative safety and low cost of barbiturates and the rapid patient recovery observed (particularly with ultrashort-acting agents) have led to the extensive use of barbiturates in small animal anesthesia. Barbiturates are commonly used as induction agents to allow endotracheal intubation, usually followed by maintenance of anesthesia with an inhalation anesthetic, such as halothane or isoflurane. A barbiturate may also be used as the sole agent of anesthesia, particularly for short procedures. Endotracheal intubation is strongly advised for all patients anesthetized with barbiturates, even for brief periods, to prevent aspiration of fluid or vomitus and to allow the anesthetist to support ventilation if necessary.

Because of the potential toxicity of barbiturates to the cardiovascular and respiratory systems and the variation in dose requirements among individual patients, these drugs are normally administered ''to effect'' (i.e., only the amount necessary to induce anesthesia is given). Most commonly, half of the calculated dosage is given, and the effect of this bolus (a portion of the dose given rapidly) is closely observed before additional drug is administered (described in more detail in the box on p. 65).

Effect on vital systems

Barbiturates may have significant adverse effects on respiration and cardiovascular function. In fact, concentrated barbiturate solutions are commonly used as euthanasia agents, a fact that illustrates the potential danger of these drugs. Once injected into an animal, there is no way to retrieve a barbiturate drug. The most important adverse effects of barbiturates on vital systems are respiratory depression and cardiac toxicity.

Respiratory depression. Barbiturates may profoundly depress respiration. This effect is especially evident immediately after IV administration of thiobarbiturates for anesthetic induction, when a short period of apnea (cessation of breathing) is commonly seen. This results from direct depression of the respiratory center in the medulla, which is the area of the brain that controls respiration. In the awake animal, the respiratory center responds to rising blood carbon dioxide levels by sending out impulses to the muscles that initiate inspiration. Barbiturates cause the respiratory center to become relatively insensitive to blood CO_2 levels, and as a result fewer nervous impulses are sent to the respiratory muscles. Respiratory rate decreases and, in some cases, respirations may cease for a short time. The patient's mucous membrane color and heart rate should be closely monitored throughout the induction period to ensure that circulation is maintained during the period of apnea. Mucous membranes should remain pink, the heart beat should be regular, and the pulse should be strong throughout the induction period. If spontaneous respiration does not resume within a few minutes or cardiovascular function appears to be threatened, ventilatory support may be necessary. This can be provided by periodic bagging (see Chapter 2) or through the use of a mechanical ventilator.

During anesthesia induced with a longer-acting agent, such as pentobarbital, the most common effect on respiration is a persistent reduction in tidal volume (shallow breaths). The effect may be short-lived, or the patient's respirations may appear shallow throughout the anesthetic period. Patients with reduced tidal volume are predisposed to respiratory acidosis and poor tissue oxygenation, particularly if barbiturates are used as the sole agent of anesthesia and oxygen delivery via an anesthetic machine is not available.

Respiratory depression is also a potential problem when barbiturates are used in cesarean surgeries. Barbiturates, like most anesthetic agents, readily cross the placenta and enter the fetal circulation and may interfere with breathing in the neonate immediately after delivery. In fact, the fetus is more susceptible than the mother to the effect of barbiturates, and fetal respiration may be completely inhibited by doses of barbiturates that do not even cause anesthesia in the mother.

Neonatal survival rates are particularly poor when a long-acting barbiturate, such as pentobarbital, is part of the anesthetic protocol for a cesarean.

Respiratory depression is not the only effect of barbiturates on the respiratory system: coughing and laryngospasm are also seen. These effects are thought to result from excessive salivation and may be minimized by the use of an anticholinergic preanesthetic, such as atropine.

Cardiac toxicity. Although less commonly seen than respiratory depression, cardiac toxicity may be significant in barbiturate anesthesia, particularly in the first 10 minutes after IV injection. It has been shown in the dog that barbiturates may directly depress myocardial cells, reducing cardiac output. The decline in cardiac function may cause blood pressure to fall immediately after barbiturate injection.

Thiobarbiturates increase the heart's sensitivity to the action of epinephrine. This hormone is released by the adrenal gland, particularly in patients that are excited or stressed. Circulating epinephrine may have profound effects on the heart, causing potentially dangerous dysrhythmias. During the induction period, it is not uncommon for cardiac dysrhythmias, such as ventricular premature contractions (VPCs), to occur as a result of the combined effect of barbiturates, epinephrine, and hypoxia. These cardiac dysrhythmias are not clinically significant in most patients; however, cardiac arrest has been reported.

Toxic side effects on the heart can be minimized by ensuring that barbiturates are given slowly (over 10 to 15 seconds in the case of thiobarbiturates) and that dilute concentrations are used (2.0%, 2.5%). Barbiturate anesthesia should be avoided in animals with known cardiac disease, because a dose of barbiturate that is well tolerated by a healthy heart may severely stress a diseased heart.

Other adverse side effects

In addition to cardiovascular and respiratory problems outlined above, barbiturates may exhibit exaggerated and potentially dangerous potency in certain animals. Classes of patients that are particularly sensitive to barbiturates include hypoproteinemic animals, acidotic animals, and very lean animals.

Effect on hypoproteinemic animals. Barbiturates are normally found in the blood both free and bound to plasma proteins. Only the free (unbound) molecules of barbiturate are able to enter the brain to induce the anesthetic effect, because the molecules bound to proteins are unable to cross cell membranes. In hypoproteinemic animals (those with total solids less than 3 g/dl, often due to renal, hepatic, or intestinal disease) there is less plasma protein to bind barbiturate molecules, and consequently, relatively more barbiturate is in the active, unbound form. The potency of barbiturates within the body is therefore increased in animals with low plasma protein levels. Dosages of barbiturates suitable for healthy animals may cause prolonged unconsciousness or death in these patients.

Effect on acidotic animals. The potency of barbiturates depends on blood pH, and these drugs have greater effect if blood pH is low (acidosis). Extreme care should therefore be used when administering barbiturates to animals with metabolic or respiratory acidosis, since a normal dose of barbiturates can produce high drug levels in the brain and an exaggerated response in these animals.

The effect of pH on the potency of barbiturates is significant in many patients. Metabolic acidosis is frequently encountered in small animal practice; it may be present in animals suffering from urinary obstruction, diabetic ketoacidosis, ethylene glycol poisoning, chronic renal failure, shock, and many other conditions. The dose of barbiturates required to anesthetize animals suffering from acidosis may be significantly less than that required to anesthetize healthy animals.

Respiratory acidosis also is encountered in veterinary patients, particularly those with significant respiratory disease, such as pulmonary edema. Respiratory acidosis may be present even in healthy patients during anesthesia, because many suffer from respiratory depression (which can result in respiratory acidosis). Barbiturates themselves, as potent respiratory depressants, may induce respiratory acidosis. After lengthy barbiturate anesthesia, a vicious cycle may be initiated in which respiratory depression caused by barbiturate administration leads to respiratory acidosis. This, in turn, increases the potency of the barbiturate and causes further respiratory depression and more severe respiratory acidosis. This cycle may be broken by supporting the animal's ventilation (by bagging or the use of a ventilator), which reduces blood carbon dioxide levels and helps reverse respiratory acidosis.

Tissue irritation. Barbiturate solutions are strongly alkaline (pH 9.5-10.5) and may cause significant tissue damage if injected perivascularly, particularly if the concentration of barbiturate exceeds 2.5%. Perivascular injection of concentrated barbiturate solutions may be followed in 24 to 48 hours by local swelling, pain, necrosis, and even tissue sloughing. The irritation caused by perivascular barbiturate injections may cause the animal to chew at the area, thereby increasing tissue damage. Tissue sloughs are impossible to reverse, are slow to heal, and usually result in permanent scarring.

To avoid perivascular injections, barbiturates are often administered through an IV catheter or butterfly. If perivascular injection occurs, the area should be immediately infiltrated with saline (in a volume equal to the volume of barbiturate injected) to dilute the barbiturate and reduce its irritating effect. Many veterinarians prefer to add 2% lidocaine without epinephrine to the saline to give a local analgesic effect.

Excitement during induction or recovery. Perivascular injection or administration of a small dose of barbiturates may result in stage II excitement during induction. This occurs if the amount of barbiturate injected intravenously (and therefore the amount reaching the brain) is insufficient to produce a deeper level of anesthesia. If excitement is exhibited, it is necessary to immediately administer more barbiturate to induce stage III anesthesia. The use of barbiturates, particularly pentobarbital, is also associated with a high incidence of excitement during the recovery period. Paddling and vocalization are commonly seen but may be relieved by administration of IV diazepam.

Drug dependence. Prolonged use of barbiturates is associated with drug dependence in humans, and for this reason the federal governments in both the United States and Canada have enacted laws regulating the purchase, storage, and use of these agents. Careful record keeping is essential in order to comply with these regulations.

Loss of potency. Thiobarbiturate agents are unstable in solution. These drugs are purchased in powdered form and are reconstituted by adding sterile saline or water to the bottle. Once reconstituted, thiopental and thiamylal have a short shelf life (a maximum of 2 weeks if refrigerated, less at room temperature). A solution should not be used if a precipitate is present.

Distribution and elimination of barbiturates

To understand the mode of action of specific barbiturate agents, it is necessary to have some knowledge of the distribution and elimination of these drugs within the body. After IV injection, the barbiturate agent is rapidly dispersed throughout the body via the bloodstream. Large amounts of the drug rapidly enter the brain, partly because of the excellent blood supply this organ receives. Also, thiobarbiturates are highly lipid soluble, and the high lipid content of the brain enhances the entry of these agents into brain tissue. The rapid penetration of barbiturates into the brain explains why anesthesia is usually seen within 1 minute of injection of a thiobarbiturate. Pentobarbital is less lipid soluble and requires several minutes to reach its full effect.

Tissues such as muscle and fat have proportionately less blood flow than the brain, and barbiturate levels in these tissues rise more slowly (Fig. 3-1). Gradually, however, the level of barbiturate in the blood falls as the drug enters muscle and fat. Once the level of barbiturate in the blood decreases below that in brain tissue, barbiturate begins to leave the brain and reenters the circulation, where it continues to be redistributed to muscle, fat, and other body tissues. (This occurs because barbiturates, like all drugs, diffuse from areas of high concentration to areas of low concentration.) The animal will show signs of recovery as the concentration of barbiturate in the brain decreases, although the barbiturate is still present in other tissues. Over the next few hours, the barbiturate is very gradually released from the muscle and fat and is eliminated from the body by liver metabolism and excretion of the metabolites in urine. Animals with hepatic or renal disease and animals suffering from hypothermia may exhibit prolonged recoveries or ''hangover'' from these agents, because metabolism and excretion are delayed.

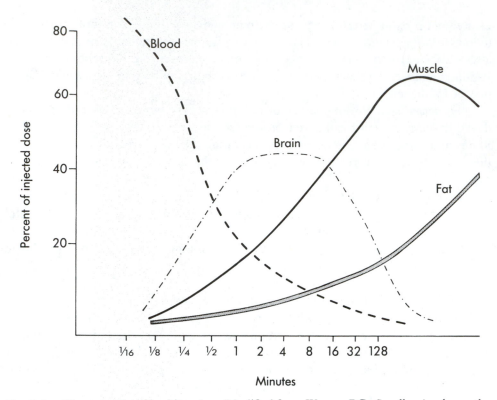

Fig. 3-1. Tissue levels of barbiturates. (Modified from Warren RG: *Small animal anesthesia,* St Louis, 1983, Mosby.)

Because of the high lipid solubility of thiobarbiturates, these agents show increased potency and duration of action in very thin animals, including sighthounds (Afghan hounds, whippets, salukis, borzoi, and greyhounds). Distribution of the agent into body fat cannot readily occur in such lean animals, and therefore barbiturate levels in the brain remain high. Hepatic metabolism of barbiturates may also be slow in sighthounds, further delaying clearance from the body. For this reason, thiobarbiturates and pentobarbital are not recommended for use in lean animals, although another barbiturate agent, methohexital, is considered to be relatively safe.

Similarly, barbiturates show greater potency in animals suffering from hypotension or shock. The body responds to lowered blood pressure by reducing the blood flow to nonessential tissues, such as fat, and increases blood flow to the brain and heart. Animals in shock can be expected to show greatly increased sensitivity to barbiturates, as the normal redistribution of these agents from the brain to body fat stores does not occur. Metabolic acidosis is also present in most animals in shock, and this condition further increases the potency of barbiturates.

Variations in lipid solubility of various barbiturate agents also help explain the differences in the duration of anesthesia for these agents. The rapid recovery of healthy animals from anesthesia with thiobarbiturates or methylated oxybarbiturates is the result of the high lipid solubility and rapid redistribution of these agents into muscle and body fat. Pentobarbital is less soluble in lipids and, as a result, remains in circulation, rather than being redistributed to body fat. Sustained blood levels of pentobarbital result in a sustained high concentration of the drug in the brain and a long duration of action.

Commonly used barbiturate drugs

The characteristics of the more commonly used barbiturate agents are summarized in Table 3-2.

Pentobarbital sodium. Pentobarbital is classified as a short-acting barbiturate. The onset of action is 30 to 60 seconds after IV injection, and the anesthetic effect lasts 30 minutes to 2 hours, depending on dosage and species.

Pentobarbital is supplied as a 6% or 6.5% solution (60 mg/ml and 65 mg/ml, respectively). It is commonly diluted with sterile water or saline to a 2% or 3% solution for use in dogs. The dosage used in dogs varies from 5 to 30 mg/kg, depending on concurrent use of other general anesthetic agents or preanesthetics. This agent must be used with caution because the euthanasia dose in healthy animals is 40 to 60 mg/kg, approximately double the dose used for surgical anesthesia.

Pentobarbital, like all barbiturates, is given to effect. One third of the calculated dose is given over 3 to 5 seconds, and the animal is observed for at least 1 minute before additional drug is given. Small increments can be given until surgical anesthesia is achieved (usually 5 to 10 minutes after the initial injection). The animal should be intubated to preserve a patent airway and to allow oxygen administration if necessary. Additional drug can be given to prolong anesthesia; however, repeated dosages may be associated with excitement during the recovery period and an extended recovery time.

Although pentobarbital is most commonly administered intravenously, intramuscular pentobarbital has been used as a premedication or sedative. It is also administered by intraperitoneal injection (particularly to rodents); however, its potency and duration of effect is variable when given by this route.

There are many problems associated with the use of pentobarbital in small animal anesthesia:

- Animals anesthetized with pentobarbital show poor muscle relaxation.
- Pentobarbital provides minimal analgesia, and pain sensitivity in the postoperative period may be increased when this drug is used.
- Recovery from this agent is prolonged, particularly in cats, which lack the necessary liver enzymes to metabolize the drug quickly. Excitement during recovery is also common in both cats and dogs anesthetized with pentobarbital.

TABLE 3-2

Characteristics of commonly used barbiturate agents

Generic name	Trade name	Classification	Time to onset of anesthesia	Duration of action	Recovery time	Method of elimination
Pentobarbital	Nembutal Somnotol	Short-acting	5-10 min	30 min-2 hr	6-24 hr	Liver metabolism
Thiopental sodium	Pentothal	Ultrashort-acting	30-60 sec	10-20 min	1-2 hr	Redistribution followed by liver metabolism
Thiamylal sodium	Surital Bio-Tal	Ultrashort-acting	30-60 sec	10-20 min	1-2 hr	Redistribution followed by liver metabolism
Methohexital	Brevital	Ultrashort-acting	15-60 sec	5-10 min	30 min	Redistribution followed by rapid liver metabolism

- If pentobarbital anesthesia is performed without the benefit of intubation and the administration of oxygen, the patient may suffer from significant respiratory depression resulting in hypercapnia (elevated blood CO_2) and respiratory acidosis.
- Anesthetic depth is difficult to control, except by injecting more agent.
- Recovery depends on adequate liver and kidney function.

Because of these disadvantages, the use of this agent for major surgical procedures is now uncommon in veterinary practice. It is still used occasionally in research, either as a sole anesthetic or in combination with nitrous oxide and a neuroleptanalgesic as part of a balanced anesthesia technique. Pentobarbital is also commonly used in the treatment of seizures arising from epilepsy, strychnine poisoning, and other causes.

Thiobarbiturates. Thiobarbiturates are probably the most commonly used induction agents in small animal anesthesia and have also found widespread use as the sole anesthetic for brief procedures. These agents, including thiopental sodium and thiamylal sodium, are classified as ultrashort-acting barbiturates. The two drugs are similar in their properties and clinical use; however, thiamylal is slightly more potent than thiopental. As mentioned previously, their onset of action is rapid (30 to 60 seconds), and duration of action is short (10 to 20 minutes). Recovery usually occurs within 1 to 2 hours. Both agents have a wide margin of safety, as the lethal dose in a healthy animal is approximately 6 times the anesthetic dose.

Thiamylal and thiopental are supplied as crystalline powder in multidose vials. Sterile water or saline is added to the vial, making a 2% or 2.5% (20 mg/ml or 25 mg/ml) or more concentrated solution. All vials should be labelled with the percent concentration and date of reconstitution as solutions remain stable for a limited time. Care should be taken to avoid injecting air into prepared solutions, as this may cause premature precipitation of the barbiturate.

The dosage used varies from 6 to 20 mg/kg, depending on concurrent use of other agents and the depth of anesthesia required. Dosages are commonly reduced by up to 80% in debilitated animals or in animals that have been heavily sedated.

As with other barbiturates, thiobarbiturates are given to effect. One method for IV induction using a thiobarbiturate is given in the box on p. 65. Additional increments may be given, extending anesthesia up to 60 minutes, but it is advisable to use an inhalation anesthetic if anything more than a brief procedure is planned.

Although relatively safe, anesthetic induction using thiobarbiturates requires care.

- Perivascular infiltration should be avoided because local necrosis may result.
- Too rapid infusion of barbiturate must be avoided during bolus induction because a dramatic drop in blood pressure may result.
- Transient apnea is commonly seen during induction, particularly if a concentrated thiobarbiturate solution is given rapidly IV. If apnea is prolonged or if cyanosis or bradycardia is observed, it may be necessary to support ventilation by inserting an endotracheal tube and administering oxygen.

- Transient dysrhythmias are commonly observed during induction, particularly if the drug is given rapidly. Cardiac dysrhythmias may be successfully treated in most cases by administration of two to three breaths of oxygen (by squeezing the reservoir bag of the anesthetic machine). Because of their dysrhythmogenic tendency, thiobarbiturates are not well suited for induction of animals with heart disease.
- Thiobarbiturates should be avoided in sighthounds, since recovery in these breeds may be prolonged (2 to 4 times that of a normal animal).
- As with pentobarbital, muscle relaxation and analgesia are poor when a thiobarbiturate is used as the sole anesthetic agent.
- Repeated administration is cumulative, and recovery can be greatly prolonged if anesthesia is maintained for more than 30 minutes.

Methohexital. Methohexital is a methylated oxybarbiturate similar to the thiobarbiturates in that the onset of action is rapid (15 to 60 seconds), duration of anesthesia is short (5 to 10 minutes), and recovery is usually prompt. In fact, animals induced with methohexital and subsequently connected to an anesthetic machine may show signs of recovery before the inhalation anesthetic has had time to take effect. The rapid induction achieved with this agent is useful when anesthetizing a patient with a full stomach, because the anesthetist can intubate rapidly, decreasing the risk of aspiration of vomitus.

As with the thiobarbiturates, methohexital is provided as a powder, which must be reconstituted. The reconstituted drug has a shelf life of 6 weeks and does not require refrigeration.

Methohexital is administered in a manner similar to thiobarbiturates. One half to three quarters of the calculated dose is given intravenously over 10 seconds. One injection is usually sufficient to allow intubation, but additional drug should be given in 30 seconds if an adequate plane is not reached. Delay will result in a poor induction because of the rapid redistribution and recovery properties.

Methohexital is used most commonly in sighthounds, as it produces faster recoveries and less hangover than the thiobarbiturates. Liver metabolism of methohexital is much faster than the other barbiturates and therefore repeated administration is not cumulative. The rapid recovery seen with this agent has made it useful in brachycephalic animals, which may experience increased incidence of respiratory distress if return to consciousness is delayed following anesthesia.

Despite these useful applications in veterinary anesthesia, methohexital should be used with caution; it may cause profound respiratory depression, and the lethal dose is only 2 to 3 times the anesthetic dose. Methohexital is also associated with excitement during recovery, particularly if it is used as the sole anesthetic agent. For this reason, premedication is always recommended. Postoperative seizures that are sometimes seen with this agent may be satisfactorily controlled with the use of IV diazepam.

Cyclohexamines

With the introduction of the injectable anesthetic phencyclidine in the late 1950s, a new class of injectable anesthetic drugs, the cyclohexamines, became available to veterinarians. Although phencyclidine (''angel dust'') has not been widely used in veterinary medicine because of its tendency to cause hallucinations, its derivatives, ketamine hydrochloride and tiletamine hydrochloride, are used to induce anesthesia in many species.

Mechanism of action

The mechanism of action of the cyclohexamines appears to be a disruption of nervous system pathways within the cerebrum and a stimulation of the reticular activating center of the brain. Unlike other general anesthetics, which cause CNS depression, cyclohexamines cause selective CNS stimulation. Nervous system stimulation may result from a suppression of inhibitory neurons by these drugs. This results in a distinctive type of anesthesia termed *dissociative anesthesia* or *catalepsy,* in which the animal appears awake but unaware of its surroundings (Fig. 3-2). Characteristics of dissociative anesthesia include the following:

• Reflex responses are exaggerated rather than depressed. For example, animals under dissociative anesthesia usually have a brisk palpebral reflex. For this reason, it may be difficult to determine the level of anesthetic depth in patients under cyclohexamine anesthesia. Patients that show signs of purposeful movement are likely too light, whereas those with very depressed respiration are too deep. The anesthetist may have some difficulty in determining where an individual patient lies between these two extremes.

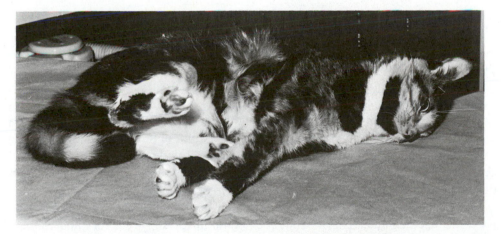

Fig. 3-2. Catalepsy induced by cyclohexamine agents. (From Warren RG: *Small animal anesthesia,* St Louis, 1983, Mosby.)

- Pharyngeal and laryngeal reflexes may persist throughout anesthesia, although they are weak. The presence of these reflexes makes endotracheal intubation more difficult; however, the use of an endotracheal tube is still advisable to ensure patient safety. This is particularly true if a dental prophylaxis or other oral procedure is planned, because blood, saliva, irrigating solutions, and other liquids present in the oral cavity may be easily aspirated if an endotracheal tube is not in place.
- Animals anesthetized with these agents may show marked sensitivity to sound, light, and other sensory stimuli.
- Muscle tone is increased, almost to the point of rigidity. The animal assumes a stiff posture, with outstretched front limbs and extended neck. Spontaneous, random movements of the head and neck may be seen, even if the animal is deeply anesthetized. This is in marked contrast to the muscle relaxation that is seen with barbiturates and inhalation agents. The concurrent use of a tranquilizing agent such as diazepam, acetylpromazine, or xylazine helps prevent excessive muscle rigidity and improve ease of intubation.
- Dissociative anesthetics provide significant analgesia to the skin and limbs, although visceral analgesia is poor. Because the analgesia provided by these agents is not adequate to relieve visceral pain, they should not be used as the sole anesthetic agent for abdominal surgery (including ovariohysterectomy), thoracic surgery, or orthopedic manipulations. A patient in dissociative anesthesia may be able to perceive pain but unable to visibly respond to it, although growling may be heard if an endotracheal tube is not in place. It is the anesthetist's obligation to ensure that pain is not perceived, through the use of supplementary anesthetic agents (opioids or inhalation anesthetics), in all major surgical procedures.

Use in practice

Unlike barbiturates, cyclohexamines may be given by either the IM or IV routes in some species. This versatility, plus the wide margin of safety of cyclohexamine drugs, has led to their widespread acceptance in veterinary anesthesia, particularly for use in cats. When given in combination with a tranquilizer (diazepam, xylazine, acetylpromazine, or zolazepam), they may be used for short procedures, such as feline castrations, or as a means of induction before intubation and inhalation anesthesia. They are also useful for chemical restraint of intractable cats, allowing examination and minor treatments to be performed without endangering hospital personnel. In dogs cyclohexamine-tranquilizer combinations (usually ketamine and diazepam) are also used for induction, usually by the IV route.

One limitation of ketamine use in veterinary practice is the lack of an effective reversing agent. Such an agent would be helpful in speeding recovery and controlling postanesthesia excitement.

Effect on vital systems

Dissociative anesthetics, such as ketamine and tiletamine, have some effect on the vital functions of anesthetized animals, but severe complications are rare.

Cardiac effects. Unlike most anesthetics, ketamine does not decrease heart rate or depress myocardial function. In fact, tachycardia may be seen, and blood pressure is often increased. These cardiovascular effects are not usually harmful to the animal; however, cyclohexamines should be used with caution in animals with cardiac dysrhythmias or preexisting cardiac disease, including cats with hyperthyroidism or cardiomyopathy. Since ketamine and atropine both may induce tachycardia, some anesthetists prefer to use glycopyrrolate rather than atropine if an anticholinergic is required.

Effect on respiration. Animals anesthetized with cyclohexamines exhibit a peculiar type of breathing pattern called *apneustic respiration*, in which inspiration is followed by a prolonged pause, and expiration is short. Respiratory rate and tidal volume may be reduced, although tissue oxygenation is usually adequate. Some animals appear to "hold their breath" when anesthetized with ketamine, but they often can be stimulated to exhale by tapping the nose or gently stroking the chest.

Other effects

Tissue irritation. Ketamine and tiletamine are irritating to tissues and many animals show transitory signs of discomfort when these drugs are given IM. Tissue necrosis and sloughing, however, do not occur with these agents.

Effect on salivation. Cyclohexamine agents may cause increased salivation. A low dose of anticholinergic, such as glycopyrrolate or atropine, may be given before use of a cyclohexamine agent to prevent profuse salivation and the resultant risk of aspiration.

Effect on CSF pressure. Ketamine may increase cerebral spinal fluid (CSF) pressure, and although this effect is not hazardous to most patients, the drug is contraindicated in cases of cranial trauma.

Effect on the eyes. Unlike conventional anesthesia, the dissociative state produced by cyclohexamine agents does not result in closure of the eyelids or eyeball rotation. The eye normally remains open, with a central and dilated pupil. The use of ophthalmic lubricant is advised to prevent corneal drying. Another unusual characteristic of dissociative anesthetics is their tendency to induce nystagmus, a repetitive side-to-side motion of the eyeball. Ketamine-induced nystagmus is more commonly seen in cats than in dogs. This condition is harmless and resolves upon recovery from anesthesia.

Ketamine causes a rise in intraocular pressure that can result in rupture of the eye if ocular injury is present.

CNS activity. Animals recovering from cyclohexamine anesthesia often show an exaggerated response to touch, light, or sound, and convulsive seizures may occur. Diazepam may be given IV (or, if IV injection is impossible, by the IM route) to reduce seizure activity. Reduction of light, sound, and other stimuli is also helpful. Some animals recovering from dissociative anesthesia may attempt to paw their faces or demonstrate other bizarre behavior, possibly a result of hallucinations induced by cyclohexamine agents. Because of the high incidence of excited recoveries seen with dissociative anesthesia, recovering patients should be closely monitored to prevent self-injury. It may be advisable that recovery take place in a hospital cage, rather than in the owner's home.

Personality changes have been reported in animals following recovery from ketamine anesthesia. Fortunately, these usually resolve spontaneously after a few days or weeks.

Because of the stimulation of the CNS seen with cyclohexamine agents, these drugs are contraindicated in animals with a history of epilepsy or other seizure disorders. Cyclohexamines should be avoided in animals that have ingested strychnine, metaldehyde, marijuana or other street drugs, organophosphates, and other toxins that affect the CNS. Cyclohexamines should also be used with caution in animals undergoing procedures involving the neurologic system, including CSF taps and myelograms, since postoperative seizures may occur after these procedures.

Cyclohexamine agents

Ketamine. Ketamine (Ketaset, Ketalean, Vetalar) is the most commonly used cyclohexamine agent and can be used to anesthetize not only cats and dogs, but also birds, horses, and exotic species. Ketamine is at present only licensed for use in cats. It is most commonly supplied as a 100 mg/ml solution.

Ketamine has a rapid onset of action after IV or IM administration. This is due to its high lipid solubility, which allows quick entry into brain tissue. Cats may lose their righting reflex within 90 seconds of IV administration of ketamine and within 2 to 4 minutes of an IM injection.

IV administration has several advantages over IM administration, as induction and recovery are more rapid, and the dose is much less if the IV route is used. The anesthetist must ensure that the dose of ketamine is correct for the route of administration used: as with most anesthetic agents, the IV dose is much less than the IM dose. If the IM dose is inadvertently given by the IV route, death may result. In dogs ketamine is given by the IV route only, because IM ketamine may cause convulsions.

Although ketamine can be administered repeatedly to maintain anesthesia, this should be done with caution. After repeated injections, large amounts of the drug accumulate in the tissues, increasing the risk of convulsions during recovery and prolonging the recovery period significantly.

Recovery from ketamine anesthesia normally occurs within 2 to 6 hours in healthy patients, depending on the dosage given and the administration route. Unlike barbiturates, redistribution to body fat does not occur with cyclohexamines. Recovery occurs as the drug gradually leaves the brain and is metabolized and excreted. Dogs appear to have faster recoveries than cats, probably because of differences in the method of ketamine excretion. Elimination of ketamine depends on hepatic metabolism in the dog, but in the cat it is primarily excreted through the kidney. Ketamine should be used with extreme caution in cats with compromised renal function or urinary obstruction and in dogs with hepatic disease.

Ketamine is usually administered in combination with a tranquilizer, such as diazepam, xylazine, or acetylpromazine. The tranquilizer may be given as a premedication or mixed with ketamine and administered simultaneously. The use of a tranquilizer aids muscle relaxation and allows smoother recovery than the use of ketamine alone. As previously mentioned, administration of an anticholinergic is also suggested when ketamine is used, to prevent excessive salivation.

Ketamine-diazepam mixtures are popular for IV induction of cats and dogs and are formulated by combining equal volumes of diazepam (5 mg/ml) and ketamine (100 mg/ml). The resulting mixture may show precipitation if stored more than 1 week and should not be used after this time. When ketamine-diazepam is given by IV administration at a dosage rate of 1 ml/7 kg, the animal loses consciousness within 30 to 90 seconds. If the mixture is given slowly (over 1 to 2 minutes), the dosage required for induction may be considerably less. The combination of ketamine and diazepam has several advantages, including minimal toxicity to the heart. Respiratory depression, however, may be greater than that seen with ketamine alone. Muscle relaxation and anesthetic recovery are superior to that seen with the use of ketamine as the sole agent of anesthesia.

Ketamine-diazepam does not work well when given by the IM route, because diazepam is poorly absorbed after IM injection. Midazolam, a water-soluble benzodiazepine, may be combined with ketamine in a manner similar to diazepam, and the midazolam-ketamine mixture is well absorbed after IM administration.

Ketamine also is commonly used with xylazine, although the combination is associated with significant cardiovascular and respiratory side effects. *Ketamine-xylazine mixtures* may be given either IM or IV, a significant advantage of this combination. IM ketamine-xylazine is a particularly convenient anesthetic combination for use in uncooperative cats. The combination induces profound catalepsy with excellent muscle relaxation and some analgesia (although the analgesia is considered inadequate for major surgery and probably lasts only 15 minutes or less). Because of the potentially adverse effect of xylazine on the cardiovascular and respiratory systems, however, this anesthetic combination does not offer the safety of ketamine-diazepam mixtures and, in the opinion of some authorities, should not be used. Patients recovering from ketamine-xylazine anesthesia should be closely monitored, as anesthetic complications and even death may result from cardiovascular collapse and respiratory depression long after the surgical procedure is finished. The combination of ketamine and xylazine is also associated with an increased risk of aspiration of vomitus, as xylazine acts as an emetic (particularly in cats), and the swallowing reflexes may not be maintained adequately. This risk may be alleviated somewhat by premedicating the patient with atropine and xylazine and allowing 10 or 15 minutes for emesis to occur before anesthesia is achieved by the administration of ketamine.

Ketamine-acetylpromazine combinations are used commonly (particularly in cats) for IV or IM administration. Atropine is usually added to the mixture to reduce salivation. There is less respiratory depression and fewer cardiovascular side effects with this combination than with ketamine-xylazine. As with other ketamine-tranquilizer combinations, the anesthesia produced is not sufficient for major surgery unless supplemented with an opioid agent or inhalation anesthetic.

Tiletamine. Tiletamine is a newer dissociative agent with effects similar to ketamine. Tiletamine is sold only in combination with zolazepam, which is a benzodiazepine agent closely related to diazepam. The use of zolazepam in combination with tiletamine reduces the risk of convulsive seizures during recovery and helps promote skeletal muscle relaxation. The product is sold as a powder, which when reconstituted, is stable for 4 days at room temperature and 14 days if refrigerated. Telazol is a class III controlled substance in the United States, and is currently unavailable in Canada.

The combination of tiletamine and zolazepam (Telazol) is similar in effect to ketamine-diazepam but offers the following advantages:
- Tiletamine appears to cause less pronounced apneustic respiration than ketamine. Respiratory depression may be present, particularly if used in combination with sedatives or anesthetics.
- Tiletamine-zolazepam may be administered by both the IM and IV routes.
- Telazol is approved for use in both dogs and cats (in the United States), although at present it is approved for IM use only.
- Because of the IM route of administration, Telazol is particularly useful for chemical restraint of aggressive dogs. A mixture of 3 mg/kg Telazol and 4 mg/kg butorphanol given IM provides adequate restraint for examination and minor procedures.

Onset of anesthesia is 2 to 5 minutes after IM injection, and duration of anesthesia is 20 to 30 minutes. As with ketamine, intramuscular injection may be painful.

In tiletamine-zolazepam anesthesia, many reflexes arc maintained throughout anesthesia, including the palpebral, corneal, laryngeal, pedal, and pinna reflexes, and depth of anesthesia may be difficult to judge. As with ketamine, there is some analgesia, but visceral analgesia is probably inadequate for major abdominal surgery unless supplemented with other agents. Cardiac dysrhythmias may be present in light anesthesia, but may be prevented by atropine premedication or by increasing the dose administered. Like ketamine, tiletamine induces marked salivation, and the patient should be premedicated with an anticholinergic agent, such as atropine or glycopyrrolate.

Tiletamine has been associated with tremors and convulsions during anesthetic recovery. As with ketamine, ataxia and increased sensitivity to stimuli are commonly observed during the recovery period. Recovery may be prolonged (up to 5 hours after IM injection), particularly if high doses are administered.

Neuroleptanalgesia

As outlined in Chapter 1, the combination of an opioid and a tranquilizing agent can be used to induce a state of profound sedation, termed *neuroleptanalgesia*. The same combination of drugs can be used to induce general anesthesia when given by IV injection. The opioid agents most commonly used for neuroleptanalgesia are morphine, meperidine, butorphanol, fentanyl, and oxymorphone. These are combined with a tranquilizer, such as acetylpromazine, diazepam, or droperidol.

Neuroleptanalgesia combinations are not suitable for routine induction of healthy young animals, because true anesthesia is unlikely to occur in these patients unless nitrous oxide or another anesthetic agent is given as well. However, neuroleptanalgesics may have a profound effect in high-risk or debilitated patients and are a useful and safe alternative to barbiturates or ketamine in these animals.

Induction with opioid-tranquilizer combinations provides a wide margin of safety in most patients, although care must be taken to either administer the drugs slowly or use a dilute solution. If opioid-tranquilizer combinations are rapidly injected, hypotension may occur as a result of sudden vasodilation. Additionally, CNS stimulation may be seen following rapid administration of these agents. The anesthetist using neuroleptanalgesia agents must also be prepared to intubate and ventilate the patient if necessary, as profound respiratory depression may occur (as with any opioid agent).

Several procedures have been described for induction of anesthesia using neuroleptanalgesics. These include:
1. Administration of atropine and a tranquilizer 15 minutes before IV opioid administration.
2. Administration of atropine, followed 15 minutes later by slow IV administration of a tranquilizer-opioid mixture. If diazepam is selected as the tranquilizing

agent, administration must be done using separate syringes, as diazepam and the opioid agent may precipitate if mixed. Small amounts of each agent can be administered alternately through an IV catheter.

3. Administration of atropine and tranquilizer, followed 15 minutes later by rapid administration of IV fluids containing the opioid agent. Administration of the fluids may be discontinued when the desired level of anesthesia is reached.

The above regimens can be safely carried out without atropine, provided the heart rate is carefully monitored. If bradycardia is noted, atropine or glycopyrrolate should be administered.

Propofol

Propofol (Diprivan, Rapinovet) is a recently introduced anesthetic induction agent that may be used as the sole agent for short procedures or for anesthetic induction before inhalant anesthesia. It is a substituted phenol with a structure unlike that of other anesthetic or preanesthetic agents. Propofol is provided as an oil in water emulsion with a concentration of 10 mg/ml. Although this agent has a milky appearance, it can be safely administered intravenously. Injections should be given by the IV route only, over a period of 20 to 60 seconds until the desired anesthetic depth is reached. When given at a dose rate of 6 mg/kg IV, onset of anesthesia is less than 60 seconds and duration of anesthesia is 10 to 20 minutes. Anesthesia may be maintained for longer periods by administering additional drug every 3 to 5 minutes. Recovery is fairly rapid even after repeated injections, but may be accompanied by vomiting in some patients.

Propofol has a rapid onset and short duration of action, similar to the thiobarbiturates. It has several advantages over other injectable agents, including a wide margin of safety in both the dog and cat. Other characteristics include the following:

- Propofol can be given repeatedly to a patient without concern that accumulated effects or poor recoveries will occur. It is one of the few injectable agents that can be safely used for prolonged anesthesia, by continuous infusion or repeated boluses. Recovery is rapid and smooth, even after multiple injections.
- Transient excitation and muscle tremors are seen occasionally during induction.
- Overall effects on the cardiovascular system are minimal, although episodes of tachycardia or bradycardia may occur.
- The effect on respiration is usually minimal, although transient apnea has been reported after rapid IV injection.
- There is no need for atropine premedication. However, preanesthetic tranquilizers are useful since they decrease the dose of propofol required.
- Recovery occurs as a result of rapid redistribution and metabolism in the liver and lung. Metabolites are excreted in the urine. Propofol appears to be safe for use in sighthounds and is suitable for patients with renal or hepatic disease.

• Some muscle relaxation occurs with this agent, although analgesia is poor.

The chief disadvantages of propofol are the high cost and poor storage characteristics of this agent. Propofol is available in 20-ml (200 mg) ampules, the entire contents of which must be used within 24 hours of opening to avoid contamination. (Unopened, the shelf life is approximately 3 years.) Propofol may exacerbate systemic infections and should be avoided in bacteremic patients.

Propofol is currently not approved for animal use in Canada or the United States.

INHALATION ANESTHETICS

Inhalation anesthesia has become so commonplace in veterinary and human anesthesia that it is difficult to imagine the impact that the introduction of the first inhalation anesthetic had on surgical practice. Before the introduction of anesthesia, every surgical procedure was associated with pain, and it was usually necessary for surgeons to work at breakneck speed while the patients were manually restrained by attendants. The introduction of diethyl ether in 1842 and nitrous oxide in 1844 allowed the performance of safe and humane surgery, marking one of the most significant advances of medical science. Indeed, inhalation anesthesia continues to be the safest and most commonly used form of surgical anesthesia.

The inhalation anesthetics in common use in small animal practice at the present time include halothane, isoflurane, methoxyflurane, and nitrous oxide. Of the many inhalation agents currently available, these four have proven to be best suited to veterinary patients, based on convenience, safety, and effectiveness. Many other inhalation agents, including diethyl ether, chloroform, divinyl ether, and trichloroethylene, have been used in the past but are now of historical interest only.

Characteristics of an ideal agent

Although each inhalation agent has desirable properties, the "ideal" inhalation agent does not exist. The characteristics of such an agent would include:
1. Minimal toxicity to the patient, particularly to the cardiovascular, respiratory, hepatic, renal, and nervous systems
2. Minimal toxicity of waste gas vapors to anesthetists and other operating room personnel
3. Ease of administration, even to fractious animals
4. Rapid and gentle induction and recovery
5. Anesthetic depth easily controlled and altered
6. Good muscle relaxation and adequate postoperative analgesia
7. Low cost
8. Adequate potency to achieve surgical anesthesia

9. Handling safety (agent should be nonflammable and nonexplosive)
10. No requirement for expensive equipment

Each of the four commonly used gas anesthetics approaches this standard in several respects. All are relatively safe for most veterinary patients. As previously mentioned, it is generally acknowledged that inhalation anesthetics provide the safest form of general anesthesia for most surgical procedures in small animal patients.

In choosing an inhalation agent to be used for a particular procedure, the veterinarian must consider several factors, including the availability of each agent, the special needs of the patient, the preference of the anesthetist and surgeon, and cost.

Classes of inhalation agents

Diethyl ether

Diethyl ether (''ether'') was for many years the most widely used anesthetic. Animals anesthetized with this agent normally maintain a relatively stable cardiac output and blood pressure, although heart rate may be slightly elevated. Ether does not sensitize the heart to the action of catecholamines, such as epinephrine, and thus there is little risk of cardiac dysrhythmias developing from this drug. It also produces good muscle relaxation and analgesia.

Despite these advantages, ether has significant drawbacks that have greatly limited its use in contemporary anesthesia. One major problem is the irritating effect of this agent on the tracheal and bronchial mucosa. This results in increased salivation and mucous secretions and an increased risk of laryngospasm and airway blockage. Recovery from ether anesthesia may be prolonged, and postoperative nausea is common. In addition, ether is highly flammable and explosive and requires an explosion-proof refrigerator for safe storage.

Nitrous oxide

Nitrous oxide, the first inhalation anesthetic agent to be introduced, is still used extensively in human anesthesia and, to a lesser extent, in veterinary anesthesia as well. In contrast to the other inhalation agents (which are liquids), nitrous oxide is a gas and, as such, is delivered directly from compressed air tanks and does not require a vaporizer for its administration.

Chlorofluorocarbons

The three most commonly used inhalation agents, halothane, isoflurane, and methoxyflurane, are chemically similar and are classified as halogenated organic compounds (chlorofluorocarbons). Each of the three agents is a liquid at room temperature, but vaporizes readily within an anesthetic machine. It is the vaporized anesthetic, mixed with oxygen, that is administered to the patient to achieve and maintain general anesthesia.

The physical properties and pharmacology of the chlorofluorocarbon agents are summarized in Tables 3-3 and 3-4.

Mechanism of action of inhalation agents

The mechanism of action of anesthetic molecules within the brain is poorly understood. It has been suggested that anesthetics exert their effects by inhibiting the breakdown of gamma-aminobutyric acid (GABA), an inhibitory neurotransmitter. According to this theory, this results in an increased level of GABA in the anesthetized patient's brain, inhibiting brain function. Another theory suggests that anesthetics dissolve in nerve cell membranes and cause the membrane to lose its ability to conduct nerve impulses. This theory suggests that anesthetics with greater lipid solubility will have a more potent effect than those with minimal lipid solubility. This observation holds true for the three inhalants in common use. Methoxyflurane, the most lipid soluble, is the most potent. Halothane has moderate lipid solubility and moderate potency. Isoflurane is the least lipid soluble and is the least potent of the three agents.

TABLE 3-3

Physical properties of the common inhalation anesthetics

	Nitrous oxide	Halothane	Methoxyflurane	Isoflurane
Formula	N_2O	$CF_3CHClBr$	$CH_3OCF_2CHCl_2$	$CF_3CHClOCHF_2$
Molecular weight	44	197	165	184
Date of first clinical use	1845	1956	1959	1981
Trade name	—	Fluothane	Metofane Penthrane	Forane AErrane IsoFlo
Saturated vapor pressure (mm Hg)	800 (psi)	243	22.5	261
Solubility coefficient Blood Oil Rubber	0.47 1.4 1.2	2.4 224 120	13 825 635	1.4 60 62
MAC in the dog (%)	188	0.87	0.23	1.2-1.3

Modified from Warren RG: *Small animal anesthesia*, St Louis, 1989, Mosby.
psi, pounds per square inch; MAC, minimum alveolar concentration.

TABLE 3-4

Pharmacologic properties of selected agents

Property	Methoxyflurane	Halothane	Isoflurane
Muscle relaxation	Excellent	Fair	Good
Effect on nondepolarizing muscle relaxants	None	Increased potency	Greatly increased potency
Analgesia	Excellent	Slight	Slight
Effect on respiration	Marked depression of rate and depth	Some depression	Some depression
Effect on heart	Mild depression	Severe depression	Slight at normal depth
Potential for causing cardiac dysrhythmias	Some	Very common	None reported
Effect on blood pressure	May decrease	Decreases	May decrease
Elimination from the body	Metabolism 50%-80% Respiration 20%-50%	Metabolism 20%-50% Respiration 50%-80%	Respiration 99%
Effect on the liver	None reported	May rarely cause hepatitis in humans	None reported
Effect on the kidneys	Toxicity reported in humans and animals	None reported	None reported
Lipid solubility	High	Moderate	Low
Maintenance range	0.25%-1.0%	0.5%-2%	1%-3%

Modified from McKelvey D: Halothane, isoflurane, and methoxyflurane, *Vet Tech* 12(1):25, 1991.

Distribution and elimination of inhalation agents

To understand the properties of the inhalation agents, it is necessary to briefly discuss their intake into, distribution within, and elimination from the body. Liquid anesthetic in the anesthetic machine is vaporized into oxygen and delivered to the patient by mask or endotracheal tube. The anesthetic travels via the air passages to the lung alveoli, where it diffuses across the alveolar cells and enters the bloodstream. The rate of diffusion is controlled by the concentration gradient between the alveolus and the bloodstream, as well as the lipid solubility of the drug. During the induction period, the concentration of the agent in the alveolus is high, and the concentration in the blood is low. This creates a steep concentration gradient, and diffusion of anesthetic from the alveolus into the blood is very rapid during this period.

Because of their relatively high lipid solubility, inhalation agents readily leave the circulation and enter the brain, inducing anesthesia. Anesthesia is maintained as long as sufficient quantities of inhalation agent are delivered to the alveoli, such that the blood, alveolar, and brain concentrations are maintained.

When the concentration of the inhalation agent administered is reduced or discontinued by adjusting the anesthetic machine vaporizer, the amount of anesthetic in the alveolus is reduced. Since the blood level is still high, the concentration gradient now favors the diffusion of anesthetic from the blood into the alveoli. The blood levels of the anesthetic are quickly reduced, provided the animal continues to breathe and eliminate anesthetic from the alveoli. The anesthetist can hasten the elimination of anesthetic by periodically bagging the animal with 100% oxygen, which removes anesthetic from the alveoli and re-establishes a steep concentration gradient between the alveoli and the blood. As the concentration of the anesthetic in the blood falls, the agent leaves the brain, and recovery from the anesthetic is achieved.

Some anesthetic agents (in particular, methoxyflurane) have very high lipid solubility and may accumulate in body fat stores, thereby escaping elimination through the lungs at the end of anesthesia. These agents rely on liver metabolism and renal excretion for their complete elimination from the body. Slower recoveries and prolonged hangover occur routinely with these agents.

Properties of inhalation agents

Isoflurane, methoxyflurane, halothane, and nitrous oxide differ considerably in their anesthetic effects, in part, because of differences in their physical and chemical properties. The properties of chief importance to the anesthetist include vapor pressure, solubility coefficient, minimum alveolar concentration (MAC), and rubber solubility. They also vary in their pharmacologic properties, including their effects on the cardiovascular, respiratory, and other vital systems.

Vapor pressure

The vapor pressure of an inhalation anesthetic is a measure of the amount of liquid anesthetic that will evaporate at 20° C. Agents with a high vapor pressure, such as halothane or isoflurane, are termed *volatile*, in that they evaporate easily. In fact, both isoflurane and halothane evaporate so readily that they may reach a concentration of over 30% in the oxygen delivered to the patient, which could cause a fatal anesthetic overdose. A special type of vaporizer called a *precision vaporizer* is required to limit the vaporization of these agents and allow their safe use for anesthesia. Precision vaporizers allow a maximum concentration of 5%, which is sufficient for all practical uses. The use of a volatile inhalation agent in a simple, nonprecision vaporizer is difficult because of the lack of control over the evaporation of the anesthetic and the increased risk of overdose. Such vaporizers exist but reduce the percent achievable by directing a high flow of oxygen through a bypass (thereby picking up no anesthetic).

Some agents, such as methoxyflurane, have relatively low vapor pressure and do not require the use of a precision vaporizer. At 20° C the maximum methoxyflurane concentration attainable in the anesthetic circuit is 4%. A simple, inexpensive, nonprecision vaporizer, such as a glass jar with a wick, is adequate for methoxyflurane anesthesia. Precision vaporizers for methoxyflurane are available on some machines; however, they are not a requirement for safe anesthesia.

Because each type of vaporizer is designed for use with a particular agent having a specific vapor pressure, it is theoretically necessary to use a different vaporizer for each agent. In practice, the similar vapor pressures of isoflurane and halothane result in similar evaporation rates, and isoflurane may be used safely in many vaporizers designed for halothane use. A new or recently serviced halothane vaporizer should deliver predictable levels of isoflurane within 10% of the dial setting, which is considered acceptable for anesthesia. Prior to use with isoflurane, a halothane vaporizer should be completely drained and the residual halothane evacuated by allowing oxygen to flow through the vaporizer for several hours. The use of halothane vaporizers for isoflurane is not recommended by anesthetic or vaporizer manufacturers for litigation reasons, as mistakes involving confusion of agents can occur if the anesthetic currently in the vaporizer is not clearly labelled.

Although it is inadvisable to combine halothane and isoflurane in the same vaporizer at one time, it is acceptable to switch from one anesthetic to another during the course of surgery if the patient demonstrates an adverse reaction to the first anesthetic. In this case, separate vaporizers must be available for each anesthetic, since time would not allow evacuation of the first anesthetic from the vaporizer.

Because of significant differences in vapor pressure, methoxyflurane cannot be used in precision vaporizers designed for halothane or isoflurane. Similarly, halothane and isoflurane cannot be safely used in a vaporizer intended for methoxyflurane.

Solubility coefficient

The blood-to-gas solubility coefficient (or partition coefficient) is a measure of the distribution of the inhalation agent between the blood and gas phases in the body. It is therefore a measure of the tendency of an anesthetic agent to exist as a gas or, alternatively, to dissolve in the blood. An inhalation anesthetic with a low solubility coefficient tends to remain in the gas phase in the pulmonary alveoli rather than dissolving into the tissues and blood. This phenomenon produces a high concentration of the agent in the alveoli and a steep diffusion gradient between the alveoli and the blood. As a result, an agent with a low solubility coefficient, although not intrinsically soluble in the blood, will quickly enter the circulation and escape into the brain, resulting in rapid induction and recovery. An example of such an agent is isoflurane, which has an extremely low blood-to-gas solubility coefficient and demonstrates rapid induction and recovery. Halothane has a slightly higher solubility coefficient and is therefore less rapid in its effect.

In contrast, an agent with a high solubility coefficient will be extremely soluble in the blood and tissues. Because the anesthetic is rapidly absorbed into the tissues ("sponge effect"), high levels of the anesthetics do not build up within the alveoli, and a concentration gradient is not established. Additionally, the highly soluble agents are trapped in the blood and tissues to a greater extent, resulting in less escape into brain tissue and wider distribution throughout the body. Therefore agents with high solubility coefficients induce anesthesia less rapidly than agents with low solubility coefficients. Methoxyflurane is an example of an agent with a high solubility coefficient and, as expected, demonstrates relatively slow induction and recovery rates.

The solubility coefficient of an inhalant agent has a significant effect on the clinical use of the agent. The rapid induction possible with isoflurane and halothane allows the use of these agents for mask induction, whereas methoxyflurane is not well suited to this induction method. Agents with low solubility coefficients (such as isoflurane) also have the advantage of allowing a rapid patient response to changes in anesthetic concentration during anesthesia. Patients anesthetized with isoflurane may respond within 1 minute to changes in the vaporizer setting. If an agent with a high solubility coefficient is used (such as methoxyflurane), the anesthetist will observe a relatively slower response to changes in the vaporizer setting.

Minimum alveolar concentration

The minimum alveolar concentration (MAC) of an anesthetic agent is the lowest concentration that produces no response in 50% of the patients exposed to a painful stimulus (for example, a clamp applied to the base of the tail). The MAC thus indicates the strength of an inhalation anesthetic: an agent with a low MAC is a more potent anesthetic than an agent with a high MAC. For example, halothane has a lower MAC than isoflurane. It can therefore be expected that a higher concentration of isoflurane will be necessary to maintain a similar anesthetic depth.

For any given inhalation anesthetic, a vaporizer setting of $1 \times$ MAC will produce light anesthesia in most patients, $1.5 \times$ MAC will produce a surgical depth of anesthesia, and $2 \times$ MAC will produce deep anesthesia. These figures are useful only as a rough guide: MAC varies with the species, age, and body temperature of the patient. Factors such as disease, pregnancy, obesity, and treatment with other drugs may also alter the potency of an anesthetic agent in any given patient. The anesthetist should also be aware that the response to an anesthetic depends on the percent of concentration of the anesthetic in the patient's brain, which is not necessarily the same as that indicated by the vaporizer, particularly early in the induction period (see Chapter 4).

Halothane

Halothane is at present the most commonly used volatile inhalation agent in veterinary anesthesia, although its use has decreased somewhat with the introduction of isoflurane.

Physical and chemical properties

The chief physical and chemical properties of halothane are as follows:

- Halothane has a relatively high vapor pressure and, as such, requires a precision vaporizer for its safe use. Halothane delivered through a nonprecision vaporizer may readily achieve a concentration over 30%, which dangerously exceeds the normal concentration required for anesthesia (1% to 2%).
- Halothane has a moderately low solubility coefficient and moderate fat solubility, allowing fairly rapid induction and recovery. Delivery of halothane by mask usually results in unconsciousness and stage III anesthesia in a tranquilized animal within 10 minutes. Recovery time from anesthesia varies with length of anesthesia, patient condition, and the concurrent use of other agents; however, sternal recumbency is usually achieved in less than 1 hour after the anesthetic is discontinued. Because of its moderate lipid solubility, a portion of the anesthetic is retained within body fat stores rather than being eliminated by the lungs during recovery. The stored halothane is subsequently metabolized by the liver, with elimination of the metabolites in the urine.
- Halothane has a moderate MAC and in terms of anesthetic potency is midway between methoxyflurane and isoflurane. It is approximately 4 times as potent as diethyl ether.
- Halothane has moderate rubber solubility. This is of concern to the anesthetist because hoses, rebreathing bags, and other anesthetic machine parts contain rubber and may absorb halothane during the course of anesthesia. Release of the agent from machine parts may delay patient recovery after the vaporizer has been turned off.
- Halothane is somewhat unstable and is available commercially only mixed with the preservative thymol. The presence of a preservative may cause a buildup of residue within the vaporizer, turning the liquid in the vaporizer yellow and, ultimately, resulting in malfunctioning of the vaporizer unless it is serviced.

Pharmacologic effects

Halothane is a relatively safe agent for veterinary use; however, it does have some adverse effects on organ function.

- Halothane affects the cardiovascular system in several ways. It sensitizes the heart to the action of catecholamines, such as epinephrine, and thus may induce dysrhythmias. Dysrhythmias may be treated by increasing patient ventilation and ensuring that anesthetic depth is adequate. If this does not alleviate the dysrhythmias, the patient may be given IV lidocaine or switched to another anesthetic (if available).
- Halothane increases vagal tone, and bradycardia may result.
- Like all inhalation anesthetics, halothane has a mild depressant effect on myocardial cells, decreasing myocardial contraction and cardiac output. Halothane also decreases peripheral resistance of the blood vessels by causing vasodilation. Vasodilation predisposes the animal to excessive heat loss (and therefore hypothermia). Vasodilation also may cause a fall in blood pressure, which roughly parallels anesthetic depth, and for this reason halothane anesthesia should be avoided in hypovolemic or hypotensive patients.
- Halothane causes some depression of respiration, and respiratory rate and tidal volume usually fall if anesthesia is prolonged. Halothane and all other inhalation anesthetics readily cross the placenta and may depress respiration in the newborn.
- Halothane is moderately lipid soluble and is retained in body fat stores and, subsequently, metabolized in the liver. It has been associated with hepatotoxicity and liver necrosis in human patients. There is no clear evidence at present that hepatotoxicity occurs with halothane use in veterinary patients; however, the use of alternative inhalation agents is probably advisable for patients with hepatic disease.
- Halothane produces adequate muscle relaxation, but only slight analgesia. Halothane and nitrous oxide may be used in combination to achieve even greater muscle relaxation and significant analgesia.
- Halothane use is associated with malignant hyperthermia, which is a rare but often fatal disorder of thermoregulation. Affected animals show increased temperature, muscle rigidity, and cardiac dysrhythmias and may die as a result. Treatment consists of removal from halothane, cooling, and administration of oxygen and specific drugs.

Isoflurane

Physical and chemical properties

Isoflurane is closely related chemically to methoxyflurane, but its properties are more similar to those of halothane. The margin of safety of this agent is apparently greater than that of halothane or methoxyflurane, which has led to its wide acceptance in veterinary anesthesia despite its considerable cost (presently this is approximately 9 times that for the same volume of halothane). Isoflurane is licensed for use only in dogs and horses, although it has gained widespread use in other species.

The chief physical and chemical properties of isoflurane are as follows:

- The vapor pressure of isoflurane is almost identical to that of halothane. Because of its volatile nature, isoflurane is normally used in a precision vaporizer. Some halothane vaporizers have been adapted successfully for isoflurane administration, although this practice is discouraged by the manufacturer.
- The solubility coefficient of isoflurane is extremely low, and this, combined with the relatively low lipid solubility of this agent, results in extremely rapid induction and recovery. Isoflurane is better suited to mask or chamber induction than are slower-acting agents, such as methoxyflurane. It is important that the anesthetist administering isoflurane refrain from turning off the anesthetic machine vaporizer until the end of surgery, as return of consciousness may occur as rapidly as 1 to 2 minutes after isoflurane administration is discontinued. The low solubility coefficient of isoflurane also allows the anesthetist to change the patient's depth of anesthesia very rapidly during the course of anesthesia. An animal that appears too deep or too light usually responds rapidly (within 1 or 2 minutes) to adjustment of the anesthetic level.
- The MAC of isoflurane is higher than that of halothane or methoxyflurane, and isoflurane is thus the least potent of the three agents. Anesthesia is maintained in most patients at a concentration of 1.5% to 2% isoflurane in oxygen.
- The rubber solubility of isoflurane is very low, and there is little absorption of this anesthetic by rubber-containing components.
- Isoflurane is stable at room temperature, and no preservative is necessary. This is an advantage, since consequently there is no preservative residue to accumulate in isoflurane vaporizers.

Pharmacologic effects

Of all the volatile anesthetics, isoflurane is considered to have the fewest adverse effects on the heart and other vital systems.

- When used at normal anesthetic levels, isoflurane maintains cardiac performance close to that of preanesthetic levels. It causes only a small decrease in cardiac output, with little or no depression of myocardial cells and little effect on heart rate. Isoflurane does not sensitize the myocardium to the effects of epinephrine and is therefore not dysrhythmogenic. Because of its minimal effect on the heart, isoflurane is considered to be the inhalation agent of choice for patients with cardiac disease. As with halothane, vasodilation and decreased blood pressure may be observed, particularly at deeper levels of anesthesia.
- Isoflurane depresses respiration. The effect of isoflurane on respiration is greater than that of halothane but less than that of methoxyflurane.

- Nearly all of the isoflurane administered to a patient is exhaled very quickly once the vaporizer is turned off. Isoflurane has low fat solubility, and consequently, there is very little retention of isoflurane in body fat stores, little hepatic metabolism, and very little renal excretion of metabolites. For this reason isoflurane is well suited to animals with liver or kidney disease. Isoflurane is also the preferred anesthetic for use in neonatal and geriatric animals, in which hepatic metabolism and renal excretion mechanisms may be inefficient compared to the healthy adult animal.
- Animals anesthetized with isoflurane show good muscle relaxation.
- Isoflurane has little or no analgesic effect in the postanesthetic period. The use of postoperative analgesics may be advisable, as the lack of analgesic effect combined with the rapid recoveries experienced with this agent may lead to pain and excitement during recovery.

Methoxyflurane

Although no longer used as often as halothane or isoflurane, methoxyflurane is a useful anesthetic agent in small animal patients.

Physical and chemical properties

The physical and chemical properties of methoxyflurane may be summarized as follows:

- The vapor pressure of methoxyflurane is significantly lower than that of halothane or isoflurane, and as a result methoxyflurane may be safely used in a nonprecision vaporizer. Since an anesthetic machine with a nonprecision vaporizer is considerably less expensive than one with a precision vaporizer, the initial equipment costs are less for methoxyflurane anesthesia than for halothane or isoflurane, both of which require precision vaporizers. Methoxyflurane itself is more expensive than halothane on a per milliliter basis but is less expensive than isoflurane.
- The solubility coefficient of methoxyflurane is considerably higher than that of halothane or isoflurane, as is the lipid solubility. These two factors combine to produce slow induction and recovery rates in animals anesthetized with methoxyflurane. Because of the slow induction rates, it is not generally advocated that this agent be used for mask induction or chamber induction, as stage II of general anesthesia may be prolonged.

Because of the high solubility coefficient of methoxyflurane, there is a considerable delay before patient response is seen after changing the inspired concentration of anesthetic. In patients undergoing surgery while under methoxyflurane anesthesia, administration of the anesthetic often can be discontinued 10 minutes before the end of surgery without danger of premature arousal.

- Methoxyflurane is the most potent inhalation anesthetic in common use, because the MAC of methoxyflurane is considerably lower than that of the other volatile inhalation anesthetics. Methoxyflurane is approximately twice as potent as halothane.
- Methoxyflurane has considerable solubility in rubber or plastics and readily dissolves in rebreathing bags, hoses, and endotracheal tubes. This may lead to deterioration of these products unless they are rinsed out immediately after use. The solubility of methoxyflurane in rubber or plastic anesthetic machine parts may also result in considerable release of methoxyflurane gas into the anesthetic circuit after the vaporizer has been turned off.
- As with halothane, methoxyflurane requires the addition of a preservative in order to extend its shelf life. The accumulation of preservative may interfere with vaporizer function; however, cleaning and maintenance procedures for nonprecision vaporizers are much easier than those for precision vaporizers.

Pharmacologic effects

Methoxyflurane has a considerable margin of safety in both the dog and cat.

- Methoxyflurane, unlike halothane, does not sensitize the myocardium to the dysrhythmogenic effects of catecholamines. However, methoxyflurane may depress myocardial cells such that the contractility of the myocardium is reduced by up to 40%. Methoxyflurane also reduces heart rate, with a resulting decrease in cardiac output. The reduction in cardiac output may cause a fall in blood pressure. Mild-to-moderate hypotension often is present in light anesthetic planes, and deeper planes of anesthesia may be associated with marked fall in blood pressure.
- Methoxyflurane is the most potent respiratory depressant of all the inhalation anesthetics. Both the respiratory rate and the tidal volume are decreased, and it is important to monitor anesthetized animals to ensure adequate ventilation. The use of a ventilator or periodic bagging by hand will help expand alveoli and prevent a state of hypercarbia (elevated levels of carbon dioxide in the blood). However, the anesthetist should avoid continuous bagging of a patient under methoxyflurane anesthesia unless the vaporizer setting is reduced. Failure to do so may lead to excessive anesthetic being delivered to the patient, as the concentration of anesthetic increases as oxygen is forced through a nonprecision vaporizer by the bagging procedure.
- Animals under methoxyflurane anesthesia may, to some extent, regulate their own anesthetic depth, although close attention on the part of the anesthetist is essential to ensure patient safety. An animal entering a lighter plane of anesthesia will begin to breathe more rapidly and more deeply. If the methoxyflurane is being delivered by a nonprecision vaporizer, more of the liquid anesthetic will be vaporized and a higher level of methoxyflurane will be delivered to the patient,

resulting in a return to a deeper plane of anesthesia. Conversely, if the patient enters a deeper plane of anesthesia, the rate and depth of respiration will decrease, resulting in less delivery of anesthetic from a nonprecision vaporizer.

- Because of its high lipid solubility, methoxyflurane is retained in body fat stores such that over half of the anesthetic delivered to the animal is eventually metabolized and excreted by the liver and kidney. The presence of toxic metabolites, such as fluoride ions, within the kidney may lead to renal damage, particularly if flunixin (Banamine) or other potentially nephrotoxic drugs are administered currently. This effect has been well documented in human anesthesia, although its occurrence in veterinary anesthesia seems to be limited to dehydrated animals with preexisting renal damage. Urine concentrating ability may be impaired for up to 3 days after methoxyflurane use, even in healthy patients.
- From the standpoint of both the patient and the operating room personnel, the persistence of methoxyflurane within the body fat raises some concern about long-term deleterious effects (see Chapter 5).
- Methoxyflurane causes marked skeletal muscle relaxation and has considerable analgesic effect. This allows surgery to proceed at relatively light planes of anesthesia, minimizing cardiovascular depression. The analgesic effect of this agent and the relatively slow recovery rate also ensure that recovery from methoxyflurane anesthesia is generally smooth, and patient distress seldom occurs.

Enflurane

Enflurane, a volatile gaseous anesthetic used in human medicine, has not found wide acceptance in veterinary anesthesia. As with the other volatile anesthetics, it is nonflammable and nonexplosive and produces good muscle relaxation. Induction and recovery are relatively rapid and smooth, with minimal effects on heart rate and no sensitization of the myocardium to catecholamines. However, enflurane causes profound depression of respiration, and spontaneous ventilation of the patient is poor under this anesthetic. In the dog, enflurane also induces significant muscle hyperactivity, and seizure-like muscle spasms may result.

Nitrous oxide

Physical and pharmacologic properties

Nitrous oxide (N_2O) is an odorless gas that can be used as an adjunct to anesthesia with other inhalation agents, particularly halothane and methoxyflurane. It is seldom used as the sole anesthetic agent in domestic animals.

The property that limits the use of nitrous oxide in veterinary anesthesia is its lack of potency (high MAC) in domestic species. The MAC of nitrous oxide in humans is approximately 100%, whereas the MAC in the dog and horse is close to

200% and in the cat approximately 250%. As these figures demonstrate, it is impossible to achieve a surgical plane of anesthesia in a healthy dog or cat using nitrous oxide alone.

Other properties of nitrous oxide can be summarized as follows:
- The use of nitrous oxide with another inhalation anesthetic (such as halothane) usually allows the anesthetist to lower the concentration of the other agent being administered. Nitrous oxide reduces the MAC (and therefore the vaporizer setting) of other anesthetics by 20% to 30%. This reduces the toxicity of the anesthetic agents and allows faster recoveries. Nitrous oxide also has been shown to speed the uptake of other anesthetic gases into the bloodstream by the "second gas effect" when used at high concentrations (50% to 70% of the total gas flow).
- Nitrous oxide has an extremely low solubility coefficient and is associated with rapid induction and recovery rates. It is therefore a helpful addition to slow-acting agents such as methoxyflurane, although it does little to enhance isoflurane anesthesia.
- Nitrous oxide has little effect on the cardiovascular, respiratory, hepatic, or urinary systems and is considered to have a wide margin of safety. Nitrous oxide offers good analgesia and excellent muscle relaxation.

Despite these advantages, the use of nitrous oxide in veterinary anesthesia has declined in recent years. One reason is the increased cost of N_2O anesthesia, compared to anesthesia with an inhalation agent alone. Another reason is the increased use of isoflurane, which provides rapid induction and recovery without the concurrent use of nitrous oxide.

Special precautions

Use of nitrous oxide is associated with several potential problems, including the following.

Risk of hypoxia. The use of nitrous oxide in an anesthetic machine limits the amount of oxygen that is delivered to the patient, in that nitrous oxide replaces oxygen in the circuit. Since the minimal amount of nitrous oxide necessary to achieve analgesic effects is 50% (and values of 60% to 66% are recommended), the use of this agent decreases the amount of oxygen delivered to the patient by 50% to 66%. The anesthetist must ensure at all times that at least 30 ml/kg/minute of oxygen is delivered to the patient and that the oxygen content of the inspired gases is at least 33%. This can be achieved by ensuring that the nitrous oxide flow (in liters per minute) is no more than twice the oxygen flow and that oxygen flow rates less than 300 ml/minute are avoided.

The patient breathing nitrous oxide is at increased risk of hypoxia and should be monitored closely for cyanosis, cardiac dysrhythmias, and other indications of hypoxia. Because of the risk of hypoxia, animals with preexisting pulmonary disease, such as pneumonia, are poor candidates for N_2O anesthesia. For all patients, care should also be taken when adjusting the flowmeters of the anesthetic machine, such that the oxygen controls are not confused with those for nitrous oxide.

Diffusion into air pockets. Because of its very low solubility coefficient, nitrous oxide is able to diffuse into trapped air pockets within the body. This diffusion may result in an increase in the amount of gas within an organ and consequent distension of an organ containing trapped gas. For this reason, the use of nitrous oxide is contraindicated in animals with intestinal obstruction, gastric torsion, pneumothorax, or diaphragmatic hernia.

Use in closed systems. Nitrous oxide should never be used in a closed anesthetic circuit (i.e., one in which there is no pop-off or other waste gas exhaust). As oxygen is removed from a closed system by the animal, the level of nitrous oxide in the circuit may increase to dangerous levels, resulting in hypoxia.

Diffusion hypoxia. During recovery from anesthesia, nitrous oxide will readily exit from the body via the respiratory system. Because of the rapid outpouring of nitrous oxide into the lungs, a state of "diffusion hypoxia" may be created. In this condition, oxygen molecules normally found in the alveoli are displaced by the large numbers of nitrous oxide molecules exiting from the body. Diffusion hypoxia can be prevented by keeping the animal on high oxygen flow rates for at least 5 minutes after the nitrous oxide has been turned off and ensuring that the animal is frequently bagged with pure oxygen.

Waste anesthetic gas hazards. Exposure of operating room personnel to waste nitrous oxide has been linked to several health disorders (see Chapter 5).

AGENTS USED IN THE POSTANESTHETIC PERIOD

Two classes of drugs, reversing agents and analeptics, are available to hasten recovery after anesthesia. A *reversing agent* is a drug that negates the effect of a specific anesthetic or preanesthetic agent (usually by competing with the anesthetic for specific receptor sites). An *analeptic* agent is a drug that causes general CNS stimulation.

Although useful, these drugs should not be substituted for careful anesthetic technique. The anesthetist should rely primarily on precise control of anesthetic depth to ensure rapid and smooth patient recovery. However, the use of reversing agents and analeptics in selected patients may be a valuable addition to an anesthetic protocol.

Doxapram

Doxapram (Dopram) is a respiratory stimulant and analeptic agent. When given intravenously, doxapram will increase respiratory rate and depth and may accelerate arousal from barbiturate or inhalation anesthesia. The dose necessary to arouse the animal is much greater for patients that have undergone injectable anesthesia than it is for patients recovering from inhalation anesthesia.

Although doxapram has a wide margin of safety, it may cause tachycardia and dysrhythmias in some patients and should be used with caution in animals with cardiac disease. Doxapram must be used only in the presence of adequate oxygen levels in the brain, otherwise CNS damage may result.

Doxapram is particularly useful for stimulating respiration in newborn puppies and kittens: two or three drops placed under the tongue may greatly increase respiration rate and depth.

Yohimbine

Yohimbine (Yobine) given at a dose of 0.1 mg/kg IV is an effective reversing agent for alpha-2 adrenoreceptor agonists, particularly xylazine. Yohimbine is a useful treatment for both dogs and cats showing excessive sedation or undesirable cardiovascular side effects arising from xylazine use. It may also be used alone or in combination with other reversing agents, such as 4-aminopyridine or tolazoline, to speed recovery. Reversal of sedation and cardiovascular effects of xylazine occurs within a few minutes of IV administration of yohimbine.

Yohimbine is associated with occasional unwanted side effects, including rapid arousal, excitement, rage, and tremors. It has been reported that tolazoline produces slower arousal than yohimbine and that the incidence of excitement during arousal is less with this agent.

Atipamezole (Antisedan) is a specific antagonist for another alpha-2 adrenoreceptor agonist, medetomidine.

Flumazenil

Flumazenil (Anexate) is a recently developed reversing agent that is effective in antagonizing sedation brought about by the use of diazepam.

Narcotic antagonists

Specific narcotic antagonists (reversing agents) are available that compete with opioid agents for receptor sites in the brain. These drugs, particularly naloxone, a pure antagonist, have received widespread use in the reversal of neuroleptanalgesia and in the treatment of animals undergoing severe respiratory depression or other side effects of opioid administration. Some narcotic antagonists (classified as agonist antagonists) may themselves cause respiratory depression (see Chapter 1).

When using naloxone to reverse neuroleptanalgesia, only the opioid effects are reversed, and the action of the tranquilizing agent is unaffected. Since the maximum duration of effect is 45 minutes or less, additional doses of naloxone may be required to continue the antagonistic effect. More information on narcotic reversing agents is found in Chapter 1.

KEY POINTS

1. Injectable anesthetics are eliminated by redistribution, liver metabolism, and renal excretion. Inhalation anesthetics are eliminated primarily by exhalation from the lungs. Some inhalation anesthetics are also subject to liver metabolism and renal excretion.

2. Both injectable and inhalation anesthetics have a wide margin of safety; however, most agents have depressant effects on the cardiovascular, respiratory, and thermoregulatory systems.

3. Injectable anesthetics include barbiturates, cyclohexamines, neuroleptanalgesic agents, and propofol.

4. Several classes of barbiturates are available for veterinary anesthesia, including short-acting barbiturates such as pentobarbital, ultrashort-acting barbiturates such as thiopental and thiamylal, and methylated oxybarbiturates such as methohexital. These classes differ in their lipid solubility, duration of effect, and distribution within the body.

5. Barbiturates are used most commonly as induction agents and are normally administered by titration to achieve the minimum effective dose.

6. Barbiturates may cause respiratory depression and respiratory acidosis. Other adverse side effects include tissue necrosis (when injected perivascularly), cardiac dysrhythmias, and excitement during anesthetic induction and/or recovery.

7. Barbiturates show unusual potency in patients that are acidotic, hypoproteinemic, or hypotensive. They may cause prolonged sleeping times in sighthounds.

8. Pentobarbital can be given intravenously or intramuscularly to achieve anesthesia, but it is seldom recommended because of poor muscle relaxation, lack of analgesia, respiratory depression, and prolonged recoveries associated with its use.

9. Thiobarbiturates have a rapid onset of action and short duration and are well suited as induction agents for dogs and cats. Transient apnea may be seen during induction. Methohexital is an alternative agent for use in sighthounds.

10. Cyclohexamine agents, such as ketamine and tiletamine, produce a state of dissociative anesthesia, which is characterized by exaggerated reflex responses, central nervous system excitement, apneustic respiration, tachycardia, and increased muscle tone. They may be given by intramuscular injection in cats or intravenous injection in cats or dogs. Concurrent use of a tranquilizer, such as

diazepam, zolazepam, acetylpromazine, or xylazine, is recommended to promote muscle relaxation and to prevent excitement during recovery. Anticholinergic agents commonly are used to prevent excessive salivation.

11. Neuroleptanalgesia is a profound hypnotic state produced by administration of an opioid and a tranquilizing agent. These agents provide safe induction in debilitated patients and also are used for short procedures in healthy young animals.

12. Propofol is a recently introduced induction agent that has a wide margin of safety and can be given by repeat injection to maintain anesthesia.

13. The four inhalation agents in common use are halothane, isoflurane, methoxyflurane, and nitrous oxide. In each case, the agent is administered by means of an anesthetic machine through either a mask or an endotracheal tube. These agents enter the body by absorption through the alveolus, at a rate that depends on the solubility coefficient of the agent and the concentration gradient between the alveolar air and the blood.

14. Anesthetic agents vary in their solubility coefficient, vapor pressure, and minimum alveolar concentration (MAC). These physical properties affect the speed of induction and recovery, the type of vaporizer that should be used, and the vaporizer setting that is required for anesthesia.

15. All inhalation anesthetics may cause respiratory depression and decrease blood pressure. In addition, halothane may potentiate cardiac dysrhythmias. Of the three chlorofluorocarbon agents, isoflurane is considered to have the greatest margin of safety and the shortest induction and recovery times.

16. Isoflurane is eliminated almost entirely through respiration. Halothane and methoxyflurane undergo some hepatic metabolism and renal excretion, as well as respiratory elimination.

17. Methoxyflurane has some analgesic properties and usually produces slow, uneventful recoveries. Its high degree of lipid retention and subsequent metabolism and excretion have raised some concerns regarding toxicity of waste gas vapors to health care personnel.

18. Nitrous oxide has few cardiovascular or respiratory side effects and is a useful adjunct to halothane or methoxyflurane anesthesia. It is too weak to be used as a sole anesthetic agent in animals. The anesthetist must be aware of the risk of hypoxia associated with this agent, particularly in the period immediately following discontinuation of the agent.

19. Reversing agents and analeptics may be given following anesthesia to hasten anesthetic recovery. Doxapram is a nonspecific respiratory stimulant that may accelerate arousal from barbiturate or inhalation anesthesia. Yohimbine, atipamezole, flumazenil, and naloxone are used as reversing agents for specific preanesthetics and opioids.

REVIEW QUESTIONS

1. Barbiturate drugs have a pH that is:
   a. Strongly alkaline (>9.5)
   b. Strongly acidic (<2)
   c. Close to normal body pH
2. Drugs that are more fat soluble are more likely to be taken up by the brain more quickly.
   True   False
3. Which of the following is an example of a dissociative anesthetic?
   a. Thiopental sodium
   b. Pentobarbital sodium
   c. Ketamine hydrochloride
   d. Propofol
4. One of the disadvantages of the drug methohexital is that animals that are anesthetized with it often may demonstrate excitement during recovery.
   True   False
5. Metabolism and elimination of ketamine hydrochloride are the same in the dog as they are in the cat.
   True   False
6. Halothane is considered to have a:
   a. High vapor pressure
   b. Moderate vapor pressure
   c. Low vapor pressure
7. Halothane may sensitize the heart to catecholamines.
   True   False
8. Halothane is moderately soluble in rubber, which may result in release of this gas from anesthetic equipment.
   True   False
9. Halothane can increase vagal tone.
   True   False
10. Which of the following have similar vapor pressures?
    a. Halothane and methoxyflurane
    b. Methoxyflurane and isoflurane
    c. Isoflurane and halothane
11. An anesthetic agent that has a low solubility coefficient will result in _____ induction and recovery time.
    a. Slow
    b. Moderate
    c. Fast
12. An example of a volatile anesthetic with a high solubility coefficient is:
    a. Halothane
    b. Isoflurane
    c. Enflurane
    d. Methoxyflurane
13. As a rough guideline, to safely maintain a surgical plane of anesthesia, the vaporizer should be set at _____ times MAC.

    a. 0.5

    b. 1.0

    c. 1.5

    d. 2.0

    e. 2.5

14. Halothane can have a direct depressant effect on the myocardial cells.

    True   False

15. Isoflurane is a more potent cardiac depressant than halothane.

    True   False

16. Methoxyflurane is considered to be a more potent respiratory depressant than either isoflurane or halothane.

    True   False

17. Isoflurane is more likely to be absorbed by the rubber or plastics of an anesthetic circuit than halothane.

    True   False

18. Rank the three inhalation anesthetics in regard to their fat solubility, beginning with the most soluble.

    a. Halothane > Methoxyflurane > Isoflurane

    b. Isoflurane > Halothane > Methoxyflurane

    c. Methoxyflurane > Halothane > Isoflurane

    d. Isoflurane > Methoxyflurane > Halothane

    e. Halothane > Isoflurane > Methoxyflurane

19. Recovery from methohexital compared to that from a thiobarbiturate will be:

    a. Faster

    b. Slower

    c. The same

20. A patient known to have pulmonary dysfunction would be considered a (an) _____ candidate to receive nitrous oxide.

    a. Excellent

    b. Good

    c. Fair

    d. Poor

21. To be considered effective, nitrous oxide should be used in concentrations of:

    a. 20%

    b. 40%

    c. 60%

    d. 90%

    e. None of the above percentages are correct

22. Anesthetic agents that have a high vapor pressure:

    a. Will evaporate quickly and easily

    b. Will evaporate slowly, with more difficulty

    c. Do not evaporate at all

    d. Will only exist in a gaseous form

For the following questions one or more answers may be correct.

23. The depressant effects that barbiturates have on the vital centers of the body are less likely to occur if:

    a. Only a dilute (e.g., 2%) solution is used

    b. Injection of the drug is not too rapid (greater than 10 seconds)

    c. Only a concentrated solution (4% or greater) is used

    d. None of the above are correct

24. Effects that halothane may have on the body include:

    a. Vasodilation

    b. Increased salivation

    c. Sensitization of myocardium to catecholamines

    d. Depression of myocardial cells

    e. Respiratory depression

25. Effects that barbiturates may have on the body include:

    a. Reduction of respiratory rate

    b. Tachycardia

    c. Cardiac dysrhythmias

    d. Decreased blood pressure

26. The concentration of barbiturate entering the brain is affected by a variety of factors such as:

    a. Perfusion of the brain

    b. Lipid solubility of the drug

    c. Plasma protein levels

    d. Blood pH of the animal

27. Effects that are commonly seen after administration of a phencyclidine drug include:

    a. Increased blood pressure

    b. Increased heart rate

    c. Increased CSF pressure

    d. Increased ocular pressure

28. Effects that isoflurane may have on the body include:

    a. Hepatic toxicity

    b. Accumulation in body fat stores

    c. Depression of respiration

    d. Convulsions during recovery

29. The phencyclidine derivative drugs may cause excitement and seizure-like activity during recovery, which may be precipitated by:

    a. Light

    b. Sound

    c. Touch

    d. Administration of diazepam

30. The rapid induction that occurs with halothane or isoflurane is the result of the:

    a. Low solubility coefficient

    b. Steep concentration gradient between the alveolus and the blood

    c. Presence of a fluoride ion

    d. High vapor pressure

31. MAC will vary with:

    a. Temperature of the patient

    b. Age of the patient

    c. Species

    d. Anesthetic agent

32. Factors that may affect the speed of the induction process with a volatile gaseous anesthetic include:
   a. Solubility coefficient of the agent
   b. Concentration of the agent
   c. MAC of the agent
   d. Concurrent use of atropine

33. Nitrous oxide may be included as part of an anesthetic protocol because it:
   a. Has good analgesic properties
   b. Will reduce the amount of volatile anesthetic needed
   c. Has minimal depressant effects on the respiratory or cardiovascular centers
   d. Can replace oxygen in the anesthetic circuit

34. When pentobarbital sodium is used as an anesthetic, which of the following may be noted:
   a. Relatively slow onset of action
   b. Respiratory depression
   c. Poor analgesia
   d. Slow recovery
   e. Easily reversed

35. Which of the following drugs may be safely given IM or IV in a cat?
   a. Thiopental sodium
   b. Telazol
   c. Ketamine hydrochloride
   d. Methohexital sodium

36. Effects that methoxyflurane may have on the body include:
   a. Depression of myocardial cells
   b. Decreased heart rate
   c. Decreased blood pressure
   d. Respiratory depression

ANSWERS FOR CHAPTER 3

1. a   **2.** True   **3.** c   **4.** True   **5.** False   **6.** a   **7.** True   **8.** True   **9.** True
10. c   **11.** c   **12.** d   **13.** c   **14.** True   **15.** False   **16.** True   **17.** False
18. c   **19.** a   **20.** d   **21.** c   **22.** a   **23.** a, b   **24.** a, c, d, e   **25.** a, c, d
26. a, b, c, d   **27.** a, b, c, d   **28.** c   **29.** a, b, c   **30.** a, b   **31.** a, b, c, d
32. a, b   **33.** a, b, c   **34.** a, b, c, d   **35.** b, c   **36.** a, b, c, d

SELECTED READINGS

Haskins SC: *Opinions in small animal anesthesia,* Philadelphia, 1992, Vet Clin North Am (Small Anim Pract) 22(2), WB Saunders.

McKelvey D: Halothane, isoflurane, and methoxyflurane: physical properties and pharmacology, *Vet Tech* 12(1):21-28, 1991.

Muir WW III, Hubbell JAE: *Handbook of veterinary anesthesia,* St Louis, 1989, Mosby.

Paddleford RR: *Manual of small animal anesthesia,* New York, 1988, Churchill Livingstone.

Short CE: *Principles and practice of veterinary anesthesia,* Baltimore, 1987, Williams & Wilkins.

Steffey EP, Woliner MU, Howland D: Accuracy of isoflurane delivery by halothane-specific vaporizers, *Am J Vet Res* 44(6):1072-1078, 1983.

Warren RG: *Small animal anesthesia,* St Louis, 1983, Mosby.

Weaver BMQ, Raptopoulos D: Induction of anesthesia in dogs and cats with propofol, *Vet Record* 23:617-620, 1990.

Anesthetic equipment

4

PERFORMANCE OBJECTIVES
After completion of this chapter, the reader will be able to:

Identify equipment that is used for the induction and maintenance of general anesthesia in the dog or cat.

Differentiate among the various types of endotracheal tubes and list the advantages and disadvantages of each.

List the advantages and disadvantages of cuffed versus noncuffed tubes.

Describe the functions and components of an anesthetic machine.

Trace the flow of a carrier gas, such as oxygen, through an anesthetic machine and patient breathing circuit.

State the difference between a rebreathing and a nonrebreathing system with regard to equipment, air flow pattern, and indications for use.

Understand the advantages and disadvantages of both rebreathing and nonrebreathing systems.

Differentiate between a precision and nonprecision vaporizer, and recognize the advantages and disadvantages of each.

Understand the importance of flow rates as they relate to anesthetic concentration within the breathing circuit, type of circuit created (closed vs. open), safety for the patient, and waste gas production.

Explain the procedure that should be followed in preparing an anesthetic machine for use.

Describe the proper maintenance procedures for anesthetic machines and associated equipment.

Before the introduction of anesthetic machines, administration of anesthesia was a relatively hazardous undertaking. Anesthetic liquids, such as ether or chloroform, were poured onto a cloth, which was held over the patient's nose and mouth until the patient achieved the desired depth of anesthesia. Alternatively, the patient was sometimes required to inhale vapors rising from a jar of liquid anesthetic. The development of modern anesthetic equipment allowed anesthetists to administer precise amounts of anesthetic under controlled circumstances, greatly increasing the safety and convenience of inhalation anesthesia.

This chapter describes the function and use of anesthetic equipment, as well as maintenance procedures that are likely to be the responsibility of the veterinary technician in practice.

EQUIPMENT NEEDED FOR ANESTHESIA

Useful equipment for routine intravenous (IV) induction and inhalation anesthesia includes the following:
- Syringes and needles for administering preanesthetic and induction agents
- Alcohol and absorbent cotton
- Plain (nonstretch) gauze for tying endotracheal tube
- Syringe for inflating endotracheal tube cuff
- Laryngoscope
- Endotracheal tube
- Stylet for small endotracheal tubes
- Electric clipper
- Intravenous catheter, administration set, and IV fluid bag
- Lubricating gel for endotracheal tubes (gel containing a local analgesic may be preferred for use in cats)
- Lidocaine spray (for use in cats)
- Ophthalmic ointment or drops
- Face mask
- Inhalation anesthesia machine with oxygen (O_2) and nitrous oxide (N_2O) tanks

- Machine connections, including hoses, Y piece, nonrebreathing circuit
- Reservoir bag
- Cylinder wrench
- Ventilator (if controlled ventilation is required)
- Emergency drugs (contained in crash kit)
- Towels, blankets, or other means of conserving patient's body heat
- Stethoscope, thermometer, penlight, and other monitoring devices
- Scavenging system
- Form for anesthesia record (if required)

Of the many types of equipment listed above, only two will be discussed in detail in this chapter: endotracheal tubes and the anesthetic machine.

ENDOTRACHEAL TUBES

Many types of endotracheal tubes are available for veterinary anesthesia. Tubes used in small animal practice are usually made of rubber, vinyl plastic, or silicone rubber.

Rubber endotracheal tubes (red in color) are relatively inexpensive and common in veterinary practice. The technician should be aware of some potential problems associated with their use.

- Rubber tubes may absorb disinfectant solutions, causing the outer surface of the tube to become dry and cracked after prolonged use.
- Rubber tubes are extremely flexible, and kinking or collapse of the tube is a potential hazard, particularly for small tubes. Specialized rubber tubes, called spiral or anode tubes, contain a coil of metal or nylon embedded in the rubber. These tubes are flexible but resist kinking or collapse from external pressure.

Tubes made of transparent *vinyl plastic* are also used commonly in veterinary anesthesia. These tubes are less porous than rubber and resist cracking. However, since they are less flexible than rubber, they tend to become stiff with age.

Silicone rubber tubes, although expensive, are well suited to veterinary anesthesia. They are smooth, flexible, nonporous, and less irritating to tissues than either rubber or vinyl plastic tubes.

Whether manufactured from rubber, silicone rubber, or vinyl plastic, endotracheal tubes are available in several shapes and sizes. Two types of tubes are used in veterinary practice, the Murphy tube and the Magill tube. Both have a beveled (slanted) end, but they differ in that the Murphy tube has an eye near the bevel, whereas the Magill tube does not (Fig. 4-1). The eye helps prevent complete obstruction of the tube if the bevel is plugged by mucus or the tracheal wall.

Unfortunately, several different systems of size classification have been used in the past, which has led to confusion when selecting tubes (Table 4-1). The classification used most commonly is based on the internal diameter of the tube, as

Murphy eye

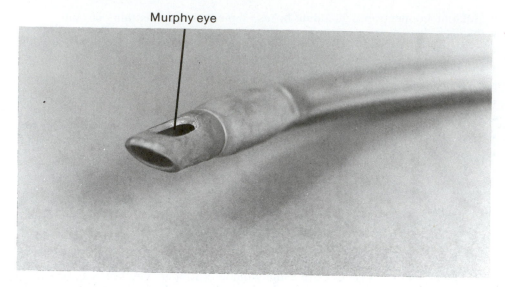

Fig. 4-1. Close-up of a Murphy endotracheal tube, showing eye. (From Warren RG: *Small animal anesthesia,* St Louis, 1983, Mosby.)

TABLE 4-1

A comparison of three systems used to classify endotracheal tubes

Magill scale	French scale	Internal diameter scale (mm)
00	13	4
0	16	5
	18	
1	20	
2	22	6
3	24	7
4	26	8
5	28	
6		9
7	30	10
8	32	11
9	34	12
10	36	

Modified from Warren RG: *Small animal anesthesia,* St Louis, 1989, Mosby.

expressed in millimeters. The internal diameter of each tube is written on its surface (Fig. 4-2). Endotracheal tubes ranging from 5 to 18 mm are suitable for use in dogs (Table 4-2). The endotracheal tubes used most commonly in cats are those with internal diameters of 3.0, 3.5, 4.0, and 4.5 mm. Very small animals may be more easily intubated with a special type of tube called a Cole catheter.

Tubes may be labeled *oral* or *nasal* according to their intended use in humans; however, endotracheal tubes are almost always passed orally in small animals to avoid damage to the sensitive nasal turbinates (the scroll-shaped passages within the nose).

Endotracheal tubes may be obtained with or without cuffs. By inflating a cuff with air, the anesthetist can obtain an airtight seal between the endotracheal tube and the trachea. The use of cuffed tubes offers three advantages over tubes without cuffs:

1. The airtight cuff helps prevent leakage of waste gas around the tube and therefore reduces operating room pollution.
2. Use of cuffed tubes reduces the risk of aspiration of blood, saliva, vomitus, and other material into the lungs.
3. Animals intubated with cuffed tubes are prevented from breathing room air, which may otherwise enter the breathing passages by flowing around the outside of the tube. Animals breathing significant amounts of room air are difficult to maintain at adequate anesthetic depth, since room air dilutes the anesthetic vapor.

Despite these advantages, cuffed tubes should be used with caution, especially in small patients. The cuff of the tube may exert significant pressure on the tracheal

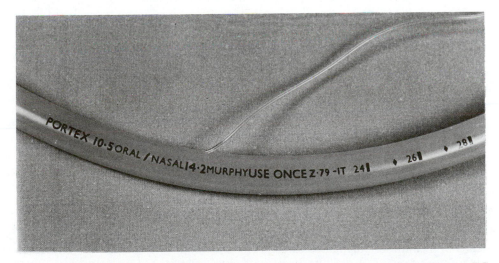

Fig. 4-2. Detail of endotracheal tube with internal diameter of 10.5 mm. (From Warren RG: *Small animal anesthesia,* St Louis, 1983, Mosby.)

TABLE 4-2

Guide for selection of veterinary endotracheal tubes according to body weight

Body weight (kg)	Internal diameter (mm)
Cats	
1	3
3	4
5	4.5
Dogs	
2	5
4	6
7	7
9	7-8
12	8
14	9-10
16-20	10-11
30	12
40	14-16

Modified from Warren RG: *Small animal anesthesia,* St Louis, 1989, Mosby.

mucosa and cause local necrosis, particularly after prolonged use. Low volume/ high pressure cuffs are of particular concern, because they exert more pressure on the tracheal mucosa than do high volume/low pressure cuffs.

The use of endotracheal tubes is outlined in detail in Chapter 2.

ANESTHETIC MACHINES

Function

The anesthetic machine (Fig. 4-3) is designed to deliver a volatile gaseous anesthetic (usually halothane, isoflurane, or methoxyflurane) to and from a patient, by means of a circuit of corrugated tubing. The anesthetic is contained within a carrier gas, which is either oxygen alone or oxygen in combination with nitrous oxide.

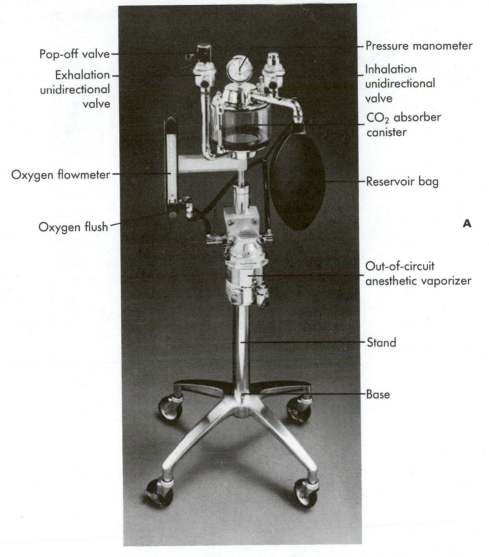

Pop-off valve

Exhalation unidirectional valve

Oxygen flowmeter

Oxygen flush

Pressure manometer

Inhalation unidirectional valve

CO_2 absorber canister

Reservoir bag

A

Out-of-circuit anesthetic vaporizer

Stand

Base

Fig. 4-3. **A,** Basic inhalation anesthesia machine with an out-of-circuit precision vaporizer. (**A, B,** and **C** from Warren RG: *Small animal anesthesia*, St Louis, 1983, Mosby.)

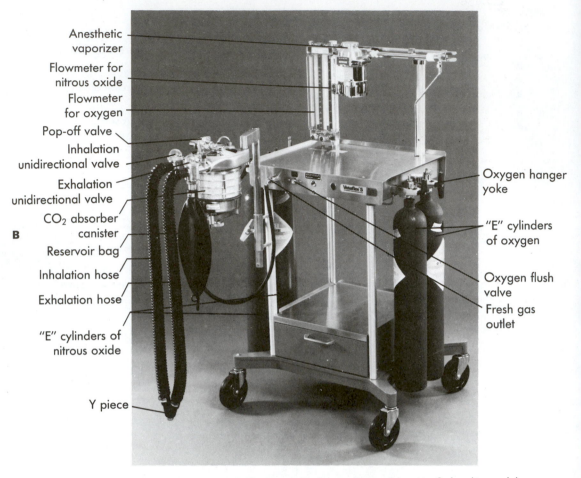

Anesthetic vaporizer

Flowmeter for nitrous oxide

Flowmeter for oxygen

Pop-off valve

Inhalation unidirectional valve

Exhalation unidirectional valve

CO_2 absorber canister

Reservoir bag

Inhalation hose

Exhalation hose

"E" cylinders of nitrous oxide

Y piece

B

Oxygen hanger yoke

"E" cylinders of oxygen

Oxygen flush valve

Fresh gas outlet

Fig. 4-3, cont'd. **B,** Two-gas inhalation anesthesia machine with out-of-circuit precision vaporizer for methoxyflurane.

To achieve this result, the anesthetic machine must perform several important functions:

- It must deliver oxygen (with or without nitrous oxide) at a controlled flow rate.
- It must vaporize a designated concentration of liquid anesthetic (isoflurane, halo-thane, or methoxyflurane), mix it with oxygen (and nitrous oxide, if used), and deliver the resulting mixture to the patient.
- It must move exhaled gases away from the patient and either dispose of them through a scavenging system or recirculate them to the patient. If the gases are reused, the machine must remove carbon dioxide from them before returning them to the patient.

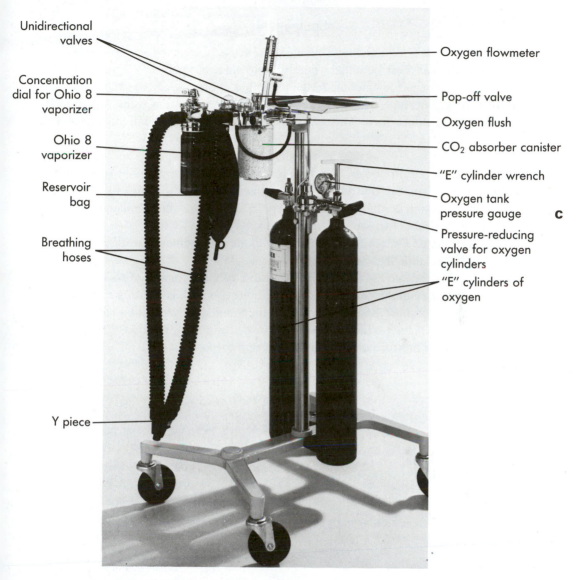

Unidirectional valves

Concentration dial for Ohio 8 vaporizer

Ohio 8 vaporizer

Reservoir bag

Breathing hoses

Y piece

Oxygen flowmeter

Pop-off valve

Oxygen flush

CO_2 absorber canister

"E" cylinder wrench

Oxygen tank pressure gauge

Pressure-reducing valve for oxygen cylinders

"E" cylinders of oxygen

C

Fig. 4-3, cont'd.   C, Inhalation anesthesia machine with an Ohio No.8 glass jar vaporizer for methoxyflurane.

Anesthetic machines are used not only for inhalation anesthesia, but also as a means of delivering oxygen to critical patients. In these situations, the machine is used with the vaporizer (anesthetic source) turned off, and the hoses are connected to a mask held over the patient's face (or to an endotracheal tube, if the patient has been intubated).

Components

The components of an anesthetic machine and the way in which an anesthetic machine works can best be understood by following the path of oxygen from the oxygen tank, through the machine to the patient, and back to the machine. For the sake of clarity, one type of anesthetic setup (the circle system using a precision vaporizer) will be described. This system is illustrated schematically in Fig. 4-4.

Gas cylinders

Oxygen must be continuously supplied to every patient throughout anesthesia. Anesthetic machines provide up to 100% oxygen, which is significantly different from room air, which contains approximately 20% oxygen. The high concentration of oxygen is desirable for two reasons:

1. The anesthetized patient has a higher metabolic requirement for oxygen than a normal awake animal.
2. The anesthetized patient has a reduced tidal volume compared to the awake animal, and the amount of air taken in with each breath is therefore smaller.

The combination of increased oxygen requirement and decreased tidal volume may result in hypoxia if high concentrations of oxygen are not provided, using either 100% oxygen or a mixture of oxygen and nitrous oxide.

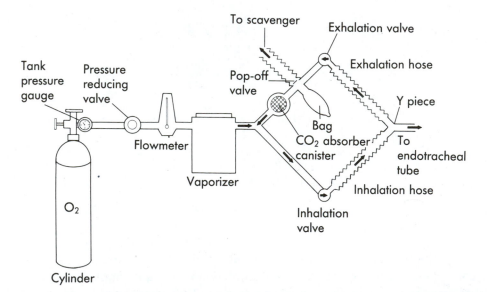

Fig. 4-4. Schematic of anesthetic machine (circle system, vaporizer in circle). (Redrawn from Hartsfield SN: Machines and breathing systems for administration of inhalation anesthetics. In Short CE (editor): *Principles and practice of veterinary anesthesia*, Baltimore, 1987, Williams & Wilkins.)

Oxygen flow from the machine to the patient not only meets the metabolic requirements of the animal but also carries the anesthetic to the patient. Anesthetic machines are designed such that no liquid anesthetic can be delivered to the patient unless oxygen is present to act as a carrier gas.

Oxygen used for anesthesia is obtained as a compressed gas, contained in metal cylinders. The gas is held under pressure in the cylinder (also called a *tank*) in order that a large amount of gas may be stored in a relatively small container. These cylinders may be small, in which case they are usually attached to the anesthetic machine (E cylinders, illustrated in Fig. 4-3). Large cylinders are also available, which stand separately from the machine (Fig. 4-5). The capacities of several types of cylinders are given in Table 4-3.

Oxygen flow into the machine occurs when the outlet valve on the top of the gas cylinder is opened in a counterclockwise direction (to the left). The flow is discontinued when the valve is turned completely to the right. The mnemonic "left loose, right tight" has been used by several generations of anesthesia students as an aid to remembering these facts.

Many anesthetic machines are designed to provide not only oxygen, but also nitrous oxide gas. Like oxygen, nitrous oxide (N_2O) is contained in a compressed gas cylinder, which may be a large freestanding tank or a smaller tank attached to the machine. Some machines have a device that discontinues nitrous oxide administration to the patient if the oxygen flow is cut off. This mechanism prevents inadvertent asphyxiation of the patient, which could occur if the patient breathed nitrous oxide in the absence of oxygen.

Gas cylinders that are part of the anesthetic machine are attached to it by a yoke (Fig. 4-6), whereas freestanding cylinders are connected to the machine by gas lines. Gas lines may take the form of flexible cords, or gas may be carried in pipes mounted within a wall.

Anesthetic machines are designed such that it is difficult or impossible to attach the wrong type of gas cylinder to the machine connections. The yokes for each gas are designed with a pin system such that an oxygen cylinder, for example, cannot be put on a nitrous oxide yoke (Fig. 4-6). In addition, cylinders and gas lines are color-coded to prevent inadvertent delivery of an incorrect gas. Oxygen cylinders are white, or green with a white shoulder, and nitrous oxide cylinders are blue (Table 4-4).

Cylinders are designed to store large quantities of gas under pressure. The volume (in liters) of gas present in any E cylinder can be calculated by multiplying the pressure (in pounds per square inch [psi]) by 0.3. For oxygen in a full cylinder, the pressure may be 15,000 kilopascals (kPa) (2200 psi), indicating that 660 liters of oxygen gas (0.3 × 2200 psi) is contained in the tank. A reading of 7500 kPa (1100 psi) indicates the tank is approximately half full and therefore contains approximately 330 liters of oxygen. If the anesthetist selects an oxygen flow rate of one liter

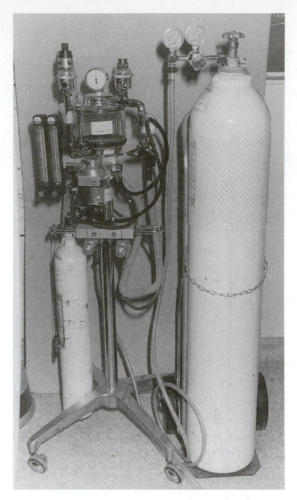

Fig. 4-5. Large cylinder connected to anesthetic machine.

TABLE 4-3

Capacity of compressed gas cylinders

Cylinder dimensions	Empty weight (kg)	Capacity (liters of oxygen)	Capacity (liters of nitrous oxide)
E Cylinder 4.25 inches OD* × 26 inches	5.9	660	1590
G Cylinder 8.5 inches OD × 51 inches	50	5331	13,836
H Cylinder 9.25 inches OD × 51 inches	59	5570-7500	15,899

* Outside diameter.
Modified from Warren RG: *Small animal anesthesia,* St Louis, 1989, Mosby.

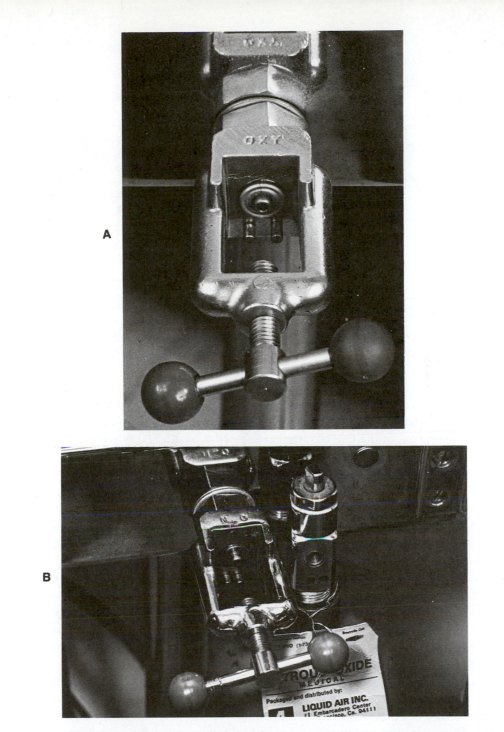

Fig. 4-6. Yokes, showing pin indexing. **A,** Pins for oxygen tank. **B,** Pins for nitrous oxide tank. (From Warren RG: *Small animal anesthesia*, St Louis, 1983, Mosby.)

TABLE 4-4
Characteristics of compressed gas cylinders

Gas	Formula	International color	Full tank pressure kPa/(psi) @ 21° C	Pressure kPa (psi) at which tank should be changed	State within cylinder
Oxygen	O_2	White (Green-USA)	15,000-18,000 (2200-2650)	680-1360 (100-200)	Gas
Nitrous oxide	N_2O	Blue	5170 (770)	Below 3400 (500)	Liquid/gas

Modified from Warren RG, *Small animal anesthesia,* St Louis, 1989, Mosby.

per minute, a full E tank will last approximately 11 hours (660 minutes), and a half-full tank will last approximately $5\frac{1}{2}$ hours (330 minutes).

The pressure of oxygen being delivered by any given tank is indicated by a pressure gauge attached to the cylinder (Fig. 4-7, *A* and *B*). The pressure gauge will read zero when the tank is empty. It also reads zero when the tank is turned off and the remaining gas in the line has been evacuated ("bled off"). When the tank valve is opened (i.e., the tank is turned on), the gauge reading rises to indicate the pressure of gas remaining in the tank. During use, oxygen is gradually released from the tank, and the pressure within the tank and therefore the reading on the pressure gauge will fall. The anesthetist may notice a considerable drop in indicated pressure during a lengthy anesthesia. The anesthetist must, of course, periodically monitor the oxygen tank pressure gauge during each procedure and change the tank when the value indicates the tank is close to empty. Because of the gradual way in which oxygen tank pressure falls, the anesthetist can rely on the gauge to roughly indicate the amount of oxygen remaining, and usually it is not necessary to change oxygen tanks until the pressure drops below 680 to 1360 kPa (100 to 200 psi), indicating only 30 to 60 liters of oxygen remaining in the tank.

Nitrous oxide is also stored in compressed air tanks, although at considerably less pressure than oxygen. The normal pressure for a full nitrous oxide tank is 5170 kPa (770 psi). Unlike oxygen, nitrous oxide exists in both the liquid and gas states in the pressurized tank. The pressure gauge reads only the pressure of the gas within the tank and not that of the liquid. As the gas leaves the tank, more liquid evaporates and enters the gas state. As a result, the pressure of the gas within the tank will not change until all of the liquid has evaporated. The anesthetist therefore should not expect the nitrous oxide tank gauge reading to change even after several hours of anesthesia, unless the tank is close to empty. It follows that the pressure

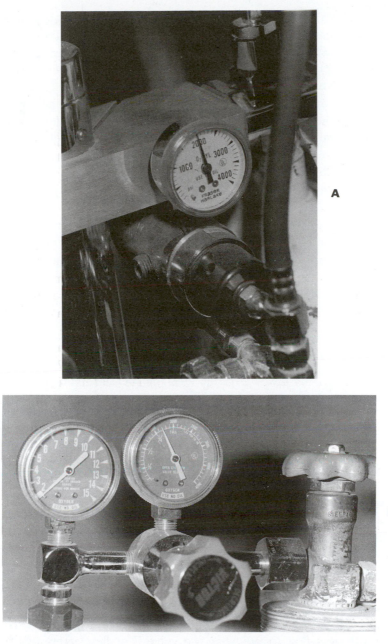

Fig. 4-7. Tank pressure gauges. **A,** Tank pressure gauge for E tank attached to anesthetic machine. **B,** Flowmeter (*left*) and tank pressure gauge (*right*) for freestanding oxygen tank.

gauge reading on a nitrous oxide tank will not tell the anesthetist how full the tank is, and this information can only be determined by weighing the tank before use. An "E" cylinder of nitrous oxide will weigh approximately 8 kg (18 lb) when full and about 5.9 kg (13 lb) when empty. (The full and empty weights are normally stamped on the outside of each cylinder.)

Usually, the anesthetist is not concerned with the exact amount of nitrous oxide present in the tank, but must be aware when the tank is close to empty and a tank change is required. Because liquid nitrous oxide is continually evaporating and maintaining the pressure of gas in the tank, the gauge reading does not fall until the liquid nitrous oxide is exhausted and the tank is nearly empty. Therefore, nitrous oxide tanks should be changed when the pressure gauge starts to drop below 3400 kPa (500 psi).

As a gas moves from a high pressure tank into the anesthetic machine, the pressure is lowered by a pressure-reducing valve, also called a pressure regulator. The use of a pressure-reducing valve allows a constant flow of gas into the machine regardless of the pressure changes within the tank and provides a safe operating pressure for the machine. Oxygen leaving a tank at a pressure of up to 15,000 kPa (2200 psi) is reduced to a pressure of 340 kPa (50 psi) before entering the anesthetic machine.

Flowmeters

From the cylinder, the pressure gauge, and the pressure-reducing valve, oxygen travels through a low pressure hose to a flowmeter (see Figs. 4-3 and 4-4). The flowmeter allows the anesthetist to set the gas flow rate, which is the amount of oxygen that travels through the machine to be delivered to the patient. Flow rates are expressed in liters of gas per minute (L/minute). If a machine is set up to use both nitrous oxide and oxygen, it is necessary to have separate flowmeters, so that the flow rates of the two gases can be monitored and adjusted separately. Some newer machines provide two flowmeters for oxygen: one for flow rates greater than 1 L/minute and one to accurately adjust flow rates less than 1 L/minute.

Each flowmeter consists of a dial attached to a glass cylinder of graduated diameter. Within the cylinder is a rotor or ball, which indicates the gas flow rate (either oxygen or nitrous oxide) on a scale that measures liters of gas per minute. Each gas enters the bottom of its respective flowmeter and exits at the top. When the dial is turned, a valve within the flowmeter opens and gas enters the cylinder. The ball or rotor rises, indicating the amount of gas flow. The anesthetist therefore can control the gas flow by adjusting the valve. For flowmeters that have a ball indicator, the center of the ball should be read to determine the flow rate. In the case of a rotor indicator, the reading should be taken at the top of the rotor.

It is the flowmeter, rather than the tank pressure gauge, that indicates the amount of oxygen or nitrous oxide being delivered to the patient. When the anesthetist opens the oxygen tank, the tank pressure gauge will indicate the pressure of gas being released from the tank; however, this does not necessarily mean that the patient receives any oxygen. Oxygen flow through the machine is indicated by the flowmeter. If it is set at zero flow, the patient does not receive any oxygen.

The flowmeters allow the anesthetist to accurately control the relative amounts of oxygen and nitrous oxide received by the animal. If the nitrous oxide flowmeter is set to deliver 2 L/minute of nitrous oxide to the patient and the oxygen flowmeter is adjusted to deliver 1 L/minute of oxygen to the patient, the resulting mixture will be a 2:1 ratio of nitrous oxide to oxygen. (This represents approximately 67% nitrous oxide and 33% oxygen.) Some machines automatically set the O_2 and N_2O proportions, and an adjustment of the flow rate of one gas will automatically change the flow rate of the other.

When using nitrous oxide, the anesthetist should ensure that the nitrous oxide:oxygen ratio never exceeds 3:1, or the patient will receive insufficient oxygen and asphyxiation may result. As mentioned in Chapter 3, it is also imperative that a minimum of 30 ml/kg/minute of oxygen flow be delivered throughout anesthesia to any patient receiving a mixture of nitrous oxide and oxygen.

As oxygen or nitrous oxide passes through the flowmeter, the gas pressure is further reduced, from 340 kPa (50 psi) to 100 kPa (15 psi). This pressure is only slightly above atmospheric pressure and is the optimum pressure for passage of gas to the patient.

Vaporizer

Oxygen gas exits at the top of the oxygen flowmeter and continues through a low pressure hose to the vaporizer (see Figs. 4-3 and 4-4). The function of the vaporizer is to convert a liquid anesthetic such as halothane or isoflurane to a gas state and to add controlled amounts of the vaporized anesthetic to the carrier gases (O_2 and N_2O) flowing through the machine. The vaporized anesthetic can only be released from the vaporizer by dialing a flow of carrier gas, which moves the anesthetic from the vaporizer into the breathing circuit of the anesthetic machine. No anesthetic is delivered to the patient if the flowmeters read zero, as there is no flow of carrier gases into the vaporizer. Anesthetic vaporizers are further discussed in a separate section of this chapter.

Fresh gas inlet

After passing through the vaporizer, oxygen (and nitrous oxide, if used) carrying the vaporized anesthetic enters a low pressure hose. The anesthetic machine is constructed such that this mixture of gases, commonly known as *fresh gas*, is not able to return to the vaporizer, but will be confined to a series of machine parts arranged in a roughly circular design. These machine parts, consisting of the flutter valves, hoses, CO_2 absorber canister, pop-off valve, and reservoir bag, together make up the anesthetic circuit.

Once fresh gas enters the anesthetic circuit, there are a variety of flow paths, depending on the type of machine used. Most commonly, fresh gas passes first through either the reservoir bag or the inhalation flutter valve.

Reservoir (rebreathing) bag

Fresh gas entering the circuit is conveyed to an inflatable rubber bag called the reservoir bag or rebreathing bag (see Figs. 4-3 and 4-4). This bag gradually fills as gases enter the circuit and is deflated when the patient breathes in. The bag therefore expands and contracts continuously, reflecting the patient's respirations.

The reservoir bag should have a minimum volume of 60 ml/kg of patient weight. Bags are available in various sizes, from 500 ml (for very small patients) to 30 liters (intended for use in horses). The most common sizes used for small animal anesthesia are 1 liter and 2 liters.

The reservoir bag serves a number of functions in addition to storing gas:

• It is easier for a patient to breathe from a reservoir bag than to rely solely on a continuous flow of air through a piece of tubing.

• The bag allows the anesthetist to observe the animal's respiration. Both the respiratory rate and the depth of respirations are indicated by the movement of the bag. Inadequate movement of the bag may indicate that the patient is breathing room air. Often this occurs because the endotracheal tube is too small or the cuff is inadequately inflated and air is passing around the tube. Alternatively, minimal movement of the reservoir bag may indicate that the patient's tidal volume is small, alerting the anesthetist to possible respiratory problems.

• Movement of the bag with the animal's respirations indicates to the anesthetist that the endotracheal tube is within the trachea (and not the esophagus) and therefore is a useful check on the location of the endotracheal tube.

• The reservoir bag allows the anesthetist to deliver oxygen (with or without anesthetic) to the patient by means of "bagging." In this procedure the reservoir bag is gently squeezed, forcing oxygen and anesthetic into the patient's lungs and causing the patient's chest to rise slightly. It is advisable to periodically "bag" an anesthetized patient in order to gently inflate the lungs with fresh oxygen and anesthetic.

There are three reasons that bagging may be beneficial to the anesthetized patient:

1. Bagging helps prevent a condition called *atelectasis,* in which the alveoli in certain sections of the lungs are collapsed and not useful for oxygen and anesthetic transfer to the patient. Bagging the patient helps reinflate the collapsed alveoli.

2. Anesthetized patients have a decreased ability to breathe, and the volume of air

inhaled with each breath may be as little as 50% of normal. By bagging the animal, the anesthetist flushes the airways and alveoli with fresh gas, removing air that has increased CO_2 content and reduced anesthetic and oxygen concentration.

3. Bagging may be a lifesaving procedure if the patient is not breathing (a condition called respiratory arrest). Bagging allows the anesthetist to continue to deliver oxygen directly to the lungs and therefore acts as an effective means of artificial respiration.

The anesthetist should ensure that the reservoir bag is properly inflated during anesthesia. The bag should not be allowed to overfill (assuming the appearance of an inflated beach ball), as this will add pressure to the breathing circuit and make it difficult for the animal to exhale. Additionally, it is difficult to monitor respiration using an overfull bag. There is also some risk that the excessive pressure may rupture alveoli in the patient's lungs. On the other hand, the bag should not be allowed to empty completely when the animal inhales, as this defeats its purpose, which is to act as a reservoir. Complete emptying of the bag indicates that the amount of gas flow is inadequate or the pop-off valve is open too widely.

Inhalation flutter valve, hoses, Y piece, and exhalation flutter valve

Fresh gas entering the anesthetic circuit passes through a one-way valve, variously called an inhalation flutter valve or unidirectional valve (see Figs. 4-3 and 4-4). The inhalation flutter valve allows gases to flow in only one direction, in this case, toward the patient.

When the patient inhales, the inhalation flutter valve opens, allowing the oxygen and anesthetic to enter the hoses. The gases travel through the inspiratory hose to the Y piece and are directed into the endotracheal tube or mask. Upon reaching the patient's lungs, oxygen and anesthetic molecules are absorbed and enter the bloodstream. At the same time, carbon dioxide and anesthetic molecules are released from the bloodstream, enter the alveoli, and are exhaled on the next breath.

Exhaled gases leave the patient and travel through another hose to reenter the anesthetic machine. At the point at which the exhalation hose attaches to the machine, there is another flutter valve, commonly called the exhalation valve or expiratory unidirectional valve (see Figs. 4-3 and 4-4). As with the inhalation valve, this valve controls the direction of gas flow and only allows gases travelling back into the anesthetic machine to pass through. It is important that gas can only flow in one direction through the circuit, to prevent expired gases from returning to the patient without first passing through the CO_2 absorber canister.

Oxygen flush valve

Many anesthetic machines have a valve marked ''oxygen flush.'' This valve, if depressed, allows oxygen to bypass the flowmeter and vaporizer and enter the machine between the flutter valves, often at the carbon dioxide absorber. Pure oxygen is thereby delivered directly to the anesthetic circuit at a flow rate of 30 to 50 L/minute. This feature is particularly useful when delivering oxygen to a critical patient and also can be used to rapidly fill a depleted reservoir bag. It is also useful at the end of the anesthetic period, when the oxygen flush allows the anesthetist to add pure oxygen to the system, thereby diluting residual anesthetic being exhaled by the animal. The oxygen flush should not be used with certain nonrebreathing systems (such as the Bain system) because a high flow rate of oxygen into this type of circuit can seriously damage an animal's lungs.

Pop-off valve

Almost all anesthetic machine circuits contain a pressure relief valve, usually in the form of a pop-off valve or overflow valve (see Figs. 4-3 and 4-4). This valve is similar to a tap in that it can be turned fully open, partly open, or closed off entirely, allowing varying amounts of gas to exit. The pop-off valve is usually kept partly open during anesthesia, allowing some gas escape. It is closed or nearly closed when the anesthetist wishes to bag the patient or when very low gas flows are used.

The pop-off valve has several uses:

- Waste gases (oxygen, nitrous oxide, inhalation anesthetic, and carbon dioxide) exit from the anesthetic circuit at this valve and enter the scavenging system.
- By venting excess gas, the pop-off valve prevents the buildup of excessive pressure or volume of gases within the circuit. If this was allowed to occur, the excess pressure would eventually reach the animal's lungs, causing the alveoli to distend and possibly rupture.
- If the pop-off valve is closed, the anesthetist can increase the pressure of gas present in the circuit, allowing the animal to be bagged.

Carbon dioxide absorber canister

Any gases that do not exit from the system through the pop-off valve are directed to the carbon dioxide absorber canister before being returned to the patient (see Figs. 4-3 and 4-4). Gas may enter the canister through the bottom or the top, depending on the design. The canister contains an absorbing chemical, either soda lime or barium hydroxide lime. In both cases, the absorbing ingredient is calcium hydroxide, $Ca(OH)_2$, which removes carbon dioxide from the gases that percolate through the canister. The chemical reaction that takes place within the canister is as follows:

$$2\ CO_2 + Ca(OH)_2 + 2\ NaOH \rightarrow Na_2CO_3 + CaCO_3 + 2\ H_2O + heat$$

The heat released by this reaction is sufficient to raise the temperature of the carbon dioxide absorber canister, and it may become warm to the touch during operation. The water that is produced by this reaction is captured in a trap that lies immediately below the absorbing granules.

Soda lime and barium hydroxide lime granules do not last indefinitely: after several hours of use the granules become exhausted and will no longer absorb carbon dioxide molecules. Use of depleted granules is inadvisable, as it may result in the delivery of excessive amounts of carbon dioxide to the patient, leading to hypercarbia. There are several ways in which the anesthetist may become aware that the granules are exhausted and must be replaced:

- Fresh granules, containing mainly $Ca(OH)_2$, can be chipped or crumbled with finger pressure, whereas granules saturated with carbon dioxide (containing mainly $CaCO_3$) become hard and brittle. This test can be used to determine the saturation of the granules before or after the anesthetic procedure.
- The color of the granules may indicate their degree of saturation. Absorber granules contain a pH indicator that causes the granules to change color when they are saturated with carbon dioxide. The color change that occurs will vary with the type of granules used: some granules become whiter in appearance when exhausted, whereas other granules are normally white or pink and turn blue when exhausted. The color reaction is time-limited, and granules that have changed color (indicating saturation with carbon dioxide) may return to the original color after a few hours, although they are still saturated with carbon dioxide. Thus it is important that the anesthetist remove any granules that have changed color as soon as possible after using an anesthetic machine.

Pressure manometer

Many machines have a pressure gauge (also called a pressure manometer) situated on top of the carbon dioxide absorber canister (Fig. 4-8). This gauge measures the pressure of the gases within the anesthetic system (expressed in centimeters of water or in millimeters of mercury, mm Hg), which, in turn, reflects the pressure of the gas in the animal's airway and lungs. Pressures over 15 cm of water (11 mm Hg) indicate a buildup of air within the machine, either because the pop-off valve is not sufficiently open or the oxygen flow rate is too high.

The pressure manometer is a useful aid when bagging an animal, as it indicates the approximate pressure being exerted on the animal's lungs when the anesthetist squeezes the reservoir bag. The pressure should not exceed 15 to 20 cm of water (11 to 15 mm Hg) during bagging.

Negative pressure relief valve

Some machines have an additional valve, called the negative pressure relief valve. This valve is designed to open and admit room air to the circuit if for some reason a negative pressure (partial vacuum) is detected in the circuit. This may happen when

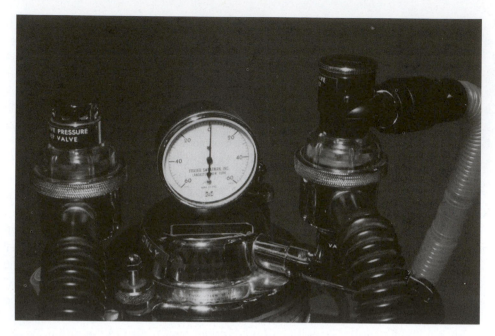

Fig. 4-8. Pressure manometer.

an active scavenging system is attached to the circuit, particularly if excessive suction is present.

Negative pressure may also develop in the circuit if the oxygen tank runs out of oxygen. By adding room air to the circuit, the negative pressure relief valve ensures that the patient always receives some oxygen. It is certainly preferable that the patient receive 21% oxygen in room air rather than none at all, as would otherwise be the case if the machine ran out of oxygen.

Anesthetic breathing systems

The anesthetist operating any anesthetic machine has a number of options regarding its use. The most important decision is the type of breathing system to be used. There are three systems in common use: total rebreathing (closed), partial rebreathing (semiclosed), and nonrebreathing (open). The choice of system to be used is important, since it will determine the following:
• Whether the patient will breathe back in ("rebreathe") the gases that have been exhaled
• Oxygen and nitrous oxide flow rates
• Position of the pop-off valve (closed or open)
• Type of equipment used (e.g., whether a Bain system will be required)

Rebreathing systems

In the system described thus far in this chapter, the gases that exit the carbon dioxide canister are directed into the reservoir bag and back toward the patient through the inhalation flutter valve. At this point, fresh oxygen and anesthetic enter the circuit from the vaporizer. The flow of gas through the anesthetic machine therefore is circular (reservoir bag, inhalation flutter valve, inspiration hose, animal, expiration hose, exhalation flutter valve, carbon dioxide canister, back to the inhalation flutter valve). The machine adapts to the patient's ventilation patterns and maintains a constant flow of gas to the patient through the use of a reservoir bag, pop-off valve, and negative pressure relief valve.

This type of system allows recirculation of exhaled gases to the patient and therefore is called a *rebreathing system*. It is also sometimes referred to as a *circle system*. The patient rebreathes its own exhaled gases, from which carbon dioxide has been removed and a small amount of fresh oxygen and anesthetic are continuously added.

Rebreathing systems are further subdivided into *total rebreathing systems* (also called *closed systems*) and *partial rebreathing systems* (also called *semiclosed systems*). In a closed, total rebreathing system, the oxygen flow rate is relatively low, providing only the oxygen necessary to meet the patient's metabolic requirements. In this type of system, it may be necessary to turn the pop-off valve to the nearly closed position to prevent gases from escaping, particularly if the suction from the scavenger is strong. A total rebreathing system recirculates all of the exhaled gases (with the exception of carbon dioxide, which is removed by the absorber), and only a small amount of fresh oxygen and anesthetic is added to the system. The amount of oxygen used by the patient is closely matched by the amount of oxygen entering the circuit from the vaporizer.

In the semiclosed, partial rebreathing system, the flow rate of fresh oxygen and anesthetic entering the system must be considerably higher than that for the closed, total rebreathing system. The pop-off valve is left partly open, allowing some exhaled gases to escape. Thus, although some of the exhaled gases are recirculated to the patient, much of the exhaled gases exits via the scavenger.

Safety concerns when using a total rebreathing system

Most patients weighing over 7 kg are anesthetized using either a partial or total rebreathing system. Because total rebreathing systems use less oxygen and anesthetic than partial rebreathing systems, total rebreathing systems are more economical. This may be an important consideration if a relatively expensive anesthetic such as isoflurane is used. However, there are serious safety concerns that must be addressed when using a total rebreathing system:

- *Carbon dioxide accumulation.* If the carbon dioxide absorber in a closed system is not operating efficiently, exhaled carbon dioxide will build up within the circuit.

This is less likely to happen in a semiclosed, partial rebreathing system, in which some CO_2 is vented to the scavenger.

- *Increased pressure in the anesthetic circuit.* In a total rebreathing system, the volume of gas in the system may increase as fresh gas enters the circuit, particularly if the pop-off valve is closed. Excessive pressure may build up in the circuit, making it difficult for the animal to exhale. In a partial rebreathing system, the pop-off valve is partly to fully open and excessive gas is vented.
- *Oxygen depletion and nitrous oxide accumulation.* In any anesthetic machine setup, oxygen is gradually depleted as the patient breathes the circulating gas. This is normally compensated by fresh oxygen entering the circuit. In a total rebreathing system, the oxygen flow rate is low and the amount of fresh oxygen added to the circuit may not entirely compensate for this loss. This is particularly serious if nitrous oxide is used in addition to oxygen, because the relative amount of nitrous oxide in the circuit may increase as the amount of oxygen decreases. As a result, the patient may breathe dangerously high levels of nitrous oxide gas. This effect is less likely to occur in a partial rebreathing system, in which nitrous oxide escapes through the pop-off valve and oxygen flow rates are higher. The use of a minimum of 30 ml/kg/minute of oxygen in the presence of nitrous oxide prevents N_2O buildup, but this flow rate is not possible in a total rebreathing system. Total rebreathing (closed) systems therefore are not recommended if nitrous oxide is part of the anesthetic protocol.

For safety reasons, many anesthetists prefer to use a partial rather than a total rebreathing setup, choosing to err on the side of wasting some gas by using higher gas flow rates rather than risking accumulation of carbon dioxide and depletion of oxygen within the circuit. Conversion from a total rebreathing system to a partial rebreathing system can be easily achieved by keeping the pop-off valve at least partially open (except when bagging the patient) and maintaining a higher oxygen flow rate.

If a total rebreathing (closed) system is used, the anesthetist should take the following active steps to ensure patient safety:

- Check the machine for leaks before use. If leaks are present, oxygen may escape from the circuit. This is not normally of critical importance to the patient; however, in a total rebreathing system the oxygen flow rate is low, and any loss of oxygen may be detrimental.
- Empty and refill the reservoir bag with oxygen 2 to 3 times during the first 15 minutes of anesthesia and every 30 minutes thereafter to help prevent patient hypoxia. Alternatively, the anesthetist may provide 5 minutes of high oxygen flow (200 ml/kg/minute) at the start of anesthesia. Thereafter, much lower flow rates (15 ml/kg/minute) can be used.
- Closely monitor the reservoir bag if a total rebreathing system is used. If the bag becomes smaller, either a leak is present in the system, the pop-off valve is open

too much, or the flow rate of oxygen is inadequate. If the bag becomes distended, either the oxygen flow rate should be reduced or the pop-off valve should be opened.

- Very close monitoring of the patient and machine is essential.
- If a rapid change in anesthetic depth is required, convert to a partial rebreathing system by increasing the oxygen flow rate and opening the pop-off valve. Because the oxygen flow rate in a total rebreathing system is low, changes in the vaporizer setting may not affect the concentration of anesthetic in the circuit for several minutes.
- The low oxygen flow rates used in a total rebreathing system may be inadequate for accurate delivery of anesthetic by some vaporizers. Consult the vaporizer manual for minimum recommended flow rates, and be aware that the anesthetic concentration indicated by the dial may be incorrect at lower flows. Total rebreathing systems should not be used at all with certain vaporizers, including the Fluothane Tek-2, Copper kettle, and Vernitrol.

In a total rebreathing system, the vaporizer concentration required may be 1% to 2% higher than that of a partial rebreathing system. (This is the case for an out-of-circle precision vaporizer only.)

Nonrebreathing systems

The total and partial rebreathing systems discussed above are well suited to many patients. However, in some circumstances the anesthetist may prefer to use a different type of anesthetic setup, called a nonrebreathing system. In a nonrebreathing system, little or no exhaled gases are returned to the patient; instead, they are evacuated by a scavenger connected to a pop-off valve or exit port. The characteristics of rebreathing and nonrebreathing systems are compared in Table 4-5.

As with the rebreathing system, the nonrebreathing system can best be understood by following the path of an oxygen molecule from the tank, to the patient, and finally to the scavenger. Just as in a rebreathing system, oxygen (and nitrous oxide gas, if used) flows from the tank, through a flowmeter, and into the vaporizer. At this point, however, gases exiting the vaporizer go directly into a hose for delivery to the patient, bypassing the inhalation flutter valve. Exhaled gases pass through another hose and may enter a reservoir bag, but do not enter a carbon dioxide canister. The gas is then released through a pop-off valve, pressure relief valve, or other mechanism connected to a scavenger. Since most of the gases exit through the scavenger and are not returned to the patient, the system is accurately described as nonrebreathing.

It is evident that several anesthetic machine parts that are used for a rebreathing system are not required in a nonrebreathing system. These include the carbon dioxide canister, the flutter valves, and the pressure manometer.

TABLE 4-5

Comparison of rebreathing and nonrebreathing systems

Parameters	Nonrebreathing	Rebreathing (semiclosed or closed system)
CO_2 absorption	Not required	Must have CO_2 absorber canister
Changes in depth of anesthesia	Quickly	Slowly
Flow rates	High flow rates—must equal or exceed the respiratory minute volume	Low flow rates—only to meet the metabolic oxygen requirement (closed)
Cost of operation	High due to volume of oxygen and anesthetic used	Low, as less oxygen and anesthetic used
Amount of waste gas produced	High	Minimal
Heat and moisture conservation (from exhaled gases)	Poor	Good
Safety to patient	Perhaps safer because depth of anesthesia can be changed more quickly; minimal danger of hypoxia and hypercarbia	Perhaps not as safe because changes in depth of anesthesia occur more slowly; some danger of hypoxia and buildup of CO_2 in circuit especially for closed system
Size of animal	Any size; limited only by the total gas flow that is delivered; generally recommended for animals under 7 kg	Only for animals over 7 kg

Most anesthetic machines are designed to be used as a rebreathing system but may be easily converted to a nonrebreathing system by the use of attachments, such as the Bain system (The Kendall Company, Boston, MA 02161) (Figs. 4-9 and 4-10, *A*), the Ayres T piece, the Mapleson A system (Magill), the Kuhn circuit (Fig. 4-10, *B*), the Norman mask elbow, an anesthetic chamber, or similar equipment. Each of these attachments delivers the fresh gas from the vaporizer to the animal and conducts the expired gases to a scavenger. Most systems have a fresh gas inlet, reservoir bag, tubing, scavenger outlet, and endotracheal tube connection, but differ in the site of fresh gas inflow, the position of the reservoir bag, and the location of the exhalation port. A partial rebreathing system using a conventional anesthetic machine (with a CO_2 absorber canister and flutter valves) can be converted to a nonrebreathing system by using a high oxygen flow rate (200 to 300 ml/kg/minute), which effectively flushes most of the exhaled gases through the pop-off valve.

Because the Bain system is a very commonly used nonrebreathing attachment, it will be discussed in more detail here. Readers are referred to more detailed reference texts or equipment manufacturers for information on other systems. The Bain system consists of an inner tubing (which conducts gas to the patient and corresponds to the inspiratory hose of a rebreathing system) surrounded by a larger, corrugated tubing (which conducts gas away from the patient and corresponds to the expiratory hose in a rebreathing system). The arrangement of the tubing into an inner and outer hose makes the setup less cumbersome and allows the incoming gases to be warmed slightly by the exhaled gases that surround them, before reaching the patient. When using or cleaning a Bain circuit, care must be

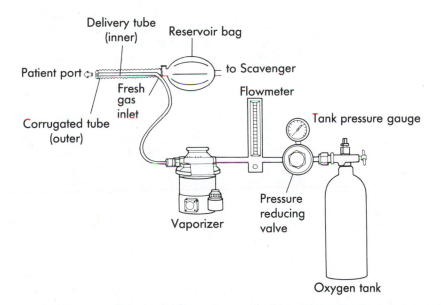

Fig. 4-9. Components of an anesthesia delivery system using a Bain circuit. (Redrawn from Hodgson DS: The case for nonrebreathing circuits for very small animals. In Haskins SC: *Opinions in small animal anesthesia*, Philadelphia, 1992, Vet Clin North Am. (Small Anim Pract) 22(2), WB Saunders.)

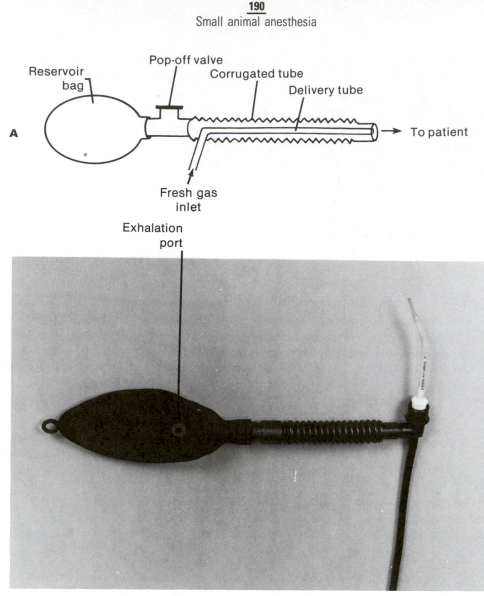

Fig. 4-10. **A,** Schematic of Bain system. **B,** Modified Mapleson E system (Kuhn circuit). Fresh gases enter near the patient end while exhaled gases exit through the hole in the reservoir bag. (Photo does not illustrate scavenger attachment.) (From Warren RG: *Small animal anesthesia,* St Louis, 1983, Mosby.)

taken to ensure that the inner tubing does not detach from the rest of the circuit, or gas will not be delivered to the patient.

Gas from the outer, exhalation tubing enters a reservoir bag. Many Bain circuits are not equipped with an overflow valve or pop-off valve, and it may be necessary to cut the tail of the reservoir bag to allow escape of waste gases. In this case, the tail of the reservoir bag should be connected to the scavenging system to allow proper disposal of the waste gas. It may be necessary to partially clamp the outlet of the reservoir bag with a paper clip or screw clamp, which acts as a pop-off valve and allows the anesthetist to control the rate at which the reservoir bag empties. Alternatively, a Bain mount is available that allows the use of an uncut bag. This mount features a pop-off valve, allowing easy scavenging and bagging.

When using a nonrebreathing system such as the Bain, the oxygen flow rate is normally high (usually at least 130 ml/kg/minute) and a large proportion of the exhaled gases enters the scavenger. Some rebreathing of gas can occur if a reservoir bag is present, particularly during peak inspiration or if the respiratory pattern is rapid. The amount of rebreathing depends on the oxygen flow rate and therefore can be controlled by the anesthetist. If the anesthetist selects a high oxygen flow rate (e.g., 2 L/minute for a 5-kg cat), there is little return of exhaled gases to the patient. The system is therefore completely nonrebreathing, and the reservoir bag outlet is kept fully open. At lower flow rates (e.g., 500 ml of oxygen/minute for a 5-kg cat), significant rebreathing of exhaled gases may occur even with a Bain circuit, and the setup would be more properly classified as a partial rebreathing system, rather than a nonrebreathing system. In the latter case, the reservoir bag outlet on the Bain would be kept partly closed to prevent rapid escape of the exhaled gases.

When using a Bain circuit, a rebreathing setup is more economical than a nonrebreathing setup, since lower oxygen flow rates can be used and therefore the amount of anesthetic vaporized is less. However, significant rebreathing of gas is not advisable when using a nonrebreathing system such as the Bain circuit. There is some risk that CO_2 levels may become dangerously high in such a system because a CO_2 absorber is not used.

Choice of rebreathing versus nonrebreathing system

The decision of whether to use a rebreathing system (such as the conventional anesthetic machine setup) or a nonrebreathing system (such as a Bain) is made on the basis of the following factors:

- *Patient size*. Nonrebreathing systems such as the Bain are most commonly used in patients weighing less than 7 kg (15 lb). Nonrebreathing systems offer little resistance to respiration, a significant advantage for small patients. If a rebreathing system is used, the flutter valves, carbon dioxide canister, and pop-off valve increase the resistance to air movement within the system. Small patients may have difficulty inhaling with enough force to draw air from such a circuit into their lungs.*

* The size of the endotracheal tube has a greater effect on resistance than does the type of circuit used. The use of an endotracheal tube that is too small results in far greater resistance to air passage than that offered by the remainder of the anesthetic circuit, even in a rebreathing setup.

- *Convenience.* In addition to offering less resistance to breathing, nonrebreathing circuits are generally lighter than the Y piece and hose assembly of a rebreathing circuit and therefore cause less drag on the endotracheal tube.
- *Cost.* As previously mentioned, total rebreathing (closed) systems are the most economical type available, because gas flows are relatively low and less anesthetic and oxygen are used. Partial rebreathing (semiclosed) systems are not as economical as total rebreathing systems but require much less oxygen and anesthetic (on a per kg basis) than nonrebreathing systems such as the Bain. For this reason, rebreathing systems (either total or partial rebreathing) are used commonly in large patients, which would require prohibitively large amounts of anesthetic and oxygen in a nonrebreathing system.
- *Control.* The speed at which the anesthetist can change anesthetic depth depends, in part, on the type of system used. A rebreathing system has a relatively slow turnover of gases, because the flow rate of fresh oxygen and anesthetic into the system is low. A nonrebreathing system allows a much faster turnover of gases, because flow rates of fresh gas are higher and a large proportion of exhaled gases exit the system through the scavenger. This means that changes made in the (precision) vaporizer setting will result in rapid changes in anesthetic concentration within a nonrebreathing system, and the percentage of anesthetic breathed by the patient is very close to that indicated by the dial. Changes in anesthetic concentration within a rebreathing system, however, require a longer time, and the concentration of anesthetic inhaled by the patient may not be the same as that indicated on the dial for several minutes after the dial setting is changed.*
- *Conservation of heat and moisture.* Rebreathing systems automatically warm and humidify inspired gases within the circle. Nonrebreathing systems may be associated with significant loss of heat and water from the patient because the warmed and humidified gases exhaled by the patient are not returned. Inspired fresh anesthetic gases in a nonrebreathing circuit have a relative humidity close to 0% and a temperature of approximately 16° C, whereas exhaled gases have a relative humidity of almost 100% and a temperature close to 25° C.
- *Production of waste gas.* Although scavenging of waste gas is strongly recommended for any anesthetic system, there may be occasions in which scavenging is impossible. In these cases, total rebreathing systems may be preferred, since oxygen flow rates are lower and exhaled gases are recirculated rather than vented through the pop-off valve.

---

* The type of volatile anesthetic used will also determine how quickly anesthetic depth can be changed, irrespective of oxygen flow rates or the type of circuit used. Anesthetics with high solubility coefficients, such as methoxyflurane, will allow only slow changes in anesthetic depth, whereas anesthetics that have a low tissue solubility, such as isoflurane and halothane, will pass quickly between the blood and the alveolus, allowing rapid changes in anesthetic depth. See discussion on pp. 144-147.

Vaporizers

Of all the components of the anesthetic machine, the vaporizer is the most complicated and often the most expensive to purchase and service. The function of the
vaporizer is to add anesthetic to the carrier gases (either oxygen alone or oxygen
plus nitrous oxide) that flow to the patient. Regardless of the type of anesthetic
used, it is purchased in liquid form and put into the vaporizer before use. When
oxygen passes through the vaporizer, the anesthetic is evaporated and conveyed to
the patient as a gas.

Anesthetic machines may be equipped with either a *precision* or *nonprecision*
vaporizer. Characteristics of these two types of vaporizers are summarized in
Table 4-6.

Precision vaporizers

A precision vaporizer is one that is designed to deliver an exact concentration of
anesthetic selected by the anesthetist. The dial of a precision vaporizer (Fig. 4-11) is

TABLE 4-6

Comparison of precision and nonprecision vaporizers

Parameters	Precision vaporizer	Nonprecision vaporizer
Temperature compensation	Yes; output usually not affected by temperature in most models	No; output affected by temperature
Flow compensation	Yes; output usually not affected over a wide range of flow rates	No; output affected by flow rate
Back pressure compensation	Yes; changes in back pressure do not affect output	No; changes in back pressure affect output
Maintenance requirements	Requires periodic factory recalibration and cleaning	Minimal; can be done by hospital staff
Cost	High	Minimal
Anesthetics commonly used	Isoflurane, halothane (i.e., those with high vapor pressure)	Methoxyflurane (i.e., those with low vapor pressure)
Control over anesthetic concentration	Precise; given as a percentage	Not precise; given as a control lever setting (1-10)
Position relative to anesthetic circuit	Out of circle (VOC)	In circle (VIC)

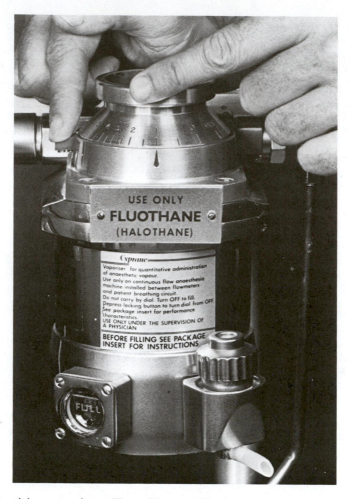

Fig. 4-11. Precision vaporizer. (From Warren RG: *Small animal anesthesia,* St Louis, 1983, Mosby.)

graduated in percent concentration (1%, 2%, etc.). For most patients, a concentration of 1.5 times the MAC (minimum alveolar concentration) of that anesthetic will result in a moderate depth of anesthesia. For example, the MAC of isoflurane in the dog is 1.30. A concentration of 2% isoflurane therefore can be expected to maintain surgical anesthesia in most dogs. This is only a rough guideline, and the anesthetist must, of course, monitor each animal's response to the anesthetic to determine the optimum setting for that individual.

Precision vaporizers are expensive, but offer the advantage of closely controlling the delivery of anesthetic. This is of particular importance if the anesthetic used has a high vapor pressure (e.g., halothane and isoflurane). These anesthetics evaporate very readily and may reach a concentration close to 30% within the anesthetic circuit if vaporization is not controlled. Since the maximum safe concentration of these agents is less than 5%, uncontrolled evaporation would obviously be dangerous for the patient. It is therefore customary to use halothane and isoflurane in a precision vaporizer, affording the anesthetist more exact control of the anesthetic concentration in the circuit. (For information on the use of halothane or isoflurane in a nonprecision vaporizer, see the next section.)

Not all anesthetics require this degree of control. For example, methoxyflurane has a low vapor pressure (i.e., does not evaporate readily) and will only produce a maximum of 4% concentration in the carrier gases. This is a safe level for anesthesia of most patients, so a nonprecision vaporizer is adequate for methoxyflurane delivery.

A variety of precision anesthetic vaporizers are available on the market. Each vaporizer is designed for use with an anesthetic with a particular vapor pressure; therefore vaporizers are labelled for use with one anesthetic only. There is one exception to this rule: halothane and isoflurane have similar vapor pressures and may be used interchangeably in some vaporizers, although this practice is not recommended by vaporizer manufacturers.

Most vaporizers have keyed filler systems that help prevent inadvertent introduction of the wrong anesthetic into the vaporizer. If the wrong anesthetic is accidentally put into a vaporizer (e.g., halothane into a methoxyflurane vaporizer), the vaporizer should be drained, flushed with oxygen, and allowed to air overnight before use.

When using an anesthetic machine, it is easy to assume that the concentration of anesthetic delivered depends only on the vaporizer setting. However, the concentration delivered may, in some cases, be affected by three other factors: temperature, carrier gas flow rate, and back pressure. Most recently manufactured precision vaporizers are compensated for all three factors and are able to deliver the concentration indicated on the dial with very little error or variation. However, technicians working with older precision vaporizers that are not automatically compensated for these factors may need to perform calculations to allow for the effect of temperature or flow rates.

Temperature compensation. Volatile anesthetics, like all liquids, evaporate more readily at a high temperature than at a low temperature. If a vaporizer is not constructed to compensate for temperature changes, the amount of anesthetic vaporized will vary with changes in room temperature. If the anesthetic in a noncompensated vaporizer is used in a cold room, the amount of anesthetic vaporized may be considerably less than that indicated on the dial. Conversely, in a warm room the amount vaporized may be greater than the reading on the dial.

Temperature compensation is also important because at high oxygen flow rates, the passage of oxygen will cause the temperature of the liquid anesthetic to fall. Unless the vaporizer has built-in compensation for this effect, this leads to decreased vaporization and decreased concentration of anesthetic in the circle. The result is that at high flow rates, a noncompensated vaporizer will deliver less anesthetic than the amount indicated by the dial.

Most precision vaporizers are temperature-compensated to prevent variation of anesthetic output. Older models that are not temperature-compensated provide a thermometer and temperature adjustment scale that allow the anesthetist to adjust the vaporizer setting to account for room temperature.

Flow compensation. Just as temperature may influence the evaporation rate of a volatile anesthetic, the amount of gas that flows over the liquid anesthetic (the carrier gas flow rate) will also affect the evaporation rate. In a vaporizer that is not flow-compensated, the concentration of anesthetic that is released at an oxygen flow rate of 3 L/minute may be different from that released at a flow rate of 500 ml/minute. Most modern precision vaporizers are compensated to prevent this variation and will vaporize the amount of anesthetic indicated on the vaporizer dial, regardless of the flow rate. Older halothane vaporizers are not flow-compensated, however, and provide a chart that estimates the dial setting required for a range of flow rates.

For any precision vaporizer, flow compensation is not unlimited, and flows that are very high (in excess of 10 L/minute) or very low (below 500 ml/minute) may affect the amount of anesthetic liquid that is vaporized even in a flow-compensated precision vaporizer. The vaporizer setting may not accurately reflect the concentration of anesthetic released at these extreme flow rates.

Although an exact percentage output is indicated by the dial or chart on the vaporizer, the amount of anesthetic received by the animal is somewhat affected by the flow of the carrier gas in the circuit, even in a compensated precision vaporizer. High flows allow the patient to achieve a percent concentration close to that dialed because a large amount of fresh gas is continuously delivered to the circuit. Lower flows result in more rebreathing of expired gases that have had some anesthetic removed by the animal on the last breath, lowering the anesthetic concentration. For example, if a 20-kg dog is connected to an anesthetic machine with a flow rate of 300 ml/kg/minute (in this case, 6 L/minute) and a vaporizer setting of 2%, the actual concentration of anesthetic being breathed by the animal is close to 2%. If the flow is reduced to 100 ml/kg/minute (in this case, 2 L/minute), then to 50 ml/kg/minute (1 L/minute), and finally to 10 ml/kg/minute (200 ml/minute), the percent concentration of anesthetic being inspired may drop to 1.8%, 1.2%, and 0.8%, respectively. The vaporizer in each case is producing a 2% concentration of anesthetic, but the lower the fresh gas flow, the more the expired gases dilute the anesthetic that is flowing into the machine.

Back pressure compensation. A vaporizer that is not back pressure compensated will release additional anesthetic if gas from the circuit passes through it under pressure. This may occur when, for example, the animal is bagged. Precision vaporizers are normally back pressure compensated, in that they are placed outside the anesthetic circuit and gas from the circuit cannot reenter the vaporizer and affect the evaporation of the anesthetic. Bagging therefore does not affect the amount of anesthetic released by these vaporizers.*

Almost all vaporizers have an indicator window at the base of the vaporizer, which allows the technician to inspect the amount of liquid anesthetic remaining in the vaporizer. This should be checked before the machine is used, and the vaporizer should be refilled if the level indicates that over half of the anesthetic has evaporated. The indicator window also allows the anesthetist to assess the color of the anesthetic: with prolonged use, excessive amounts of preservative may accumulate within a halothane vaporizer, resulting in a yellow discoloration of the liquid. Servicing or vaporizer flushing is recommended if this discoloration is apparent because vaporizer function may be impaired by high levels of preservative (see p. 206).

Nonprecision vaporizers

Not all machines are equipped with precision vaporizers. Nonprecision vaporizers are available that are much simpler in design and much less expensive than precision vaporizers. They are acceptable for use with anesthetics that have a low vapor pressure (e.g., methoxyflurane) and under certain circumstances may be used with anesthetics with a high vapor pressure (e.g., isoflurane, halothane).

The most commonly used nonprecision vaporizer is the Ohio No.8 vaporizer, which consists of a glass jar containing a wick. The wick absorbs anesthetic contained in the jar, and as oxygen gas flows past the wick, the anesthetic is vaporized. In a nonprecision vaporizer, the concentration of anesthetic delivered to the patient is not known exactly and therefore cannot be given as a percentage and is indicated only by a control lever setting (Fig. 4-12). The anesthetist varies the amount of anesthetic that is delivered to the patient by opening or closing the control valve, basing this decision on the patient's depth of anesthesia. This type of control is adequate for methoxyflurane, which has a low vapor pressure and will only achieve a maximum of 4% concentration even if the vaporizer is fully open. However, many anesthetists have traditionally felt that this control is inadequate for more volatile anesthetics such as halothane or isoflurane, which can achieve very high concentrations in such a system, resulting in rapid increase in patient depth. Recently, machines have become available that feature a nonprecision vaporizer that can be used with isoflurane or halothane (Stephens Universal Vaporizer). The

---

* Despite back pressure compensation, an increased amount of anesthetic may be delivered to a patient that is bagged continuously. This occurs because the volume of gas entering the lungs in a bagged animal is greater than that breathed by an anesthetized patient breathing on its own. It is therefore important to reduce the setting of a precision vaporizer when continuous bagging is administered, particularly if patient depth seems excessive.

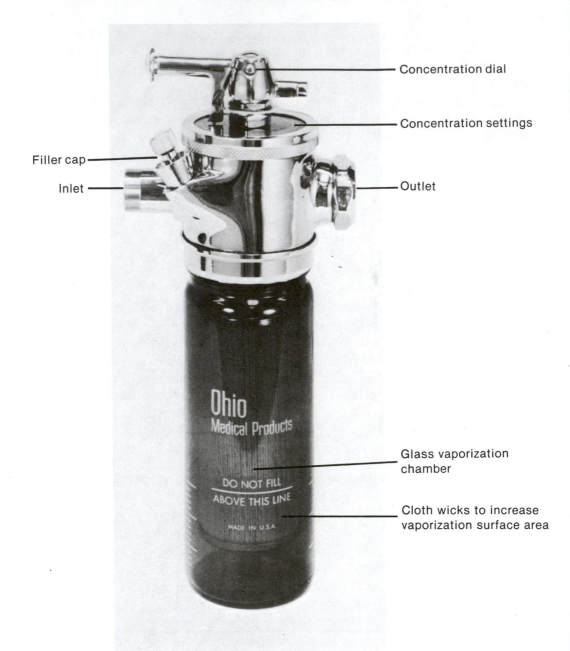

Concentration dial

Concentration settings

Filler cap

Inlet

Outlet

Glass vaporization chamber

Cloth wicks to increase vaporization surface area

Fig. 4-12. Nonprecision vaporizer. (From Warren RG: *Small animal anesthesia,* St Louis, 1983, Mosby.)

vaporizer of this machine is made inefficient by removal of the wick, allowing halothane or isoflurane to be delivered at a concentration suitable for anesthesia. The two advantages of this system are:

1. It can be used with low flow rates and is therefore economical.
2. The initial cost is somewhat less than for a precision vaporizer.

The chief disadvantage of any nonprecision vaporizer is that it is not compensated for temperature, carrier gas flow rates, or back pressure. This has several serious implications that must be understood by the anesthetist using this type of vaporizer, particularly if isoflurane or halothane is to be administered.

- *Lack of temperature compensation.* At any given setting, the vaporizer will deliver a greater concentration of anesthetic in a warm room than in a cold room.
- *Lack of flow compensation.* The amount of anesthetic delivered to the patient will increase if the patient breathes more deeply. Increased respiration rate results in increased flow of gas through the vaporizer and thus will increase evaporation of the anesthetic. Eventually the high flow rates will cause the temperature of the anesthetic in the vaporizer to fall, and the concentration of anesthetic may decrease. The variation in anesthetic output with flow rate does not occur in a flow-compensated precision vaporizer, in which anesthetic output will not vary despite changes in respiratory rate or depth or changes in oxygen flow rate.
- *Lack of back pressure compensation.* Most importantly, because nonprecision vaporizers are not backpressure compensated, a buildup of pressure within the circuit (as may occur when the patient is bagged or a ventilator is used) may result in increased evaporation of anesthetic. The increased delivery of anesthetic to the patient being bagged may result in excessive anesthetic depth. Controlled ventilation therefore is difficult with these vaporizers: the anesthetist must ensure that the vaporizer setting is greatly reduced (or the vaporizer is turned off) when bagging the animal or when delivering intermittent positive pressure ventilation by means of a ventilator. In contrast, it is not normally necessary to turn off a precision vaporizer when bagging because of the back-pressure compensation of these vaporizers.
- *Monitoring.* The use of a nonprecision vaporizer with a volatile anesthetic such as isoflurane offers less precise control over anesthetic depth than does a standard precision vaporizer. Close monitoring of the patient is essential, particularly during the first 5 minutes of anesthesia, when patient depth increases rapidly.
- *Use with nonrebreathing systems.* This setup is difficult to adapt to nonrebreathing systems such as the Bain circuit.

VOC versus VIC

The anesthetist may occasionally find an anesthetic machine referred to as VOC or VIC. The letters *VOC* are an abbreviation for *vaporizer out of circle* and indicate that the vaporizer is not placed within the anesthetic circuit itself (Fig. 4-13*A*). (As

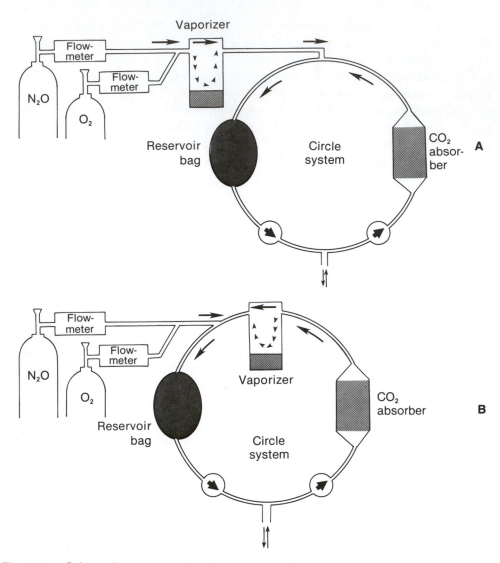

Fig. 4-13. Schematic representation of anesthetic system, **A,** out of circle and **B,** in circle. (From Warren RG: *Small animal anesthesia,* St Louis, 1983, Mosby.)

previously mentioned the circuit includes the flutter valves, hoses, carbon dioxide absorber canister, pop-off valve, and reservoir bag.) This is the type of setup described earlier in this chapter and applies to all anesthetic machines with precision vaporizers. The letters *VIC* indicate a *vaporizer in circle* (Fig. 4-13*B*). In this type of machine (e.g., the Ohio No.8), the carrier gases enter the circuit directly from the flowmeter. The vaporizer (which is nonprecision in this case) is part of the circuit, and exhaled gases reenter the vaporizer each time they flow through the circuit.

It is reasonable to ask at this point why precision vaporizers are always found out of circle and nonprecision vaporizers are found in circle. The position of a vaporizer in circle or out of circle is governed by the resistance it offers to the passage of gases. Nonprecision vaporizers offer little resistance to gas flow and do not impede the passage of gases around the circuit. Precision vaporizers, however, offer a high resistance to gas flow and must be placed out of circle.

Carrier gas flow rates

For each anesthetic procedure, the anesthetist is faced with the problem of deciding how much flow (or volume) of carrier gas is required. Usually, the carrier gas is oxygen alone, but if both oxygen and nitrous oxide are used, flow rate determinations must consider the total flow of gas, as well as the individual flow rates of each gas. Thus it may be decided that for a particular patient and machine setup, a total flow of 1 L/minute is required. The 1 liter may consist of pure oxygen or some combination of nitrous oxide and oxygen, for example, 600 ml/minute of nitrous oxide and 400 ml/minute of oxygen. If nitrous oxide is used, the nitrous oxide flow should be 1.5 to 2.0 times the oxygen flow rate.

The calculation of the flow rate to be used for each anesthetic procedure is based on several factors, including the period of anesthesia (induction, maintenance, or recovery) and the type of circuit. These factors are summarized in the box on p. 202.

Flow rates during induction

It is customary to use higher flow rates during induction than during the maintenance period. This is particularly true if mask induction or chamber induction is used. Use of high flow rates in the induction period allows the anesthetist to saturate the anesthetic circuit with carrier gas and anesthetic and dilute the expired gases of the patient. Once the animal reaches the desired plane of anesthesia, flow rates are decreased.

- For mask induction it is generally agreed that a flow rate equal to 30 times the tidal volume is adequate. Since the tidal volume of most animals is approximately 10 ml/kg/minute, the recommended flow rate is approximately 300 ml/kg/minute. For animals under 10 kg, 1 to 3 liters is usually adequate, and 3 to 5 L/minute is suggested for animals over 10 kg.
- A flow rate of 5 L/minute is recommended for chamber induction.
- For animals induced with an injectable anesthetic and subsequently intubated and connected to an anesthetic machine, the minimum flow rate during the initial anesthetic period is the respiratory minute volume, which is the tidal volume (10

Recommended flow rates

Induction
Chamber induction

- 5 L/minute

Face mask induction

- 300 ml/kg/minute, or 1-3 L/minute for animals under 10 kg, 3-5 L/minute for animals over 10 kg

Intravenous induction

- 200 ml/kg/minute (500 ml to 5 L/minute depending on patient size)

Maintenance
Nonrebreathing systems

- Bain: 130-200 ml/kg/min
- Other systems: 200-300 ml/kg/minute

Rebreathing systems

- Total rebreathing (closed) system: minimum of 15 ml/kg/minute; use of N_2O is inadvisable at this flow rate
- Partial rebreathing (semiclosed system): 25-50 ml/kg/minute
- Semiclosed system with minimal rebreathing: 150-200 ml/kg/minute

Recovery

- 200 ml/kg/minute (500 ml to 5 L/minute, depending on patient size)

Flow rates in excess of 2 L/minute should be avoided when using nonprecision vaporizers. Many vaporizers deliver inaccurate amounts of anesthetic at flow rates less than 500 ml/minute or greater than 10 L/minute.
When using nitrous oxide, a minimum oxygen flow of 30 ml/kg/minute must be provided. Nitrous oxide flow rate should be 1.5 to 2 times the oxygen flow rate.

ml/kg) times the number of breaths per minute. A figure of 200 ml/kg/minute is commonly used, which results in a flow rate between 500 ml and 5 L/minute, depending on the size of the animal.

Flow rates in the maintenance period

Once the animal achieves a satisfactory level of anesthetic depth, the flow rate may be safely reduced to a maintenance level. This value depends on the type of system used (total rebreathing, partial rebreathing, or nonrebreathing).

Nonrebreathing systems require relatively high flow rates, on a per kg. basis, since the expired gases are evacuated by the scavenger and, for the most part, are not returned to the patient. Fresh gas must be continuously provided, because there is minimal rebreathing of exhaled gases. The recommended flow rate for a Bain circuit is 130 to 200 ml/kg/minute. For a 5-kg animal, this flow rate is 650 ml to 1 L/minute of pure oxygen. If nitrous oxide is used, flow rates of 600 ml nitrous oxide and 400 ml of oxygen per minute (a ratio of 1.5:1) would be appropriate.

For other types of nonrebreathing circuits, flow rates of 200 to 300 ml/kg/minute are generally accepted.

Rebreathing systems require relatively low flow rates compared with nonrebreathing systems, because carbon dioxide absorption is available and the expired gases are returned to the patient. Provided the carbon dioxide absorber canister is effective, the carrier gas and anesthetic can be recycled continuously and only a small amount of fresh gas is required. For a total rebreathing (closed) system, the oxygen flow must only equal the oxygen requirements of the animal. The minimum oxygen requirement for an animal is approximately 10 ml/kg/minute, although to account for leaks within the circuit, a value of 15 ml/kg/minute is usually recommended. The anesthetist should be aware that flow rates less than 500 ml/minute will not allow accurate delivery of the dialed vaporizer concentration by most precision vaporizers.

Flow rates of 25 to 50 ml/kg/minute are recommended for partial rebreathing systems. If minimal rebreathing is preferred, a flow rate of 150 to 200 ml/kg/minute can be used.

Flow rates at the end of anesthesia

It is recommended that the flow rates be increased immediately after the vaporizer is turned off. During this time, anesthetic gas is exhaled by the patient and may accumulate within the circuit, particularly if a rebreathing system is used. In order to evacuate this anesthetic and to allow the patient to breathe pure oxygen, a flow rate similar to that used during induction is recommended. The anesthetist should periodically remove expired gases from the circuit by opening the pop-off valve and evacuating the reservoir bag. The bag can be refilled using the oxygen flush control.

Summary

Within the guidelines given above, there is considerable leeway for the anesthetist to use his or her judgment when determining the flow rate for any particular procedure. See the box on p. 204 and the box on p. 202 for a summary of currently recommended flow rates and sample flow rate calculations. In many cases, the ultimate decision may be based on economic factors: high gas flow rates are less economical than low flow rates, since more oxygen, nitrous oxide, and anesthetic are used. It is evident, therefore, that nonrebreathing systems are less economical than rebreathing systems. If the patient is small, the flow rate, even with a nonrebreathing system, is unlikely to be greater than 1.5 L/minute, and the cost of

Examples of flow rates

1. Given a 5-kg cat and an anesthetic machine with a precision vaporizer, what type of circuit and flow rate would normally be used? Calculate the flow rates for oxygen alone and for oxygen and nitrous oxide used together.
   Answer: Since the cat weighs less than 7 kg, a Bain or other nonrebreathing system is preferred. The flow rate recommended for the Bain system is 130 to 200 ml/kg/minute. Thus the anesthetist could select 200 ml × 5 kg = 1000 ml or 1 liter of gas flow per minute. Note that if nitrous oxide is used for this animal, a 2 : 1 ratio of $N_2O : O_2$ should be provided. For a 1 liter total flow of gas, this is equal to:

   Oxygen: $\frac{1}{3}$ of 1 L/minute = 333 ml/minute

   Nitrous oxide: $\frac{2}{3}$ of 1 L/minute = 667 ml/minute

   If nitrous oxide is used, the anesthetist must ensure that the animal receives adequate oxygen (30 ml/kg/minute). For this cat, the minimum is 30 ml oxygen/minute × 5 kg = 150 ml of oxygen/minute. (Therefore 333 ml is safe.)

2. Given a 25-kg dog and a precision vaporizer, what type of circuit and flow rate would be preferred?
   Answer: For economic reasons, the type of circuit used would probably be a circle system. If a total rebreathing system is used, the minimum oxygen flow rate is 15 ml × 25 kg per minute, which is 375 ml per minute. (For many vaporizers, this flow rate is too low and should be increased to a minimum of 500 ml/minute.) If, as is more common, a partial rebreathing system is used, the flow rate should be 25 to 50 ml/kg/minute. For this animal, the flow rate would therefore be 625 ml to 1.25 liters of oxygen per minute. If the anesthetist wishes to increase the flow rate to achieve a nonrebreathing system, the flow rate would be calculated as 150 to 200 ml/kg/minute, which is 3.75 to 5 L/minute in this patient.

   The oxygen flow rate therefore can be set at a minimum of 500 ml/minute and at a maximum of 5 L/minute (if the pop-off valve is completely open and the animal is not rebreathing any expired gases). Many anesthetists would choose a flow rate midway between these two extremes, approximately 1 to 1.5 L/minute.

3. Given a 15-kg dog anesthetized with a nonprecision methoxyflurane system, what would be the recommended flow rate?
   (a) If a semiclosed, partial rebreathing system is used
   (b) If minimal rebreathing is desired
   Answer: If the dog is on a semiclosed system, the flow rate should be 25 to 50 ml/kg/minute. For this animal, the flow rate therefore would be 375 to 750 ml/minute.

   If minimal rebreathing is desired, the anesthetist should use a flow rate of 200 ml/kg/hr, which is 3 L/minute. However, since the vaporizer in this example is not compensated for flow rate, it would be inadvisable to use a flow rate over 2 L/minute.

anesthetic and oxygen is relatively minor. Economic considerations are more important when considering whether to use a total or partial rebreathing system for a larger animal. Partial rebreathing systems use higher flow rates (see discussion above) and, for this reason, may be considerably more expensive than total rebreathing systems.

CARE AND USE OF ANESTHETIC EQUIPMENT

Setting up anesthetic equipment

Prior to use, the anesthetic machine should be assembled and thoroughly checked for problems. The following is a checklist of procedures to be followed when setting up anesthetic equipment:
- Assemble all needed supplies.
- Inflate the endotracheal tube cuffs and record the amount of air required.
- Check the laryngoscope bulb.
- Draw up and label the injectable preanesthetic and anesthetic agents.
- Mix and warm intravenous fluids to be used.
- Rotate the vaporizer dial to ensure smooth function.
- Check the amount of anesthetic in the vaporizer and replenish as necessary.
- Turn on the gas tanks using a cylinder wrench or similar device. Tanks should be opened slowly and turned to full open position for use. The oxygen tank should be changed if the tank pressure gauge indicates a pressure less than 680 kPa (100 psi). A cutoff of 1360 kPa (200 psi) is advisable if a long anesthesia is planned or high flow rates are to be used. A nitrous oxide tank should be changed if nitrous oxide pressure is less than 3400 kPa (500 psi).
- Check the flowmeter controls, with the oxygen tank open, to ensure proper function.
- Assemble the appropriate circuit (nonrebreathing circuit or hoses and Y piece) and connect to the machine. The gas flow should be mentally traced from the tank to the patient and back to the machine and scavenger to ensure that connections are correctly assembled.
- Attach the reservoir bag to the machine or nonrebreathing circuit.
- Change the carbon dioxide absorber canister contents if necessary. This procedure is best done immediately after machine use, when color changes are most evident.
- Test the machine for leaks (see Chapter 5).

Maintenance of anesthetic equipment

As with any piece of equipment, the anesthetic machine requires periodic maintenance to ensure proper performance. A routine maintenance checklist includes the items listed below.

Oxygen and nitrous oxide tanks

Following use, the outlet valve of each tank should be closed by turning it clockwise (i.e., to the right). Failure to turn off the gas valve will result in excessive pressure on the regulator and, in some cases, leakage of gas from the tank.

Oxygen pressure remaining in the machine after closure of the tank (line pressure) should be removed using the oxygen flush valve or by turning the flowmeter to a high rate of flow. Failure to evacuate line pressure may damage the pressure gauge and regulator.

Petroleum or petroleum distillate products (grease, gasoline) should not be used on oxygen tanks or their connections. An explosion may occur when the tank is opened and these materials contact oxygen released from the tank.

Flowmeters

The dial of each flowmeter should be returned to the off position (full clockwise) for storage. Failure to do so may result in a sudden rush of air into the flowmeter when the oxygen tank is opened, which may jam the float or ball at the top of the flowmeter tube. Care should be taken not to overtighten the flowmeter knob when turning the flowmeter off.

Flowmeter accuracy can be assessed easily by setting the flow at, for example, 2 L/minute and ensuring that a 2-liter bag connected to the machine fills in approximately 1 minute.

Vaporizer

It is not necessary to routinely empty the anesthetic from the vaporizer after each anesthetic procedure. However, precision vaporizers designed for halothane or methoxyflurane should be emptied of anesthetic every 6 to 12 months and flushed to help remove the buildup of preservative within the vaporizer. Isoflurane is supplied without a preservative, and periodic flushing is not usually necessary.

To perform the flushing procedure, the drained vaporizer is filled with ethyl alcohol and left standing for 30 minutes, then emptied. The ethyl alcohol flush may be repeated until the alcohol appears free of residue. Before refilling the vaporizer with anesthetic, the machine should be flushed with oxygen at a flow rate of 3 to 5 L/minute for 30 to 40 minutes.

Despite periodic flushing, a precision vaporizer may eventually become clogged with preservative and other residue. When this occurs, the anesthetic levels produced by the vaporizer will not correlate with the percentage indicated by the dial. The anesthetist may become aware of the problem when patients can no longer be maintained at a satisfactory anesthetic depth even at high vaporizer settings. To prevent this problem, precision vaporizers should be cleaned and recalibrated by the manufacturer or other qualified personnel every 12 to 24 months. Usually, the vaporizer is removed from the anesthetic machine and sent away for servicing. Many companies provide a "loaner" replacement during the servicing period.

Carbon dioxide absorber canister

Barium hydroxide lime or soda crystals should be checked after each anesthetic procedure. Crystals that change color or cannot be crushed with finger pressure should be replaced. When replacing the granules, it is important to ensure that they are not tightly packed. At least 1 centimeter (one half inch) of air space should be left between the granules and the top of the canister to allow unimpeded air flow out of the canister. Gentle shaking of the canister after filling helps prevent channels from forming in the granules, which could reduce the efficiency of the absorber.

When replenishing soda lime or barium hydroxide lime granules, the technician must ensure that dust does not enter the tubing or hoses of the machine, as it may be inhaled by the patient and is corrosive to mucous membranes.

Water may collect in the trap below the CO_2 canister and should be periodically removed.

Flutter valves

Flutter valves require periodic removal and cleaning with a disinfectant to prevent a buildup of water vapor, mucus, dust from the soda lime or barium hydroxide lime, and other material. Access to the valves is obtained by unscrewing the plastic caps that lie over the valves. Valves that are not cleaned may become sticky and adhere to the machine housing, impeding air flow through the circuit.

Other machine parts

After each anesthetic procedure, removable machine parts, such as the hoses, Y piece, Bain circuit or other nonrebreathing system, and the reservoir bag, should be washed in a mild soapy solution and thoroughly rinsed with water. A surgical scrub brush or bottle brush is useful in cleaning equipment surfaces. After cleaning, the equipment should be air dried. Other machine parts (compressed air tanks, pop-off valve, CO_2 canister) should be wiped with a disinfectant solution on a weekly basis.

In some cases anesthetic equipment will require more effective disinfection. This is particularly true of equipment that contacts the patient's airway or oral cavity, including the endotracheal tube, laryngoscope blade, esophageal stethoscope, and face mask. If used on a patient harboring certain viruses or bacteria (including feline rhinotracheitis virus, *Bordetella,* and other respiratory pathogens), the equipment may easily spread infection to the next patient. To prevent disease transmission between patients, these items should be soaked in a disinfectant solution such as 2% glutaraldehyde or sterilized in an ethylene oxide system or autoclave (if the material allows this). Gauze, adhesive tape, and the adapter should be removed from an endotracheal tube before disinfection.

Unfortunately, there is no ideal agent for cleaning anesthetic supplies. Agents such as chlorhexidine are relatively harmless to tissues but are not effective against all microorganisms and spores. Glutaraldehyde solutions (2%) are effective against many microorganisms but are stable for only 2 to 4 weeks and must be periodically replaced. Glutaraldehyde solutions also are irritating to the skin, and the technician should wear rubber gloves when working with this substance. All items exposed to any chemical solution should be thoroughly rinsed with water after cleaning. Some chemicals may be absorbed by rubber and, if not completely removed by rinsing, may cause burns when in contact with the patient's airway or skin. Ethylene oxide is particularly well absorbed by materials being sterilized, and endotracheal tubes exposed to this substance have been known to cause tracheal necrosis.

After prolonged use rubber items deteriorate and must be replaced. Autoclaving causes rubber surfaces to become brittle and crack. Prolonged exposure to disinfectants or rubber-soluble anesthetics, such as methoxyflurane, may also cause rubber surfaces to deteriorate. Endotracheal tubes, masks, and reservoir bags should be periodically checked for wear and discarded if necessary. Endotracheal tubes with leaking or nonfunctional cuffs should also be discarded.

KEY POINTS

1. Many different types and sizes of endotracheal tubes are available for use in veterinary patients.

2. The anesthetic machine delivers volatile gas anesthetic and carrier gases (oxygen with or without nitrous oxide) to the patient and moves exhaled gases away from the patient. If gases are reused, the machine removes carbon dioxide from them before returning them to the patient.

3. Anesthetic machines can be used as a source of oxygen for emergencies.

4. Compressed oxygen cylinders contain oxygen gas under high pressure (up to 2200 psi or 15,000 kilopascals). Various sizes of cylinders are available, which may be freestanding or attach to the anesthesia machine, but are always white or green in color. Large cylinders contain more liters of oxygen and function for a longer time than small cylinders. For all oxygen cylinders, tank pressure is gradually reduced as the cylinder empties. Cylinders should be changed when the pressure reaches 100 to 200 psi.

5. Nitrous oxide cylinders are blue in color and contain nitrous oxide gas and liquid at a pressure up to 770 psi (5170 kilopascals). As the tank empties, tank pressure is maintained until most of the nitrous oxide is gone: tanks therefore should be changed when the pressure starts to drop below 500 psi.

6. The pressure regulator (pressure-reducing valve) allows a constant flow of gas

to enter the machine and provides a safe operating pressure (50 psi) for the machine.

7. For each type of carrier gas, the flow rate is set by its respective flowmeter. Flows are generally expressed in liters per minute. The flow rate indicates to the anesthetist how much gas is being delivered to the patient at any given time. When using nitrous oxide, the anesthetist should set a nitrous oxide:oxygen ratio of 2:1 to 3:1.

8. Liquid anesthetic is evaporated and added to the carrier gas in the vaporizer. The combination of vaporized anesthetic, oxygen, and nitrous oxide (if present) is called *fresh gas.* Vaporizers may be precision or nonprecision, based on their construction. Precision vaporizers are commonly used with anesthetics with high vapor pressures, which require compensation for variations in temperature, gas flow rate, and back pressure. Precision vaporizers are found outside of the anesthetic circuit (VOC), whereas nonprecision vaporizers are found inside the anesthetic circuit (VIC).

9. The reservoir bag (rebreathing bag) can be used to monitor the animal's respiration and to deliver oxygen (with or without anesthetic) to the patient by a process called *bagging.*

10. Inhalation and exhalation valves allow one-way passage of gas through the machine.

11. Waste gas exits the machine at the pop-off valve, which is usually connected to a scavenger. The pop-off valve is usually kept open unless the patient is being bagged.

12. Carbon dioxide is removed by the circuit in an absorber canister containing granules. Most types of granules exhibit a color change when they have become depleted and require replacement.

13. The pressure manometer measures the pressure of gases within the anesthetic circuit.

14. Anesthetic circuits may be classified as *rebreathing* (either closed or semi-closed) or *nonrebreathing.* Rebreathing systems use lower flow rates but must provide for carbon dioxide absorption. Total rebreathing systems may be less safe than partial rebreathing systems because of increased risk of oxygen depletion and carbon dioxide accumulation within the circuit. Nonrebreathing systems, such as the Bain system, are considered effective and safe. However, they are associated with relatively high flow rates and are commonly used only in small patients.

15. Carrier gas flow rates vary with the period of anesthesia and type of anesthetic circuit used (rebreathing or nonrebreathing). High flow rates are used during induction and recovery and also during the maintenance period if a nonrebreathing system is used.

16. Anesthetic equipment requires routine cleaning, care, and maintenance.

REVIEW QUESTIONS

1. When the oxygen tank is half full, the pressure gauge will read approximately:
   a. 1000 psi
   b. 2000 psi
   c. 500 psi
   d. 2200 psi
   e. None of the above
2. The pressure gauge of a nitrous oxide tank will read _____ psi when the tank is full.
   a. 750
   b. 2200
   c. 1000
   d. 500
3. When the nitrous oxide tank is half full, the pressure gauge will read _____ psi.
   a. 750
   b. 350
   c. 100
   d. 500
4. Nitrous oxide exists in the tank as a _____.
   a. Liquid
   b. Gas
   c. Liquid and a gas
5. The amount of oxygen an animal is receiving is indicated by the:
   a. Oxygen tank pressure gauge
   b. Flowmeter
   c. Pressure manometer
   d. Vaporizer setting
6. Flowmeters that have a ball for reading the gauge should be read from the _____ of the ball.
   a. Top   b. Bottom   c. Middle
7. The best flow rate to use with nitrous oxide and oxygen would be a combination of _____.
   a. 50% oxygen and 50% nitrous oxide
   b. 33% oxygen and 67% nitrous oxide
   c. 23% oxygen and 77% nitrous oxide
   d. 77% oxygen and 23% nitrous oxide
8. The minimum size for the reservoir bag can be calculated as _____.
   a. 20 ml/kg
   b. 60 ml/kg
   c. 80 ml/kg
   d. 100 ml/kg
9. The term *atelectasis* means:
   a. The animal is not ventilating
   b. Some of the alveoli have collapsed
   c. The heart is not pumping
   d. The patient's blood pressure is falling

10. An animal that is under a general anesthetic may have its tidal volume decreased by as much as:
    a. 15%
    b. 25%
    c. 50%
    d. 75%
11. The flutter valves on an anesthetic machine help _____.
    a. Control the direction of movement of gases
    b. Maintain a full reservoir bag
    c. Remove carbon dioxide
    d. Vaporize the liquid anesthetic
12. The pop-off valve is part of the anesthetic machine and helps:
    a. Vaporize the liquid anesthetic
    b. Prevent excess gas pressure from building up within the breathing circuit
    c. Keep the oxygen flowing in one direction only
    d. Prevent waste gases from reentering the vaporizer
13. When the pressure manometer reading exceeds _____ cm of water pressure, it indicates there is a buildup of pressure within the circuit that could be dangerous.
    a. 5
    b. 10
    c. 15
    d. 20
14. Which of the following circuits must have a carbon dioxide canister as part of the circuit?
    a. Circle system
    b. Bain system
    c. Ayres-T system
15. Rebreathing systems are best reserved for animals over 7 kg.
    True   False
16. Rebreathing is determined primarily by the:
    a. Fresh gas flow
    b. Design or type of circuit
    c. Presence of a reservoir bag
    d. None of the above
17. Nonrebreathing systems should have flow rates that are:
    a. Very high ($\geq$130 ml/kg/minute)
    b. Very low (10 ml/kg/minute)
    c. Moderate ($\geq$ 50 ml/kg/minute)
18. At room temperature it is possible for halothane to vaporize up to 33%, and therefore it is administered most safely by a precision vaporizer.
    True   False
19. Anesthetics with low vapor pressures can be delivered from a _____ vaporizer.
    a. Precision
    b. Nonprecision
    c. Precision or nonprecision

20. For mask induction purposes, the minimum suggested flow rate should be
_____ times the tidal volume.
   a. 10
   b. 20
   c. 30
   d. 40
   e. 50
21. The tidal volume of an animal is considered to be _____ ml/kg of
body weight.
   a. 5
   b. 10
   c. 15
   d. 20
22. During the induction period, _____ flow rates are considered preferable.
   a. High
   b. Moderate
   c. Low
23. Acceptable flow rates in rebreathing systems may be as low as
_____ ml/kg/minute.
   a. 5
   b. 15
   c. 25
   d. 50

For the following questions, more than one answer may be correct.

24. A reservoir bag that is not moving may indicate:
   a. The endotracheal tube is not in the trachea
   b. The animal has a decreased tidal volume
   c. There is a leak around the endotracheal tube
   d. The vaporizer is empty
25. The anesthetist will know when the granules in the carbon dioxide absorber have
been depleted because the:
   a. Anesthetist will smell waste carbon dioxide
   b. Granules will be brittle
   c. Granules may change color
   d. Granules may be hard
26. An increase in the depth of anesthesia can be achieved quickly by:
   a. Having high flow rates
   b. Having high vaporizer settings
   c. Bagging the animal with the vaporizer on
   d. Using a closed anesthetic system
27. The concentration of anesthetic delivered from a nonprecision vaporizer may depend
on the:
   a. Temperature of the liquid anesthetic
   b. Flow of the carrier gas through the vaporizer
   c. Back pressure

28. The advantages of a nonprecision vaporizer include:
  a. It is economical to buy
  b. It can be readily used with all anesthetics
  c. It is easy to clean and service

ANSWERS FOR CHAPTER 4

1. a	**2.** a	**3.** a	**4.** c	**5.** b	**6.** c	**7.** b	**8.** b	**9.** b	**10.** c
11. a	**12.** b	**13.** c	**14.** a	**15.** True	**16.** a	**17.** a	**18.** True	**19.** c	**20.** c
21. b	**22.** a	**23.** b	**24.** a, b, c	**25.** b, c, d	**26.** a, b, c	**27.** a, b, c	**28.** a, c		

SELECTED READINGS

Bednarski RM, Gaynor JS, Muir WW, III: Vaporizer in circle for delivery of isoflurane to dogs, *JAVMA* 202(6):943-948, 1993.

Dyson DH: Influence of oxygen flows during anesthetic management, *Can Vet J* 32:752-754, 1991.

Haskins SC: *Opinions in small animal anesthesia*, Vet Clin North Am (Small Anim Pract) 22(2), Philadelphia, 1992, WB Saunders.

Ludders JW, Stafford KL: Basic equipment for small animal anesthesia: use and maintenance. II. *Compendium* 12(1):35-40, 1981.

Muir WW, III, Hubbell JAE: *Handbook of veterinary anesthesia*, St Louis, 1989, Mosby.

Paddleford RR: *Manual of small animal anesthesia,* New York, 1988, Churchill Livingstone.

Short CE: *Principles and practice of veterinary anesthesia*, Baltimore, 1987, Williams & Wilkins.

Warren RG: *Small animal anesthesia,* St Louis, 1983, Mosby.

Workplace safety

5

PERFORMANCE OBJECTIVES
After completion of this chapter, the reader will be able to:

Describe both the short-term and long-term effects of waste anesthetic gas on the operating room personnel.

Recognize ways in which the release of waste anesthetic gases may be minimized.

Describe proper procedures for handling and transporting compressed gas cylinders.

Understand WHMIS regulations as they relate to materials used in small animal anesthesia.

A veterinary technician may participate in the anesthetic management of several thousand animals during the course of his or her career. It is therefore essential that he or she be familiar with the human safety considerations involved in veterinary anesthesia. These can be divided into the following categories:

- Hazards of waste anesthetic gas
- Workplace Hazardous Materials Information System (WHMIS) considerations
- Hazards involved in handling compressed gas cylinders

This chapter outlines the precautions that the anesthetist can take to reduce as much as possible the health risks of working with anesthetic equipment and gases.

HAZARDS OF WASTE ANESTHETIC GAS

Concerns have been raised regarding possible adverse effects resulting from exposure of hospital personnel to waste anesthetic gas. The term *waste anesthetic gas* refers to the nitrous oxide, halothane, isoflurane, or methoxyflurane vapors that are breathed out by the patient or that escape from the anesthetic machine. These vapors are inadvertently breathed by all personnel working in areas in which animals are anesthetized or recovering from inhalation anesthesia. Significant exposure to anesthetic vapors also occurs when the technician empties or fills anesthetic vaporizers. In addition, short-term exposure to very high levels of anesthetic vapors can occur as the result of an accidental spill of liquid anesthetic.

Since the first study of waste anesthetic gas was published in 1967, many investigators have attempted to determine the toxicity of halothane, methoxyflurane, nitrous oxide, and other anesthetic agents to operating room personnel. Although some of the evidence is contradictory, it is generally accepted that exposure to waste anesthetic gas is associated with a higher than normal incidence of some health problems. The suspected health hazards can be divided into two categories: (1) short-term problems that occur during or immediately after exposure to these agents and (2) long-term problems that may become evident days, weeks, or years after exposure.

Short-term problems

Short-term problems associated with breathing waste gas vapors appear to arise from a direct effect of anesthetic molecules on brain neurons. Symptoms such as fatigue, headache, drowsiness, nausea, depression, and irritability have been reported by persons working in environments in which a high level of waste gas is present. Although these symptoms usually resolve spontaneously when the affected person leaves the area, frequent occurrence of these symptoms may indicate that excessive levels of waste gas are present and a potential for long-term toxicity exists.

Long-term effects

Long-term inhalation of air polluted with waste gas appears to be associated with serious health problems, including reproductive disorders, liver and kidney damage, and chronic nervous system dysfunction. The mechanism of long-term anesthetic gas toxicity is not fully understood, but may be the result of toxic metabolites produced by the breakdown of anesthetic gases within the liver and their subsequent excretion by the kidneys. These metabolites include inorganic fluoride or bromide ions, oxalic acid, and free radicals, all of which are known to have harmful effects on animal tissues.

It is widely accepted that anesthetic agents that are retained by the body and metabolized will have greater long-term toxicity than those that are eliminated through the lungs. For this reason, isoflurane is believed to be the least toxic inhalation agent in common use (0.2% of the amount inhaled is retained and metabolized). In contrast, 20% to 50% of halothane and 50% to 80% of methoxyflurane administered to a patient are retained within body fat, metabolized, and excreted through the kidneys. Although the patient may appear completely recovered from anesthesia induced by these agents, this indicates only that the level of anesthetic in the brain is very low. Significant amounts of anesthetic may linger in the liver, kidney, and body fat stores. Metabolites of halothane have been recovered from the urine of patients as long as 20 days after anesthesia, and anesthetists may show traces of halothane in their breath 64 hours after administering this gas to a patient.

Effects on reproduction

The most convincing evidence of waste anesthetic gas toxicity has emerged from numerous studies into the adverse effects of these agents on reproduction. A comprehensive survey of nurse and physician anesthetists, undertaken by the American Society of Anesthesiologists, found that the risk of spontaneous abortion in this group was 1.3 to 2 times that of the normal population. Another study showed that the frequency of spontaneous abortion among working hospital anesthetists (18.2%) was higher than that observed among nonworking anesthetists (13.7%) and a control group (14.7%). The same study showed that 12% of the working anesthetists interviewed were infertile, compared to 6% of the control group.

Exposure to anesthetic gases also has been linked to an increase in congenital abnormalities in the children of pregnant operating room personnel. One study reported a 16% incidence of congenital abnormalities in children of practicing nurse-anesthetists, compared to a 6% incidence in a control group. Other studies have failed to show a statistically significant correlation between waste gas exposure and an increased incidence in congenital abnormalities.

It is difficult to interpret or compare the results obtained by these and other studies, because there are wide variations in the types of anesthetics used, amount of waste gas exposure, and control measures (such as the availability of scavengers). In most cases, operating room personnel were exposed to several agents simultaneously, and it is difficult to determine which agent or combination of agents was responsible for the adverse effects. It appears, however, that nitrous oxide may be at least partially responsible for the reproductive hazards associated with waste anesthetic gas. Experimentally, exposure of rats to high levels of nitrous oxide results in abnormalities in sperm morphology, reduced ovulation, and retarded fetal development. The adverse reproductive affects associated with exposure to nitrous oxide also were evident in a survey of dentists and dental assistants. Female dental assistants that had been exposed to nitrous oxide for more than 9 hours per week showed a 1.7 to 2.3 times increase in spontaneous abortion rates compared to the normal population. An increase in the rate of spontaneous abortions also was noted in the wives of male dentists who administered nitrous oxide to their patients. Given the weight of this evidence, it is prudent for pregnant women to avoid exposure to high levels of waste anesthetic gas (particularly nitrous oxide) during pregnancy.

Oncogenic effects

Given that waste anesthetic gases may exert their adverse reproductive effects by altering DNA, investigators have attempted to determine whether these agents have a potential to cause other DNA-related changes, such as cancer. Several studies undertaken in the 1970s appeared to suggest that operating room personnel suffer from an increased incidence of some types of cancer. These studies, however, have been criticized for inappropriate data collection and statistical analysis, and it is now generally believed that none of the commonly used anesthetic agents is carcinogenic at the levels found in veterinary hospitals.

Hepatic effects

Several studies have investigated the incidence of liver disorders in personnel exposed to waste anesthetic gas. Halothane, in particular, is recognized as being potentially hepatotoxic. Metabolism of halothane in certain rare anesthetized individuals produces toxic by-products that may result in "halothane hepatitis" caused by massive hepatic necrosis. The possible adverse effects of waste anesthetic gas on the liver were revealed by a study showing that the risk of liver disease in hospital operating room personnel is 1.5 times that of the general population. However, it is difficult to say with certainty whether the increased incidence of liver disease is associated with exposure to waste anesthetic gas or results from other occupational hazards.

Renal effects

It is well established that methoxyflurane has the potential to cause renal toxicity in humans anesthetized with this agent, but the risk to operating room personnel has been more difficult to assess. Studies have indicated that there is a 1.2- to 1.4-fold increase in renal disease in female operating room personnel and a 1.2- to 1.7-fold increase in renal disease in female dental assistants compared to the general population. It has not been determined whether this increase is the result of the effect of methoxyflurane, nitrous oxide, other anesthetic agents, or other occupational factors working alone or in combination.

Neurologic effects

Because the mechanism of action of anesthetic agents involves their effect on neurons, various studies have investigated the effect of waste anesthetic gas on the central nervous system. Chronic exposure to nitrous oxide has been associated with increased risk of neurologic disease: a study of female dental assistants exposed to high levels of nitrous oxide showed them to have a 1.7- to 2.8-fold increase in the incidence of neurologic diseases compared to the normal population. Dentists and dental assistants exposed to high levels of waste nitrous oxide reported muscle weakness, tingling sensations, and numbness. It appears likely that exposure to high levels of anesthetics produces a decline in performance of motor skills and short-term memory. However, the threshold at which they begin to affect performance has not been established.

Assessment of risk

Despite the alarming list of potential health hazards, the average veterinary technician working in a veterinary clinic is not necessarily at high risk. It is difficult to determine a clear-cut assessment of risk for several reasons:

- Caution must be used in interpreting the epidemiologic evidence provided by these studies. The evidence produced by various studies (or within one study) is sometimes contradictory. For example, some studies have failed to show any association between the incidence of spontaneous abortion or congenital abnormalities and a history of exposure to waste gas, whereas other studies suggest the opposite.
- Although many epidemiologic studies indicate an increased incidence of health problems in people working in an environment where exposure to waste gas occurs, it does not necessarily follow that the anesthetic gases themselves are the causative agents. Other chemicals or other factors present in the operating room or dentist's office may contribute to increased incidence of health disorders.

• Many studies into the adverse effects of waste anesthetic gases did not measure the level of waste gas present in the working environment. Epidemiologic studies do not give information regarding the use of scavengers and procedures that reduce waste gas pollution. Without this information, interpretation of the studies is difficult.

Despite the difficulties noted here, most authorities and regulatory agencies agree that exposure to high levels of waste anesthetic gas should be avoided and that controls should be introduced to reduce exposure. The safe level of anesthetic gas in the working environment has not yet been determined. After reviewing the available literature, the U.S. National Institute for Occupational Safety and Health (NIOSH) recommended that the concentration of halothane, methoxyflurane, or isoflurane not exceed 2 parts per million (ppm) when used alone and not exceed 0.5 ppm when used with nitrous oxide. (The concentration at which the odor of halothane can be detected by the average person is 50 ppm or more, which is 25 times the maximum recommended level.) It is also suggested the nitrous oxide concentration not exceed 25 ppm. These levels were chosen because they were believed to be the lowest levels realistically achievable given current technology. The NIOSH levels have been adopted by most state and provincial regulatory bodies.

Surveys of veterinary hospitals reveal a wide variation in the level of waste anesthetic gas present in different locations within the clinic (Tables 5-1 and 5-2). As expected, air samples taken from surgery suites, surgical preparation rooms,

TABLE 5-1

Waste anesthetic gas (halothane) concentrations in various locations within the veterinary hospital (semiclosed circuit, <1 L/minute oxygen flow)

Sampling site	Level of contamination (ppm)
Personnel breathing zone	
With scavenging	1.45
No scavenging	2.00
Nose and mouth of patient just removed from anesthetic	
chamber	>10
Air around unscavenged anesthetic chamber	>10
Nose and mouth of anesthetized patient	
Intubated, cuff inflated	3.25
Intubated, cuff not inflated	6.10
Air outside recovery cage door	1.07
Nose of patient in recovery cage	5.43

Modified from Short CE, Harvey RC: Anesthetic waste gases in veterinary medicine, *Cornell Vet* 73(4):363-374, 1983.

TABLE 5-2

Sources of anesthetic gas contamination

Technique or situation	Level of contamination (ppm)
Room air when filling vaporizer	>10
Reservoir bag emptied into room air	2.5->10
Room air after spill of agent	>10
Hands of personnel filling vaporizer	2.5->10
After washing	0
Clothing of personnel filling vaporizer	5.0-8.75
Residues in unwashed rubber components	1.8->10

Modified from Short CE, Harvey RC: Anesthetic waste gases in veterinary medicine, *Cornell Vet* 73(4):363-374, 1983.

and anesthetic recovery rooms are more likely to contain waste gas than samples taken elsewhere in the clinic. During the anesthetic period itself, the level of waste gas is highest immediately adjacent to the anesthetic machine, but the actual level varies with the duration of anesthesia, the flow rate of the carrier gas, the type of anesthetic system used (rebreathing or nonrebreathing), and most importantly, whether an effective scavenging system is used. The halothane concentration in the air of unscavenged surgery suites in human hospitals has been reported to be as high as 85 ppm, and concentrations of nitrous oxide have been measured as high as 7000 ppm. In contrast, a more recent (1981) survey of veterinary hospitals indicated that levels of waste anesthetic gas in unscavenged veterinary surgeries were much lower than those reported in human hospitals, ranging from 1 to 21 ppm.

Reducing exposure to waste anesthetic gas

Given the potential health hazards associated with exposure to waste anesthetic gas, it is obviously in the technician's best interest to minimize exposure as much as possible. If proper equipment, techniques, and procedures are used, it is possible to reduce waste gas exposure to a level well below the NIOSH standards. This can be achieved through several means: using a gas scavenging system, testing equipment for leaks, and practicing techniques and procedures that minimize exposure to waste gas.

Use of a scavenging system

The installation and use of an effective gas scavenging system is the single most important step in reducing waste gas exposure. A 1982 survey of veterinary hospitals showed that scavenging reduces waste halothane concentrations by 64% to

94%. A scavenger consists of tubing attached to the anesthetic machine pop-off valve (or in the case of a nonrebreathing system, to the outlet port or tail of the reservoir bag). The function of a scavenger is to collect waste gas from the machine and conduct it to a disposal point outside the building.

Scavenging systems may be passive or active (Figs. 5-1 and 5-2). An active system uses suction created by a vacuum pump or fan to draw gas into the scavenger, whereas a passive system uses gravity and the positive pressure of the gas in the anesthetic machine to push gas into the scavenger. Both active and passive scavenging systems appear to be effective when correctly assembled and operated. The most efficient system, however, appears to be an active one with a dedicated vacuum pump.

Normally, use of a scavenging system with an anesthetic machine does not alter the operation of the machine. The anesthetist should, however, be aware of two potential difficulties that can occur when a scavenging system is present.

1. When using an active scavenging system, it is important to prevent the negative pressure (vacuum) from the scavenger from entering the breathing circuit. If this is allowed to occur, the reservoir bag will collapse and suction may be transmit-

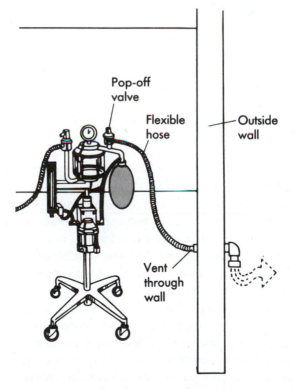

Fig. 5-1. Passive scavenging system.

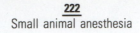

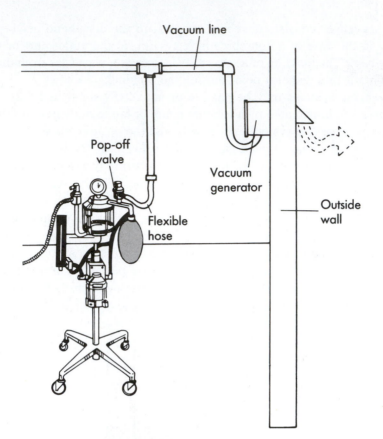

Fig. 5-2. Active scavenging system.

ted to the patient's lungs. Many machines are equipped with a negative pressure relief valve adjacent to the pop-off valve, which opens automatically if negative pressure is detected in the circuit. The open valve admits room air to the circuit, thereby ensuring that a vacuum does not develop. When using a machine that is not equipped with a negative pressure relief valve, it is important to ensure that the reservoir bag is at least partially inflated with air at all times.

2. Regardless of whether a passive or an active scavenging system is in use, the anesthetist must be aware of the potential for blockage of the entry of waste gas into the system. If a blockage of this type occurs, gas will accumulate within the anesthetic circuit. This situation is analogous to operation of a machine with a closed pop-off valve and may result in excessive pressure developing within the circuit. To prevent this occurrence, many machines are equipped with a positive pressure relief valve, which opens automatically if excessive pressure starts to build within the circuit.

It is not difficult to assemble an effective scavenging system in a veterinary hospital. Scavenger parts may be purchased or can be readily assembled using simple materials. The hose or tubing of the scavenger may be constructed from plastic tubing, PVC pipe, or other flexible, gas impermeable material. Most modern anesthesia machines are equipped with adapters to allow connection to a scavenging system. Older machines can be retrofitted with pop-off valves that can be connected to a scavenger hose.

The most commonly used type of passive system discharges waste gas to the outdoors through a hole in the wall. Another type of passive system can be set up by placing the end of the transfer hose adjacent to the room ventilation exhaust or nonrecirculating air conditioning system. This is acceptable provided the air is not recirculated within the building and the transfer hose is no more than 10 feet in length. Since anesthetic vapors are heavier than room air, the transfer hose should travel a downward course toward the exhaust.

Once the waste gas is collected, it must be expelled outside of the building. Waste gas collected in the tubing should be totally confined within the scavenger hose from the pop-off valve to the point of discharge and must not be recirculated into the building air. Scavenger hoses that end on the floor of a room, in an attic or basement, or that conduct the waste gas into a recirculating central vacuum system or recirculating ventilation exhaust merely contaminate all building rooms with the waste gas.

Regardless of whether an active or passive system is used, the anesthetist must be able to connect an anesthetic machine or anesthetic chamber to a scavenger in every room in which the machines are used. In some circumstances in which the installation of scavenging equipment is not practical, waste gas absorption may be achieved through the use of activated charcoal cartridges. In order to be effective, however, these cartridges must be replaced after 12 hours of use. An additional drawback of these units is their inability to filter nitrous oxide.

Equipment leak testing

Although the installation of a scavenging device is the most important step in reducing anesthetic gas pollution, there are many other procedures and techniques that significantly reduce the anesthetist's risk of exposure. One of these is leak testing of anesthetic machines. Leakage of gas from anesthetic machines is a significant source of operating room pollution and it is *not* reduced by a scavenging system. Leakage may occur from any part of the machine in which nitrous oxide or gas anesthetic (methoxyflurane, isoflurane, halothane) is present. The potential sites for leakage include:

• Connections for nitrous oxide gas lines
• O rings, washers, and other seals joining nitrous oxide gas tanks to the machine hanger yokes

- Connection between the flowmeter and the vaporizer
- Unidirectional valves
- Carbon dioxide absorber canisters (Often leaks are caused by improper positioning of the canister or by the presence of absorber granules on the seals around the canister.)
- Holes in the reservoir bag or hoses
- Pop-off valves
- Connection sites of the hoses, reservoir bag, or endotracheal tube

The anesthetist should routinely perform leak tests to determine the presence and location of waste gas leaks. There are two types of tests:

1. High pressure tests for nitrous oxide or oxygen leakage. High pressure leaks arise between the nitrous oxide tank and the flowmeter, in which the pressure is 50 pounds per square inch (psi) or greater.
2. Low pressure tests for the escape of anesthetic gas from the anesthetic machine itself. The pressure of gas within the machine is approximately 15 psi. Low pressure leaks may arise between the flowmeter and the patient, or within the anesthetic circuit and attachments.

High pressure system tests. One test of the high pressure system is to turn the nitrous oxide tank on and place a 10% detergent solution on all tank connections and joints. Each location is then observed for bubble formation, which would indicate a leak.

Another useful high pressure test is conducted by first turning on the nitrous oxide cylinder, noting the reading on the tank pressure gauge, and then turning the cylinder off. Throughout this procedure the flowmeter is set to zero, maintaining the pressure in the system (i.e., line pressure is not evacuated). The tank pressure gauge should be checked again in 1 hour. If the pressure gauge reading is unchanged, the high pressure system is leak-free. If the pressure is at or near zero, there is a leak somewhere between the cylinder and the flowmeter, and nitrous oxide is escaping into the room air. The most likely location of the leak is at the connection of the cylinder to the machine yoke.

It is also possible to check for high pressure leaks of oxygen by following the same procedure as that outlined for the nitrous oxide. Although the escape of small amounts of oxygen obviously poses little or no health problems to the anesthetic machine operator, it may lead to premature emptying of the oxygen tank.

Low pressure system tests. Low pressure leaks are best detected by securing all connections, closing the pop-off valve, and placing a hand over the Y piece, thus closing off all avenues of gas escape from the machine. The oxygen tank is turned on and the flowmeter is adjusted to supply a flow rate of at least 2 L/minute, and the reservoir bag is allowed to gradually fill with oxygen. The anesthetist should be able to squeeze the inflated bag with significant pressure without causing escape of air from the bag. Since the only exits from the system (the pop-off valve and the Y piece) are closed, any escape of air indicates that a leak is present. Alternatively, the anesthetist can close the pop-off valve and occlude the Y piece and use the pressure manometer and the oxygen flowmeter to adjust the oxygen flow such that a circuit pressure of 30 cm of water for 30 seconds is maintained. If the oxygen flow required is over 200 ml/minute, there is significant leakage from the machine. The location of leaks may be determined by listening for the hiss of escaping air or by using a detergent solution as previously described.

High pressure leak testing should be performed at least weekly if nitrous oxide is in use. Low pressure leak testing should be done every time the machine is assembled. If leaks are detected that cannot be resolved by the technician, the machine should be serviced by a manufacturer's representative or other qualified person.

Anesthetic techniques and procedures

The anesthetist, by his or her choice of anesthetic techniques, has considerable control over the amount of waste gas released into the room air. Faulty work practices were found to account for 94% to 99% of waste anesthetic gas released in scavenged operating rooms in one survey of human hospitals.

The following procedures are recommended in order to minimize waste gas release:

- Use caution when inducing an animal in an anesthetic chamber. Anesthetic chambers were the greatest source of anesthetic pollution noted in a 1983 survey of veterinary facilities. Not only are large amounts of waste gas released when the chamber is opened, but also the fur of the patient is saturated with anesthetic gases. If a chamber is used, a scavenging system should be connected to it, and anesthetic gas in the chamber should be evacuated before the animal is removed from the chamber. The chamber should be washed with soap and water after each use to remove residual anesthetic.

- Avoid using masks to maintain anesthesia. Significant amounts of anesthetic gas may escape from around the diaphragm of the mask, entering the room air. If the situation dictates the use of a mask, it should be fitted tightly over the animal's face and the animal should be intubated as soon as an appropriate depth is reached.

- Use cuffed endotracheal tubes, when possible. Endotracheal tubes significantly reduce the escape of waste gas into room air, as compared to masks. To be effective, however, the tube must be of adequate size, and the cuff must be inflated and in good repair. Prior to use, inflate cuffs with air to check for leaks. After intubation of the patient and cuff inflation, check the fit of the endotracheal tube within the trachea by closing the pop-off valve and gently squeezing the reservoir bag. If a loud hiss is heard, the cuff should be inflated further or a larger endotracheal tube should be selected. To prevent overinflation of the patient's lungs, ensure that the circuit pressure displayed on the manometer does not exceed 20 cm of water when applying pressure to the bag to check the cuff.

- When using a rebreathing system, ensure that the reservoir bag inflates and deflates regularly with the patient's respirations. If this does not occur, one should suspect either an air leakage around the endotracheal tube or esophageal intubation. Significant release of waste gas can occur in both cases. (It is also likely that the patient will wake up, since a significant amount of room air enters the lungs in either case.)

- The use of closed rebreathing systems may help to minimize waste gas pollution. Anesthesia using open systems and high gas flows (greater than 3 L/minute) is associated with greater release of waste gas, particularly if effective scavenging is not available.

- Do not turn on the vaporizer or nitrous oxide flowmeter until the anesthetic machine is connected to the endotracheal tube and the cuff is inflated. The practice of filling the machine and reservoir bag with anesthetic gas before connecting the machine to the patient is discouraged.

- Once the anesthetic procedure is under way, avoid disconnecting the patient from the breathing circuit unnecessarily. If the patient is to be disconnected from the machine, the vaporizer setting should be turned to zero.

- Do not release the contents of the reservoir bag into the room air. If it is necessary to empty the reservoir bag, leave it attached to the machine and evacuate the contents into the scavenger.

- Maintain the connection between the animal and the machine, having the animal breathe pure oxygen, for several minutes after the vaporizer is turned off. This allows expired anesthetic to enter the scavenging system rather than the room air.

- Be sure all rooms in which anesthetic gases are released (prep room, operating room, recovery room, radiography room, etc.) have adequate ventilation, providing at least 15 air changes per hour.

- Have anesthetic machines serviced annually or biannually to ensure minimal leakage through machine components.

- Inspect equipment frequently. Hoses, reservoir bags, and endotracheal tubes that are cracked or worn should be discarded. Endotracheal tubes with nonfunctional or leaking cuffs should not be used.

- Wash hoses, reservoir bags, masks, endotracheal tubes, and all other rubber components of the anesthetic circuit with soap and water and allow them to air dry after each procedure. These components may absorb considerable amounts of anesthetic during use. Washing not only removes absorbed waste gas, but also reduces transfer of microorganisms between patients.

- Fill vaporizers in a well-ventilated area (ideally, outside of the building). If vaporizers are filled inside the building, the procedure is best done just before leaving work in the evening. Emptying and filling vaporizers may release significant amounts of anesthetic vapor into the surrounding air. Anesthetics also may be spilled onto the technician's hands and clothing (see Table 5-2). Using a funnel or other filling device can help avoid spills. Use of an approved respirator, gloves, and other protective equipment will also minimize exposure to anesthetic liquid or vapors. If gloves are not worn, hands should be washed immediately after filling a vaporizer, since liquid anesthetics are readily absorbed through intact skin.

• If liquid anesthetic is spilled, high concentrations of anesthetic vapor will be present in the immediate area of the spill. Accidental spillage of even 1 ml of liquid anesthetic will vaporize up to 200 ml of gas with a concentration of 1,000,000 ppm. If a spill occurs, increase ventilation as much as possible during the cleanup, by opening windows or using fans. All personnel not involved in the cleanup should leave the area, and the remaining staff should wear approved respirators, protective clothing, and gloves. Remove all contaminated articles (including lab coats). Pour absorbent material such as kitty litter on the spill, such that the liquid is completely absorbed. Dispose of the litter in an airtight container, preferably outside the clinic. If the spill is large or if protective equipment is not available, all personnel should leave the building and the local fire department should be notified.

• Cap empty anesthetic bottles when discarding them, because residual anesthetic in the bottle may evaporate into the room air. Store vaporizer filling devices between uses in a sealed plastic bag.

Monitoring waste gas levels

It is possible to periodically monitor waste anesthetic gas levels to ensure that the NIOSH levels are not exceeded. If professional monitoring is required, an occupational hygienist may visit the hospital to evaluate ventilation and scavenging techniques and to interview the anesthetist regarding procedures used to minimize waste gas release. Air samples should be collected from all areas in which anesthetics are used, and the level of waste gas in the collected air should be determined using an infrared spectrometer. The cost of such a visit varies between $250 and $700.

It is also possible for clinic employees to monitor waste gas levels using detector tubes or badges. Badges may detect only one chemical, such as halothane, isoflurane, or nitrous oxide, or may be sensitive to all halogenated anesthetics. The badges are worn by personnel in the operating room during a timed period when anesthetic gases are being used. Alternatively, the badge may be placed in a room for area monitoring. After use, the badge is returned to the supplier (usually an industrial health and safety supply house or a company specializing in OSHA compliance) for analysis. Results are given as a time-weighted average in parts per million. Cost, including analysis, is approximately $40 to $50 per badge.

WHMIS CONSIDERATIONS

The Workplace Hazardous Materials Information System (WHMIS) is intended to ensure that staff working in veterinary hospitals and other workplaces are aware of the dangers associated with the use of certain chemicals and take appropriate precautions with their use. Chemicals and gases used in anesthesia that are covered by WHMIS regulations include carbon dioxide absorber (soda lime and bara lime), nitrous oxide, and oxygen. In some jurisdictions, potentially hazardous pharmaceuticals, such as xylazine and halothane, are also covered by WHMIS regulations.

WHMIS materials are subject to certain requirements, although these may vary with state and provincial regulations. The requirements generally include the following:

- All staff handling these materials must be made aware of the hazards associated with their use, including dangers associated with inhalation, ingestion, eye contact, and skin contact with the materials.
- Staff must be trained in the safe use of WHMIS materials, including the use of protective equipment such as respirators, where applicable. The employer must provide appropriate safety equipment and training in its use.
- The veterinary hospital must have on hand a material safety data sheet (MSDS) for each WHMIS chemical that is used on the premises. These sheets are provided by the companies that supply the WHMIS materials. MSDS sheets must be collected and made available for staff use at all times. The information contained on the sheets includes details on toxicity, procedures for cleaning up accidental spills and emissions, and handling precautions.
- WHMIS materials are subject to special regulations regarding labeling and hazard warnings. These labels are provided by the supplier for use on the original container. If the material is taken out of the original container, it may be necessary to devise a new label, called a workplace label. This label must include at minimum the following information: the name of the substance, the chief hazards associated with its use, and the statement that a MSDS is available.

Although it is the employer's responsibility to provide all necessary safety equipment and to train staff in the safe handling of WHMIS materials, the employee should make every effort to familiarize himself or herself with the hazards associated with the use of WHMIS materials and pharmaceuticals in the hospital and to use these materials with care. For example, xylazine has the potential to cause abortion and can be absorbed through the skin. The pregnant technician is well advised to use care in handling this material.

In the case of oxygen and nitrous oxide, the hazards are briefly outlined below. Further information on these and other WHMIS materials can be obtained by consulting the appropriate material safety data sheet.

SAFE HANDLING OF COMPRESSED GASES

Oxygen and nitrous oxide are classified as WHMIS (Workplace Hazardous Materials Information System) substances in some jurisdictions, and gas cylinders are supplied with WHMIS labels.

WHMIS information: oxygen

It is unlikely that the anesthetist would be exposed to sufficient concentrations of oxygen to be at risk of oxygen toxicity. However, prolonged exposure to high concentrations of oxygen have been reported to cause cramps, nausea, dizziness, hypothermia, blindness, respiratory difficulties, bradycardia, fainting spells, and convulsions capable of leading to death.

WHMIS information: nitrous oxide

As previously mentioned, chronic low-level exposure to nitrous oxide gas may be associated with significant health problems. Inhalation of high levels of nitrous oxide over a short time may be hazardous also, since dizziness, nausea, and unconsciousness may result. Giddiness also may result from inhalation of nitrous oxide, and this agent is commonly known as ''laughing gas.'' These effects are thought to arise in part because nitrous oxide inhalation prevents an adequate supply of oxygen from reaching the brain.

Use and storage of compressed gas cylinders

Oxygen and nitrous oxide are not flammable; however, both support combustion and should not be used in the same room as an open flame. It is recommended that no sources of ignition (matches, lighters, Bunsen burners, etc.) be present in any room in which oxygen or nitrous oxide cylinders are stored or used. Smoking must be prohibited in all rooms in which oxygen is stored or used. Even static electricity can cause fires in areas in which oxygen and flammable materials are used together. (This is one of the reasons that ether, which is extremely flammable, is no longer used in anesthesia.)

Cylinders containing compressed air should be handled with great care, because pressurized gas may be dangerous if suddenly released. It is foolish to attempt to stop a high pressure leak of gas with hand pressure because serious injury may result.

Explosion or sudden release of gas may occur if a cylinder is damaged or knocked over and the regulator (pressure-reducing valve) detaches from the tank. The force of the gas escaping from the tank may cause the tank to move in a rocket-like fashion through walls and other objects. To prevent this occurrence, large cylinders should be chained or belted to a wall and should always be stored in an upright position. To protect the regulator from damage, valve caps should be used on all large cylinders that are not connected to gas lines.

Gas cylinders should be stored away from emergency exits or areas with heavy traffic. If a cylinder must be moved to another location, a hand cart should be used, rather than simply rolling the cylinder.

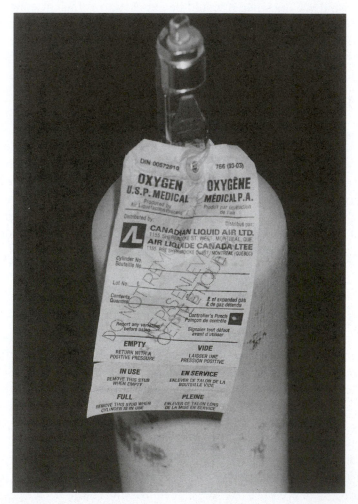

Fig. 5-3. Label for compressed gas tanks. Current status of tank is shown by printing at the bottom of the label. Label shown is from newly purchased tank and reads "FULL." When tank is connected to machine, lower portion of the label is removed, such that remaining label reads "IN USE." When tank is empty, "IN USE" stub is removed, leaving the label that reads "EMPTY."

Full tanks should be kept separate from empty tanks and also should be clearly labeled for quick identification. The use of tear-off labels helps eliminate confusion regarding the empty, in-use, or full status of a given compressed air cylinder. In reading these labels, the current status of the tank is given on the outermost section of the label (Fig. 5-3). Cylinders should be used in the order that they are received (i.e., first in, first out).

KEY POINTS

1. Anesthesia presents several potential health risks to hospital personnel, including exposure to waste anesthetic gas, use of chemicals controlled by WHMIS regulations, and handling of compressed gas cylinders.

2. Waste anesthetic gas vapors are breathed by all personnel working in areas in which animals are anesthetized or recovering from inhalation anesthesia. Filling or emptying vaporizers and cleanup of accidental spills also may result in significant exposure.

3. Exposure to waste anesthetic gas is associated with short-term problems such as fatigue, headache, drowsiness, nausea, depression, and irritability.

4. Long-term exposure to waste anesthetic gases may be associated with reproductive disorders, liver and kidney damage, and nervous system dysfunction. The evidence of epidemiologic studies is sometimes contradictory and difficult to interpret. Most authorities recommend that exposure to high levels of waste anesthetic gas be avoided, particularly by pregnant women.

5. Anesthetics, such as methoxyflurane, that are eliminated significantly by hepatic metabolism and renal excretion are considered to be a greater hazard than anesthetics eliminated by respiration.

6. Waste anesthetic gases apparently do not have oncogenic (cancer-causing) effects.

7. The NIOSH recommendations for waste anesthetic gas concentrations limit exposure to 2 parts per million (ppm) or less for halothane, isoflurane, and methoxyflurane (0.5 ppm or less if nitrous oxide is concurrently used). Surveys of veterinary clinics show concentrations from 1 to 85 ppm, depending on the sampling site, scavenging system, and anesthetic techniques used.

8. Installation and use of an effective gas scavenging system greatly reduces waste gas exposure. Caution should be used to prevent negative pressure from the scavenger from entering the breathing circuit.

9. Equipment leak testing should be done on a daily basis to detect and allow correction of leakage from the anesthetic machine and compressed air cylinders. Tests should be done on both the high pressure and low pressure components of the machine, particularly if nitrous oxide is in use.

10. Certain anesthetic techniques are associated with excessive waste gas release, including use of anesthetic chambers, masks, and uncuffed endotracheal tubes. Procedures such as turning off the vaporizer before disconnecting the animal from the machine are helpful in reducing waste gas contamination of hospital air.

11. Vaporizers should be filled and emptied with care, using appropriate protective equipment.

12. Waste gas levels may be monitored by professional occupational hygienists or by the use of detector tubes or badges.

13. WHMIS materials used in the hospital are subject to special regulations and control to ensure the safety of persons handling them.

14. Compressed air cylinders should be transported, used, and stored with care. Special hazards include risk of fire in areas in which cylinders are stored and risk of sudden release of pressurized gas from cylinders.

REVIEW QUESTIONS

1. Waste anesthetic gases are a potential hazard to personnel, but problems that arise are really only of a short-term nature.
   True   False

2. Long-term toxicity of inhalation anesthetics is thought to be caused by the release of toxic metabolites during the breakdown of these drugs.
   True   False

3. The anesthetic thought to be the least toxic is:
   a. Isoflurane
   b. Halothane
   c. Methoxyflurane
   d. Nitrous oxide

4. In the United States, the National Institute for Occupational Safety and Health recommends that the levels of waste anesthetic gases for anesthetics such as isoflurane, halothane, or methoxyflurane should not exceed _____ ppm.
   a. 2
   b. 20
   c. 200
   d. 2000

5. The odor of halothane may be detected by a person when the levels reach
_____ ppm.
   a. 5
   b. 50
   c. 500
   d. 5000
6. Anesthetic gases are considered to be heaver than air.
   True   False
7. It is recommended that for a passive scavenger system, the hose be no longer than
_____ feet.
   a. 1.0
   b. 10
   c. 25
   d. 50
8. A test for low pressure leaks should be done:
   a. Each time the machine is used
   b. At least once per week
   c. At least once per month
   d. When the anesthetist smells anesthetic gases
9. The safest way to transport a high pressure tank, such as an oxygen tank, is by:
   a. Carrying it
   b. Rolling it along the floor
   c. A hand cart
   d. Dragging it by the neck
10. Rooms in which waste anesthetic gases are at risk of being released should have a
minimum of _____ air changes per hour.
   a. 5
   b. 10
   c. 15
   d. 20

For the following questions more than one answer may be correct.

11. Long-term hazards that may occur from exposure to anesthetic waste gases may
include:
   a. Reproductive disorders
   b. Liver damage
   c. Kidney damage
   d. Nervous system dysfunction
12. A technician may reduce the amount of waste gases by:
   a. Using cuffed endotracheal tubes
   b. Ensuring the anesthetic machine has been tested for leaks
   c. Using an induction technique other than mask or chamber
   d. Using high fresh gas flows
13. To conduct a low pressure test on an anesthetic machine, you must:
   a. Close the pop-off valve and occlude the end of the circuit
   b. Pressurize the circuit with a volume of gas
   c. Compress the reservoir bag
   d. Turn off the oxygen tank

ANSWERS FOR CHAPTER 5

1. False   **2.** True   **3.** a   **4.** a   **5.** b   **6.** True   **7.** b   **8.** a   **9.** c
10. c   **11.** a, b, c, d   **12.** a, b, c   **13.** a, b, c

SELECTED READINGS

Ad Hoc Committee of the American Society of Anesthesiologists: Occupational disease among O.R. personnel: a study, *Anesthesiology* 41:321-340, 1974.

Gross ME, Branson KR: Reducing exposure to waste anesthetic gas, *Vet Tech* 14(3):175-177, 1993.

Harvey RC: *Anesthetic waste gas management in veterinary medicine,* Knoxville, 1991, University of Tennessee, (unpublished).

Lietzemayer DW: Current methods for removal of anesthetic gas, *Vet Tech* 11(4):213-220, 1990.

Paddleford RR: *Manual of small animal anesthesia,* New York, 1988, Churchill Livingstone.

Purdham JT: *Anaesthetic gases and vapours,* Hamilton, Ontario, Canada, 1986, Canadian Centre for Occupational Health and Safety.

Short CE: *Principles and practice of veterinary anesthesia,* Baltimore, 1987, Williams & Wilkins.

Short CE, Harvey RC: Anesthetic waste gases in veterinary medicine, *Cornell Vet* 73(4):363-374, 1983.

Anesthetic problems and emergencies

6

PERFORMANCE OBJECTIVES
After completion of this chapter, the reader will be able to:

Give reasons why anesthetic emergencies occur, including problems arising from human error, equipment failure, adverse effects of anesthetic agents, and variations in patient status and breed.

Describe ways in which errors in anesthetic administration may be prevented or corrected.

Explain the role that the veterinary technician can take in emergency care.

Explain the appropriate action to be taken in response to common emergencies, including cardiac arrest and respiratory arrest.

General anesthesia is not a high-risk procedure in most patients, when performed by capable personnel using an anesthetic protocol appropriate to the animal. Emergencies are uncommon, and the overwhelming majority of patients recover from anesthesia with no lasting ill effects. A survey of British veterinary clinics revealed a mortality rate of 1 death for every 870 anesthetic procedures in healthy dogs and 1 death for every 552 procedures in healthy cats. Mortality rates for dogs or cats with systemic disease was approximately 1 to 30 patients.

After successfully anesthetizing hundreds of patients, it is easy for the technician to be lulled into a false sense of security. However, it is vitally important that the anesthetist remembers that every anesthetic procedure has the potential to cause the death of the animal. The anesthetist must remain watchful for problems that may arise in even the most routine anesthetic procedure.

The focus of this chapter is anesthetic problems, ranging from minor (such as maintaining appropriate anesthetic depth) to major, including respiratory arrest and cardiac arrest. Appropriate responses to various anesthetic emergencies are presented, and the reasons the anesthetic problems may arise (and procedures for their prevention) are emphasized. The challenges associated with anesthesia of patients with special problems such as heart disease or brachycephalic conformation are also discussed.

CAUSES OF ANESTHETIC PROBLEMS AND EMERGENCIES

Although an awareness of the correct response to an anesthetic emergency is essential, it is even more important to understand why emergencies arise and how they may be prevented. Most anesthetic emergencies are the result of one or more of the following factors: human error, equipment failure, adverse effect of anesthetic agents, and patient variation factors.

Human error

Human error is unfortunately a contributing factor in some anesthetic deaths. No anesthetist is immune to error, but in general it is not the beginning anesthetist or very experienced anesthetist (both of whom tend to be very cautious) who encounters anesthetic emergencies. More often, it is the technician with a small amount of experience and a great deal of self-confidence who runs into trouble. In aviation, this has been documented as the ''200 hour syndrome,'' as airplane pilots suffer the greatest accident rates when they have between 150 and 200 hours of experience.

The most common human errors committed by anesthetists are a failure to obtain an adequate history or physical examination on the patient, inadequate experience with the anesthetic machine or anesthetic agents being used, failure to devote sufficient time or attention to the anesthetized patient, fatigue, and failure to recognize and respond to early signs of patient difficulty.

Failure to obtain an adequate history or to perform an adequate physical examination

Ideally, a complete physical examination and a thorough history should be obtained. In practice, this is not always possible. Animals are sometimes dropped off at the veterinary clinic by owners who are in a hurry and are reluctant to stop to answer questions about their pet. Animals may be brought in by neighbors or friends of the owner who are unfamiliar with the animal's history. The receptionist or other person admitting the animal to the hospital may fail to ask important questions or may not transmit the information to the anesthetist or veterinarian. The physical examination is sometimes cursory or omitted entirely. The net result is that significant information may be overlooked. For example, the anesthetist may be unaware that a patient has not been fasted or that an animal scheduled for surgery is dehydrated due to vomiting and diarrhea. An anesthetic protocol that is safe for a healthy patient could be inappropriate for these animals, and an anesthetic problem or even death of the patient could result.

Lack of familiarity with the anesthetic machine or drugs being used

It is the responsibility of the veterinarian to ensure that his or her personnel are sufficiently trained and knowledgeable to perform competently all required procedures. Some simple anesthetic tasks, such as adjusting a vaporizer setting, can be done by unskilled personnel working under a veterinarian's direct supervision. More demanding tasks, such as induction of anesthesia and monitoring of anesthetized patients, are best assigned only to personnel (veterinarians or technicians) who have sufficient training, knowledge, and experience to recognize abnormalities and danger signals and who can respond appropriately.

Incorrect administration of drugs

Most anesthetic agents have a narrow margin of safety between therapeutic and toxic doses. Incorrect administration of drugs may arise in several ways, any of which may have fatal results. These errors include:

- Failure to weigh the patient and calculate an accurate dose
- Mathematical errors (particularly decimal errors, which can result in a 10× or 100× error in the amount of drug given)
- Use of the wrong medication (i.e., calculating a dose of acetylpromazine and drawing up xylazine instead)
- Use of the wrong concentration of a medication. This is a common problem with drugs that are available in several different concentrations (atropine, acetylpro-

mazine). Obviously, the concentration used in calculating the dose must be the same as that drawn up into the syringe.

• Administration of anesthetics by the incorrect route (e.g., administration of the intramuscular dose of ketamine by the intravenous route)

• Confusion between syringes drawn up for two different patients, involving either a failure to label the syringes or a failure to read the labels correctly

Personnel who are preoccupied or in a hurry

Although efficiency is desirable in any anesthetic procedure, it is not necessary or advisable that the anesthetist feel hurried. A technician who is feeling rushed is more likely to inject barbiturates perivascularly or insert an endotracheal tube into the esophagus. Unfortunately, it is common for the technician working in a busy practice to feel pressured and distracted. The technician responsible for anesthesia may be simultaneously called on to restrain patients for examination or procedures, answer the phone, perform laboratory tests, take radiographs, discharge animals, clean soiled kennels, and similar tasks. However, when an animal is anesthetized, the technician's top priority must be monitoring that patient, as failure to satisfactorily perform this duty may result in the death of the animal. Although the technician may not have the luxury of being constantly by the animal's side throughout the procedure, the anesthetist should return to check the patient at least every 5 minutes or more frequently if the patient's status requires close monitoring. If necessary, other tasks must be temporarily set aside to allow the anesthetist to return to the patient.

Fatigue

Fatigue is an ailment common to many veterinarians and technicians, particularly at the end of a busy day. Anesthetic emergencies may arise when personnel are tired and less alert than normal, possibly because minor problems that occur are not detected and corrected at an early stage. If possible, surgeries that are lengthy or difficult should be scheduled early in the day.

Inattentiveness

One of the most serious human errors in anesthesia is failure to monitor and recognize danger signals. It is obviously better for the patient and easier for the anesthetist if anesthetic problems are detected and addressed early, rather than late. For example, an animal experiencing respiratory depression while under an inhalation anesthetic will show a gradually decreasing respiratory rate, from 12 breaths per minute to 8 breaths per minute (at which point the anesthetist should consider adjusting the vaporizer to a lower setting), then from 8 breaths per minute to 4 (at which point the vaporizer should be turned off and the animal bagged with oxygen), then from 4 breaths per minute to 0 (at which point cardiac arrest is likely to occur).

The anesthetist's attitude toward patient care is a key factor in the safety of anesthesia. The conscientious anesthetist will frequently monitor the animal to assure himself or herself that the patient is not in trouble. The best attitude is one of low-level anxiety, which is relieved only when a quick examination of the patient reveals that all vital signs are within acceptable limits.

Equipment failure

Equipment failure is an uncommon cause of anesthetic emergencies, but it does occur. In many cases, failure of the anesthetic machine is, in fact, a failure of the operator to maintain and monitor the machine properly. The importance of a preanesthetic check of the anesthetic machine, as described in Chapter 4, cannot be overemphasized.

The following anesthetic machine problems are occasionally encountered in routine anesthesia.

Carbon dioxide absorber exhaustion

Patients on a rebreathing system rely on the carbon dioxide absorber to remove expired CO_2 from the circuit, preventing inhalation of excessive levels of this toxic gas. If CO_2 is not removed from the circuit, the patient will experience hypercarbia (elevated blood CO_2). Signs of this disorder include tachypnea (rapid respiration), tachycardia, and cardiac dysrhythmias. Examination of the CO_2 absorber crystals will reveal an obvious color change, if exhaustion has occurred.

Empty oxygen tank

Failure to deliver oxygen to the patient is one of the most serious and yet one of the most easily prevented mistakes that an anesthetist can make. The oxygen tank pressure and flowmeter should be checked every 5 minutes during anesthesia. The anesthetist must ensure that either oxygen or room air is continuously provided to the patient. If the oxygen flowmeter is to be turned off (e.g., when the patient and the machine are moved from a preparation room to surgery), the patient should be disconnected from the machine before the oxygen flow is stopped, particularly if a Bain circuit or similar nonrebreathing system is in use. If a circle system is in use, the reservoir bag should be full, since it allows several minutes of oxygen supply without fresh delivery by the flowmeter.

It is important to be able to recognize when the machine is no longer delivering oxygen to the patient. If the oxygen flowmeter reads zero flow, the system is not receiving any oxygen, regardless of the oxygen tank pressure. Occasionally, the situation arises in which the oxygen tank pressure gauge reads zero, but the flowmeter indicates some oxygen flow: in this case the tank is still delivering oxygen, but loss of oxygen pressure is imminent and the tank should be changed immediately.

The anesthetist must be aware of the proper response when oxygen delivery to the patient is stopped, whether because of machine malfunction or the tank running out of oxygen. If the oxygen flow stops (i.e., the flowmeter reads zero despite the efforts of the anesthetist to establish flow), the anesthetist should immediately disconnect the Y piece from the endotracheal tube, allowing the patient to breathe room air until the oxygen delivery is reestablished.

Misassembly of the anesthetic machine

It is essential that the person handling the anesthetic machine be familiar with every connection, hose, dial, and component of the machine. Before using an unfamiliar machine, the anesthetist should take a few minutes to examine it carefully for the location of the controls and to understand the direction and path of gas flow within the machine. Every time a connection, such as a Bain circuit, is added or removed, the anesthetist must trace the flow of gas, ensuring that the correct pattern of flow is maintained and that all connections are secure.

Endotracheal tube problems

Although, strictly speaking, not a part of the anesthetic machine, the endotracheal tube is a critical component of the anesthetic delivery system and is subject to many problems. Endotracheal tubes may become blocked during anesthesia, cutting off the flow of anesthetic gas and oxygen to the patient. Blockages may be due to twisting or kinking of the tube, accumulation of material such as blood, mucus, or saliva within the tube, or inappropriate positioning of the tube (as may occur when the tip is advanced to the bifurcation of the trachea). Because endotracheal tube blockage (if complete) results in a cessation of oxygen flow to the patient, signs of dyspnea are seen, and eventually respiratory arrest may occur. The anesthetist usually becomes aware of the problem by observing the patient's exaggerated breathing pattern or by noting that the reservoir bag no longer inflates and deflates with the patient's respirations. If a problem is suspected, the anesthetist should quickly check the endotracheal tube function in two ways:
1. Attempt to bag the patient and note if the chest rises. If the endotracheal tube is blocked, no chest movement will be seen, and there will be considerable resistance to the passage of air into the patient.
2. Disconnect the animal from the machine, with the endotracheal tube still in place, and feel for air coming out of the tube. If no air movement is felt and dyspnea is apparent, a blockage may exist. In this case, the tube should be removed and a mask or other endotracheal tube used to deliver oxygen to the patient.

Vaporizer problems

A potentially disastrous problem can arise if the wrong anesthetic is put into a vaporizer. In particular, the inadvertent use of isoflurane or halothane in a nonprecision vaporizer designed for methoxyflurane may result in delivery of extremely high concentrations of anesthetic gas to the patient.

Occasionally, a vaporizer dial may stick or become jammed. If the dial cannot be adjusted, the patient should be transferred to another machine.

Pop-off valve problems

Occasionally, an anesthetist inadvertently leaves the pop-off valve in a closed position. If the oxygen flow rate is greater than the patient's requirement (in other words, a semiclosed or nonrebreathing system is being used and the oxygen flow rate is greater than the metabolic oxygen consumption, approximately 10 ml/kg/minute), pressure within the circuit will rapidly rise. The reservoir bag will expand, as will the patient's lungs. This may cause respiratory difficulty and also decrease the venous return to the heart. This, in turn, may decrease cardiac output and cause blood pressure to fall rapidly, leading to death within a short time. In extreme cases, alveolar rupture may occur.

To detect the problem at an early stage, the anesthetist should frequently monitor the reservoir bag size and attempt to maintain it no more than two-thirds full of gas during anesthesia. The reservoir bag size is easily adjusted by changing the oxygen flow rate or by opening or closing the pop-off valve.

Anesthetic agents

Each injectable or inhalation agent has the potential to harm a patient and, in some cases, cause death. Several strategies are used to reduce this potential:

- The anesthetic protocol must be chosen to reflect the special needs of the patient. For example, acetylpromazine is a poor preanesthetic for patients with low blood pressure, as this agent may cause vasodilation, further decreasing the blood pressure. Similarly, halothane is not the preferred inhalation agent for patients suffering from cardiac disease because of its potential to cause cardiac dysrhythmias. In each case, the veterinarian might choose to use an alternative agent.
- The anesthetist must be familiar with the adverse side effects and contraindications associated with the preanesthetic and general anesthetic agents used in the hospital. For example, the anesthetist who administers xylazine should be aware of its potential to cause bradycardia, cardiac dysrhythmias, vomiting, bloating, abortion, and respiratory depression.
- Multidrug use to achieve balanced anesthesia can be safer than anesthesia using a single drug, provided that the dosages of the individual drugs are appropriately reduced. For example, the concentration of halothane needed to anesthetize an

animal is greatly reduced if the animal is premedicated with acetylpromazine and butorphanol, compared to an animal given halothane alone. If the same percent halothane concentration was used in both situations, the multidrug regimen could be very dangerous for the patient.

A detailed description of the pharmacology and physiologic effects of preanesthetic and general anesthetic agents is given in Chapter 1 (preanesthetic agents) and Chapter 3 (general anesthetic agents).

Patient variation factors

As discussed in Chapter 2, animals presented for anesthesia may be suffering from systemic abnormalities that considerably increase anesthetic risk. Patients with a preoperative status of class III or class IV are particularly difficult to anesthetize successfully. Challenging patients routinely encountered in veterinary practice include geriatric animals, neonates, brachycephalic animals, sighthounds, and obese animals. Cesarean delivery of puppies or kittens also places unique demands on the anesthetist as he or she must consider the response of both the dam and the offspring to anesthetic agents. Animals suffering from recent trauma may be presented for emergency surgery, and the anesthetist must be prepared to deal with shock, respiratory difficulties, and cardiac dysrhythmias in these patients. Animals with cardiac problems such as heartworm disease or congestive heart failure may require anesthesia for diagnostic or therapeutic procedures. Similarly, animals may require anesthesia despite the presence of renal or hepatic disease. Although a detailed discussion of the anesthetic challenges posed by these and other patients is beyond the scope of this book, it is desirable that the technician be familiar with some of the special problems encountered when anesthetizing these animals. These are summarized in Table 6-1.

Geriatric patients

A geriatric patient is one who has reached 75% of the average life expectancy for that species and breed. In these patients, function of critical organs, such as the heart, lungs, kidneys, and liver, is reduced compared to the healthy young patient. Geriatric animals have less functional reserve than do younger animals and a relatively poor response to stress. In addition, geriatric animals are frequently affected with degenerative disorders such as mitral valve insufficiency and resulting heart failure, diabetes mellitus, cancer, and chronic renal disease, all of which are of concern to the anesthetist. Because of the high incidence of health problems in these animals, the importance of a thorough history and physical examination cannot be overemphasized. Preoperative tests such as a blood chemistry panel, chest radiographs, and an electrocardiogram may be advisable for selected patients.

TABLE 6-1

Patient factors that increase anesthetic risk

Patient factor	Anesthetic problems encountered	Strategies used to decrease risk
Geriatric patients	Reduced organ function; poor response to stress; degenerative disorders common; increased risk of hyperthermia and overhydration	Reduce anesthetic dosages by 30%-50%; allow longer time for response to drugs; administer fluids at reduced rate; keep patient warm
Neonatal patients	Increased risk of hypothermia and overhydration; inefficient excretion of drugs; difficult intubation and intravenous catheterization	Avoid heat loss; avoid prolonged fasting; administer 5% dextrose IV at reduced rates; weigh accurately; dilute injectable drugs; reduce anesthetic dosages; inhalant agents preferred to injectable agents
Brachycephalic dogs	Conformational tendency toward airway obstruction; abnormally high vagal tone	Include anticholinergic in anesthetic protocol; preoxygenate; induce rapidly using IV agents; delay extubation; observe closely during recovery period
Sighthounds	Increased sensitivity to barbiturates	Use alternative agents
Obese animals	Accurate dosing is difficult; may have respiratory difficulties; difficult to maintain adequate depth of anesthesia	Dose according to ideal weight; preoxygenate; induce rapidly; assist ventilation; observe closely during recovery period
Cesarean patients	Dam: increased work load to heart; respiration may be compromised; increased tendency to vomit or regurgitate; increased risk of hemorrhage Offspring: anesthetic agents cross placenta and reduce respiratory and cardiovascular function	Dam: administer intravenous fluids; clip patient before induction; avoid dorsal recumbency; use lowest effective dose of general anesthetic; preoxygenate; avoid pentobarbital Offspring: use reversing agents and doxapram; administer oxygen by face mask; administer atropine for bradycardia
Trauma patients	Respiratory distress common; cardiac dysrhythmias seen for 72 hours after incident; shock and hemorrhage common; internal injuries often present	Stabilize before anesthesia; obtain thoracic radiographs and ECG; thorough physical examination for concurrent injuries

Continued.

TABLE 6-1, cont'd
Patient factors that increase anesthetic risk

Patient factor	Anesthetic problems encountered	Strategies used to decrease risk
Cardiovascular disease	Circulation is compromised; pulmonary edema common; increased tendency to develop dysrhythmias and tachycardia	Alleviate pulmonary edema with diuretics; preoxygenate for 5 minutes before induction; avoid agents that depress myocardium or cause dysrhythmias; avoid overhydration
Respiratory disease	Poor oxygenation of tissues; patient may be anxious and difficult to restrain; respiratory arrest common	Avoid stress and unnecessary handling; preoxygenate; avoid nitrous oxide; induce with injectable agents; intubate rapidly and control ventilation if necessary; monitor closely during recovery
Hepatic disease	Delayed metabolism of anesthetic agents; decreased synthesis of blood clotting factors; may be hypoproteinemic; dehydration common; may be anemic and/or icteric	Preanesthetic blood chemistry tests; may omit preanesthetic medication; inhalation anesthetics preferred over injectable; expect prolonged recovery
Renal disease	Delayed excretion of anesthetic agents; electrolyte imbalances common including hyperkalemia, hyperphosphatemia, and metabolic acidosis; dehydration usually present	Rehydrate before surgery; obtain renal function tests and electrolyte values; reduce dosages of anesthetic agents; use caution with barbiturates; maintain on intraoperative and postoperative fluids
Urinary obstruction	Dehydration, acidosis, uremia, and hyperkalemia common; bradycardia may be present; stress may cause dysrhythmias and/or cardiac arrest	Inhalation agents or ketamine/diazepam preferred; use local analgesics in very depressed patients; treat for hyperkalemia if present

Geriatric animals typically have reduced anesthetic requirements, and doses of all anesthetic agents are often decreased by one half to one third compared to the healthy young patient. In the case of barbiturates, dose requirements may be as little as one twentieth of the normal dose. Response to drugs is slower, and the technician should allow 30 minutes to elapse after a subcutaneous injection before concluding that the injected drug has had no effect. Recovery from anesthesia also may be prolonged in geriatric animals, partly because of decreased renal and hepatic function (and hence, decreased ability to excrete drugs). These patients also have an increased tendency to develop hypothermia, as they have reduced ability to regulate body temperature.

The use of intravenous fluids is generally advocated in geriatrics, since they have less tolerance for hypotension and often a reduced ability to concentrate urine. Geriatric animals are at increased risk for developing overhydration problems such as pulmonary edema, however, and intravenous fluids should be given with care.

Neonatal patients

A veterinary patient under 3 months of age is generally considered to be at increased risk when anesthetized, compared to a mature animal. When working with these patients, the anesthetist must be aware of special considerations during preanesthesia, the anesthetic period, and recovery.

Preoperative fasting of the neonatal patient may be inadvisable, because hypoglycemia and dehydration can occur after even a short period of fasting. Oral fluids are usually allowed up to 1 hour before induction. Many veterinarians use 5% dextrose for intravenous fluid therapy of anesthetized neonates in an attempt to prevent hypoglycemia during surgery. The fluid administration rate should not exceed 5 ml/kg/hr unless shock or dehydration is present, because these animals are prone to overhydration if fluid administration is rapid. The use of pediatric minidrips (60 drips/ml) and a burette is helpful in preventing inadvertent overinfusion of fluid.

To calculate drug dosages, it is necessary to obtain an accurate weight. For animals weighing under 5 kg, a pediatric or lab animal scale gives more reliable weights than does a conventional scale. Injectable agents may require dilution, since otherwise the dose may be too small to measure or administer accurately.

The dose of injectable anesthetics given to neonatal animals is often one third to one half less than that for a mature animal, because very young animals have less plasma protein binding of drugs and lack an efficient mechanism to metabolize drugs within the liver. As a result, injectable anesthetic agents that require liver metabolism for inactivation (e.g., acetylpromazine, xylazine, or pentobarbital) can be expected to have a prolonged effect and should be avoided if possible. Renal function is also inefficient compared to the adult animal, and excretion of drugs by this route may be slow.

Many veterinarians prefer to anesthetize neonatal patients with inhalant agents, such as isoflurane, because administration and elimination of these agents are accomplished through the respiratory tract and patient recovery tends to be very rapid.

Certain anesthetic procedures such as intubation and intravenous catheterization are difficult in neonates because of their small body size. The larynx is difficult to see, and use of a laryngoscope may be required. It is often necessary to cut endotracheal tubes short to avoid bronchial intubation.

Monitoring of neonatal patients is similar to adults, although there are some minor differences. The anesthetist should be particularly watchful for bradycardia, which is associated with poor cardiac output in the anesthetized neonate. Premedication with atropine may not be effective because response to atropine is unpredictable in patients less than 14 days old.

Neonatal patients are prone to hypothermia due to their lack of subcutaneous fat, relatively large surface area, and inability to shiver. Particular care should be taken to avoid heat loss during surgery through the use of warmed intravenous fluids and circulating warm water heating pads.

Brachycephalic dogs

Technicians are frequently called on to anesthetize brachycephalic dogs, such as English bulldogs, pugs, Boston terriers, and Pekingeses. Because of their conformation, these animals may suffer from one or more anatomic characteristics that impede air exchange, including very small nasal openings, an elongated soft palate, and a small diameter trachea. Any anesthetic agent that depresses respiration or reduces muscle tone in the laryngeal area may cause increased respiratory difficulty. In some cases this may be fatal, particularly if the animal is not intubated and an open airway cannot be maintained. These problems are most evident in animals undergoing surgery to correct conformation defects in the pharyngeal region (e.g., soft palate resection) because postoperative swelling or hemorrhage may occur, increasing the risk of respiratory difficulty.

In addition to their respiratory problems, many brachycephalic animals also have abnormally high parasympathetic tone, resulting in bradycardia. Use of atropine or glycopyrrolate in these patients is helpful in increasing heart rates before surgery.

The induction period is particularly difficult for brachycephalic dogs. If possible, the anesthetist should preoxygenate brachycephalic patients for 5 minutes before induction. This is done by gently restraining the animal and administering oxygen through a face mask or oxygen chamber. This procedure helps maintain adequate blood oxygen levels and provides an increased reserve of oxygen in the lungs. This gives the animal an extra margin of safety during the induction period that follows.

Induction should be rapid, and for this reason intravenous induction agents are generally preferred over mask induction. The dog must be adequately anesthetized to allow rapid and efficient intubation. Difficulties may be encountered because of the large amount of redundant tissue in the pharynx that reduces visibility of the laryngeal opening, and the use of a laryngoscope is very helpful in these patients. The anesthetist may find that the endotracheal tube that fits the trachea is smaller than that expected, considering the size and weight of the dog.

Anesthesia usually can be safely maintained through the use of an inhalation anesthetic. With the help of an endotracheal tube, breathing during anesthesia may, in fact, be superior to that of the normal awake brachycephalic animal.

During recovery the patient should be observed closely until it is extubated and breathing well. Vigilance is necessary well into the recovery period, since patients have suffered airway obstructions even after attempting to stand. Removal of the endotracheal tube should be delayed because the animal will usually maintain an open airway as long as the tube is in place and oxygen should be delivered until the patient is extubated. The administration of butorphanol (0.2 mg/kg IM or IV) or another opioid agent may help the animal tolerate the endotracheal tube well into the recovery period. Once the endotracheal tube is removed, the animal's head and neck should be extended, and the animal should be watched very closely for dyspnea and cyanosis. If dyspnea is seen, administration of oxygen by mask or even reintubation may be necessary. It is advisable to have supplemental oxygen and supplies for reintubation (a laryngoscope, an endotracheal tube, and the appropriate dose of an inducing agent) readily available in the recovery area, in case dyspnea occurs.

Excitement and stress in the recovery period should be minimized as much as possible, especially if airway surgery was performed. Some patients may require mild tranquilization or the use of opioid analgesics to reduce the rapid respirations that can worsen laryngeal swelling.

Sighthounds

Several canine breeds, including the greyhound, saluki, Afghan hound, whippet, and Russian wolfhound, show increased sensitivity to anesthetic agents, particularly tranquilizers and barbiturates such as thiopental. The reason for this increased sensitivity is not entirely understood but may involve a lack of body fat for redistribution of the drug and inefficient hepatic metabolism of many drugs. Fortunately, many inducing agents, including diazepam and ketamine, methohexital, propofol, and the inhalation agents, can be safely used as alternatives to thiobarbiturates in these animals.

Obese animals

Some patients presented for anesthesia have a high percentage of body fat. As the blood supply to fat is relatively poor, anesthetics are not efficiently distributed to fat stores. The target organ (the brain) is no greater in size in an obese animal than it is in a lean animal of the same breed. Obese dogs, therefore, require less anesthetic on a per kilogram basis than do normal dogs. It is advisable to decrease the dose of preanesthetic and anesthetic agents such that the animal is dosed according to its ideal weight rather than its true weight.

Obese animals also may suffer from some degree of respiratory difficulty, further complicating the anesthetic process. Dogs that show respiratory difficulties should receive oxygen by face mask for 5 minutes before induction and may require the use of induction techniques similar to those used in brachycephalic dogs.

Obese dogs and toys frequently exhibit rapid shallow respirations during anesthesia. This breathing pattern delivers less oxygen and anesthetic vapor than is optimal for the patient. As a result, some patients are difficult to maintain at adequate anesthetic depth. The anesthetist who observes persistent rapid and shallow respirations should assume control over respiration by bagging the patient once every 5 seconds, until increased anesthetic depth and slower respirations are observed.

Cesarean sections

The anesthetist for animals undergoing cesarean surgery must be aware of the special needs not only of the patient undergoing the surgery, but also of the neonates being delivered. It is essential that the patient receive adequate anesthetic agent to provide immobilization and analgesia for the surgery; however, care should be taken to use minimal doses of those agents that could depress respiration in the puppies or kittens. Essentially, all anesthetic drugs administered to the pregnant patient (with the exception of neuromuscular blocking agents and local anesthetics) will readily cross the placenta and affect the newborn.

The pregnant female patient is at increased anesthetic risk for several reasons. Advanced pregnancy greatly increases the work load of the heart, particularly when the patient is in dorsal recumbency and the vena cava is compressed by the gravid uterus. Additionally, respiratory function may be compromised by the pressure of the abdominal organs on the diaphragm. Pregnant animals are prone to vomiting because of pressure from the uterus on the stomach. (Studies have shown that in human cesarean procedures inhalation of vomit causes approximately 50% of maternal anesthetic deaths.) Additionally, the patient may be exhausted before the surgery starts, particularly if the owner has delayed bringing the animal in for veterinary attention.

Hemorrhage from the uterus is a common complication of cesarean surgery, and even nonhemorrhaging patients have an increased risk of shock. It is therefore advisable that an intravenous catheter and intraoperative fluid administration be routinely used in cesarean patients.

It is helpful to do as much preoperative preparation of the cesarean patient as possible, thereby reducing the anesthesia time. If possible, clipping and prepping should be initiated in the awake patient. Whether awake or anesthetized, it is advisable that patient clipping and prepping be done as much as possible with the patient gently restrained in left lateral recumbency rather than in dorsal recumbency. The latter position may cause the heavy uterus to compress the vena cava, decreasing venous return to the heart.

Various anesthetic techniques are used for cesarean surgeries, depending on the preference of the veterinarian.

- Epidural anesthesia combined with a tranquilizer or neuroleptanalgesic is popular because the technique once mastered provides inexpensive but effective anesthesia with minimal depression of the patient or the neonates.
- General anesthesia using a variety of injectable and inhalant agents is also commonly used, with anesthetics given at the lowest effective dose in order to maintain anesthesia without unnecessarily depressing neonatal respiration. Because of the dam's increased sensitivity to medications, the dose of inhalant anesthetic required is often reduced by up to 40% during pregnancy.
- Preoxygenation is helpful, regardless of the anesthetic agents used, as it increases the oxygen tension in the lungs.
- Opioid agents are favored by some veterinarians for cesarean anesthesia because of their reversibility in both the dam and the neonates through the use of naloxone or other reversing agent.
- Use of nitrous oxide may be helpful to supplement opioids or inhalation agents, because it reduces the amount of other agents required and has minimal effects on fetal respiration, if used for a short time. The anesthetist should be aware of the possibility of diffusion hypoxia in newborn animals delivered from mothers receiving nitrous oxide, and oxygen should be administered to each puppy or kitten immediately after delivery.
- Pentobarbital is considered to be a high-risk agent because neonatal mortality may approach 100%.
- Use of diazepam should be avoided because this agent is poorly metabolized by neonatal animals.

Often puppies or kittens delivered by cesarean section show signs of reduced respiratory and cardiovascular function when first delivered. If respiration appears inadequate or cyanosis is present, oxygen should be administered by face mask. If necessary, the newborn animal can be intubated with a 16- or 18-gauge intravenous catheter and gently bagged with oxygen every 5 seconds. Techniques such as aspiration of fluid from the mouth and nose with an eyedropper or bulb syringe and swinging the newborn in a head-down position (supporting the head and neck) may also be useful. The use of reversing agents and doxapram (one or two drops from a tuberculin syringe with a 22-gauge needle, instilled under the tongue) is common. If bradycardia is present, a drop of dilute atropine (0.25 mg/ml) administered under the tongue may be helpful.

The newborn should be allowed to nurse as soon as the mother appears to be recovered from anesthesia (or, with supervision, during the recovery period). The dam may be disoriented and should be closely watched to ensure the safety of the newborn puppies or kittens. Anesthetic agents excreted in the milk appear to have little effect on nursing ability or neonatal viability.

Trauma patients

Animals that have recently undergone trauma, such as being hit by a car, may be suffering from numerous ailments that greatly increase anesthetic risk. Respiratory difficulties caused by pneumothorax, pulmonary contusions and hemorrhage, or diaphragmatic hernia may be present. Cardiac dysrhythmias are common in the period 12 to 72 hours after chest trauma. Shock is also very common in animals that have undergone significant trauma, particularly if hemorrhage has been severe. Serious internal injuries, such as fractures and herniated or ruptured organs, may pose further difficulties for the veterinarian and anesthetist.

Very few trauma patients require anesthesia immediately after the accident, and as a general rule, it is wise to stabilize these animals for several days before anesthesia is administered. Delaying anesthesia offers two advantages: it allows time for a thorough workup to assess the extent of the injuries, and it provides some time for the animal to begin the recovery process. It is advisable to obtain thoracic radiographs before anesthesia for repair of internal injuries (such as fractures) resulting from trauma, since studies have shown that one third of patients with forelimb, hind limb, or pelvic injuries have concurrent thoracic injuries that could jeopardize the safety of anesthesia. It is obviously advisable to identify and treat a disorder such as pneumothorax before anesthetizing an animal for the repair of a fractured femur. The veterinarian also may request an electrocardiogram as part of the preanesthetic workup, because cardiac dysrhythmias may be seen as long as 3 days after chest trauma. Fortunately, many thoracic injuries improve with cage rest, and if anesthesia can be delayed for several days after the traumatic incident, the anesthetist usually encounters fewer problems.

Cardiovascular disease

The most common cardiovascular disorders found in patients presented for anesthesia include anemia, shock, cardiomyopathy, hyperthyroidism, and congestive heart disease resulting from mitral valve insufficiency. In some geographic areas, heartworm disease is also common. Many animals with heart disease have concurrent pulmonary disease, such as pulmonary edema, which further complicates anesthesia. Diuretics such as furosemide (Lasix) may be helpful in alleviating pulmonary edema before anesthesia.

As with patients that have undergone recent trauma, it is generally advisable to stabilize the patient's condition before initiating anesthesia, by treating cardiovascular and respiratory disease to alleviate the symptoms as much as possible. Preoxygenation using a face mask or oxygen chamber for 5 minutes immediately before induction is also extremely helpful in reducing anesthetic risk in animals with cardiovascular or respiratory difficulties.

The veterinarian and anesthetist should ensure that anesthetic agents that depress the myocardium or exacerbate dysrhythmias (xylazine, halothane) are avoided as much as possible in these animals. Opioid agents, diazepam, and isoflurane offer the advantage of relative lack of toxicity to the heart.

When anesthetizing animals with cardiovascular problems, the anesthetist should be aware of the increased risk of overhydration through excessive or too rapid administration of intravenous fluids. Even an infusion rate of 10 ml/kg/hr may be dangerous for these animals. It is advisable to frequently monitor the anesthetized patient for signs of pulmonary edema, including increased lung sounds, ocular or nasal discharge, and increased respiratory rate.

Respiratory disease

Of all the animals presented for anesthesia, those with respiratory problems are perhaps the most difficult challenge for the anesthetist. Examples of these patients include animals with pleural effusion (free fluid present in the chest cavity), diaphragmatic hernia, pneumothorax, pulmonary contusions resulting from trauma, pneumonia, tracheal collapse, and pulmonary edema. Poor oxygenation is often present in these animals, and many show signs of tachypnea, dyspnea, and cyanosis. If possible, anesthesia should be delayed until respiratory function has improved. If surgery is absolutely required (e.g., to place a chest tube), local analgesia and gentle manual restraint may be preferable to general anesthesia.

Nitrous oxide should be avoided in patients with respiratory distress, as the administration of 100% oxygen is usually necessary to maintain adequate oxygenation. In the case of patients with a diaphragmatic hernia, nitrous oxide is inadvisable, as it may diffuse into the displaced stomach and intestines, causing distension of these organs and further compromising respiration.

Before anesthesia, it is often helpful to evaluate the animal and, if possible, to find the cause of the respiratory distress. Radiographs and thoracocentesis are particularly helpful. Thoracocentesis is useful not only in diagnosis, but also may be therapeutic if large volumes of air or fluid can be removed from the chest.

One of the most common procedures requiring anesthesia of an animal in respiratory distress is surgical repair of a diaphragmatic hernia. When preparing to anesthetize these patients, as with all patients showing signs of dyspnea, it is advisable to preoxygenate for 5 to 10 minutes before surgery. Head-down positions should be avoided before and during anesthesia, because this may result in further movement of abdominal contents into the thorax. If possible, an induction method that allows rapid intubation (i.e., use of an injectable agent) is preferred over mask induction. After induction, some patients may show signs of respiratory depression and even respiratory arrest, and the anesthetist must be prepared to intubate rapidly and assist or control ventilation. Ventilatory assistance may be provided by periodic or continuous "bagging" of the patient or a ventilator may be used. The animal should be closely observed for cyanosis. Arterial blood gas determination is also helpful, if available.

These patients require very close observation during the recovery period. Administration of oxygen may be helpful if signs of respiratory distress are seen.

Hepatic disease

Animals with liver disease are subject to increased anesthetic risk because of the central role that organ plays in drug metabolism, synthesis of blood clotting factors and other serum proteins, and carbohydrate metabolism. Some animals with liver disease are hypoproteinemic, which may lead to increased potency of barbiturate agents. Patients with chronic liver failure are also commonly dehydrated, thin, and icteric, and may be anemic.

Preanesthetic medication should be given with care or omitted from the protocol, since most of these agents require hepatic metabolism before excretion. Xylazine and acetylpromazine in particular may have long-lasting effects in patients with compromised hepatic function. Induction and maintenance of anesthesia are best achieved using inhalation agents such as isoflurane, which do not require hepatic function for their excretion.

Renal disease

The kidneys are the organs most involved in maintaining the volume and electrolyte composition of body fluids. This helps explain why animals with renal disease are often dehydrated and may have severe electrolyte imbalances including metabolic acidosis, hyperkalemia, and hyperphosphatemia. General anesthesia may be particularly stressful for these patients, because renal blood flow is decreased during anesthesia and renal function is thereby further compromised. An additional consideration is the requirement that the kidney be able to excrete many anesthetic agents and their metabolites. For this reason, animals with compromised renal function can be expected to show prolonged recovery after anesthesia with almost any injectable agent.

The patient with renal disease should be rehydrated as much as possible before surgery, and electrolyte problems should be identified and addressed. The veterinarian may elect to induce diuresis before anesthesia, using furosemide, mannitol, or dopamine and IV saline. Renal function tests such as urine specific gravity, BUN, and creatinine may be useful in obtaining an accurate picture of renal function. Preoperative fasting may not be advisable in some patients with renal disease, because dehydration may occur rapidly after withdrawal of oral fluids.

Reduced dosages of anesthetic drugs, including acetylpromazine, xylazine, diazepam, opioid agents, ketamine, and barbiturates, are often used in these patients. It should be recalled that barbiturates have increased potency in acidotic and uremic animals and should be used with great caution in patients with renal disease. Inhalation agents, particularly isoflurane, have some advantages over injectable agents, although halothane and methoxyflurane are both excreted in part through renal mechanisms. Intravenous fluids should be administered throughout anesthesia and during the recovery period, until the animal is able to drink unassisted.

Animals with urinary blockages (including male cats with urethral obstruction caused by struvite crystals) pose similar problems to the anesthetist. Many of these cats are depressed, dehydrated, uremic, acidotic, and hyperkalemic. Hyperkalemic animals are at particular risk of cardiac failure. These animals may sometimes be identified by auscultation, because bradycardia is often seen in this condition. Treatment of hyperkalemia may require the use of sodium bicarbonate, 10% calcium gluconate, and/or dextrose and should be done only with close supervision and guidance from the veterinarian. Conditions stressful to the animal should be avoided as much as possible because the release of epinephrine from the adrenal glands may potentiate cardiac dysrhythmias.

The administration of inhalation agents (particularly isoflurane) to cats with urinary blockages may be less hazardous than the use of injectable drugs, since renal excretion is not required for patient recovery. Ketamine-diazepam may be used intravenously with caution and at reduced dosages. Obstructed cats showing extreme depression may not require general anesthesia, particularly if a local anesthetic such as lidocaine gel is administered as part of the urethral catheterization procedure.

RESPONSE TO ANESTHETIC PROBLEMS AND EMERGENCIES

Despite every precaution, the veterinary technician is likely to encounter anesthetic emergencies several times during the course of his or her career. The nature of the technician's response may mean the difference between life and death for the anesthetized patient.

Role of the veterinary technician in emergency care

Ideally, emergency response is a team effort involving the veterinarian, technician, and other hospital staff. Normally the veterinarian acts as the team leader, directing the staff in emergency procedures. However, the veterinarian may be performing surgery on the patient at the time an anesthetic emergency arises and therefore has other pressing concerns besides anesthesia. In such a situation, the technician must be prepared to take an active role in resuscitating the patient and not rely solely on the already-busy veterinarian. Constant communication between the veterinarian and the technician is obviously important under these circumstances.

It is a good idea to conduct periodic "dress rehearsals" or mock resuscitations in which all staff participate. Everyone in the hospital should be familiar with the location of the crash kit, IV fluids, and emergency drugs. Procedures such as warming towels in a clothes dryer, making up hot water bottles, and drawing up drugs into a syringe can be readily taught to hospital staff and, once mastered by them, will free the veterinarian and technician to perform more demanding tasks.

Occasionally an emergency arises when the veterinarian is absent from the hospital or unavailable to assist. For example, seizures may occur in the postoperative recovery period. Most provincial and state regulations allow the technician to undertake emergency care if the veterinarian is absent. To protect the veterinarian and technician from liability, however, it is advisable to discuss in advance the procedures that the veterinarian will authorize the technician to do in an emergency. It is helpful to have written instructions available, in the form of an emergency protocol authorized by the veterinarian. Some acts, including the administration of unauthorized emergency drugs in the veterinarian's absence, may be difficult to justify from a legal point of view even though they may be in the patient's best interest.

General approach to emergencies

It cannot be assumed that every anesthetic emergency should be treated in the same way. For example, the veterinarian and animal owner may elect not to resuscitate a severely ill or debilitated animal that undergoes cardiac arrest during anesthesia. Cost considerations may influence the treatment given in some cases. Emergency care is labor-intensive and treatment costs (including drugs) may be considerable. Most veterinarians, however, will not stop to consider cost if the emergency arises during a routine surgery, such as a spay, and will do everything possible to revive the animal.

When responding to an emergency, the technician should bear in mind several principles of emergency care:

- The technician should take a few seconds to think before doing anything. After consulting with the veterinarian, the technician should mentally list the most important things to be done and undertake them in order of priority.
- Every veterinary practice should have a well-stocked crash kit for use in emergency situations within the hospital. A list of supplies that may be useful in a crash kit is given in Appendix C.
- Useful emergency drugs are listed in Tables 6-2 and 6-3. Doses for emergency drugs should be posted or listed on a paper kept in the crash kit. Emergency drugs kept in the crash kit should be periodically checked to ensure that they have not

expired. In particular, epinephrine has a short shelf life and should not be used if a brown discoloration is present.

• Above all, the technician should do no harm. In an emergency it is easy to panic and do things that are not only unnecessary but also potentially harmful to the animal, including performing cardiac compressions on an animal whose heart is still beating. Sometimes the best course of action is to watch, monitor, and wait.

After an anesthetic emergency, the technician, veterinarian, and hospital staff should discuss the reasons the emergency arose and determine what could be done to prevent the same thing from happening again. The adequacy of the resuscitation efforts should be analyzed, and if a problem exists, it should be addressed.

TABLE 6-2

Drugs used in treating anesthetic emergencies in cats and dogs

Drug	Dosage for IV use	Indications for use
Atropine	0.025 mg/kg; can give 2× dose I.T.	Treatment for bradycardia
Dexamethasone (Azium)	4-8 mg/kg	Corticosteroid use in treatment of shock
Diazepam (Valium)	0.2-0.5 mg/kg	Treatment of seizures
Dobutamine (Dobutrex)	5-10 μg/kg/min, infusion in 5% dextrose	Increases force of myocardial contractions
Dopamine (Intropin)	2-10 μg/kg/min, infusion in lactated Ringer's	Increases force of myocardial contractions
Doxapram (Dopram)	5-10 mg/kg	Respiratory and CNS stimulant
Epinephrine (Adrenalin)	0.1 mg/kg; can give 2× dose I.T.	Increases rate and force of cardiac contractions
Lidocaine without epinephrine (Xylocaine)	Dog: 2.0 mg/kg; can give 2× dose I.T.	Antidysrhythmic agent
Naloxone (Narcan)	0.01-0.02 mg/kg	Narcotic antagonist
Prednisolone sodium succinate (Solu-Delta-Cortef)	10-30 mg/kg	Corticosteroid used in treatment of shock
Sodium bicarbonate	1.0 mEq/kg	Treatment of metabolic acidosis
Yohimbine (Yobine)	0.13 mg/kg	Reversing agent for xylazine

TABLE 6-3

Doses of emergency drugs used in cardiopulmonary resuscitation of cats and dogs

Emergency drug	Dose	3 kg (6.6 lb)	5 kg (11 lb)	10 kg (22 lb)	15 kg (33 lb)	20 kg (44 lb)	25 kg (55 lb)	30 kg (66 lb)	40 kg (88 lb)	50 kg (110 lb)
Epinephrine 1:1000 1 mg/ml	0.1 mg/kg	0.3 ml	0.5 ml	1.0 ml	1.5 ml	2.0 ml	2.5 ml	3.0 ml	4.0 ml	5.0 ml
Atropine 0.54 mg/ml	0.025 mg/kg	0.1 ml	0.2 ml	0.5 ml	0.7 ml	0.9 ml	1.2 ml	1.4 ml	1.8 ml	2.3 ml
Lidocaine 20 mg/ml (dog only)	2.0 mg/kg	0.3 ml	0.5 ml	1.0 ml	1.5 ml	2.0 ml	2.5 ml	3.0 ml	4.0 ml	5.0 ml
Sodium bicarbonate 1 mEq/ml	1.0 mEq/kg	3 ml	5 ml	10 ml	15 ml	20 ml	25 ml	30 ml	40 ml	50 ml
Prednisolone sodium succinate	30 mg/kg	90 mg	150 mg	300 mg	450 mg	600 mg	750 mg	900 mg	1200 mg	1500 mg

From Robello D, Crowe T: Cardiopulmonary resuscitation: current recommendations, *Vet Clin North Am* 19(6), Nov, 1989.

Potential emergency situations during anesthesia

Although anesthetic emergencies are by their nature unpredictable, certain problems occur with some frequency. The following situations will be addressed in detail:

Animals that will not stay asleep

Animals that are too deeply anesthetized

Pale mucous membranes

Prolonged capillary refill

Cyanosis and dyspnea

Tachypnea

Abnormalities in cardiac rate and rhythm

Respiratory arrest

Cardiac arrest

Animals that will not stay asleep

Occasionally, the anesthetist will have difficulty in maintaining a patient at sufficient anesthetic depth. Often, the technician becomes aware of the problem when the patient shows signs of movement in response to surgical stimulation. If depth appears inadequate, the anesthetist should answer the following questions:

- Has the vaporizer been turned off, or is the setting too low to maintain anesthesia?
- Has the vaporizer run out of anesthetic?
- Is the endotracheal tube in the esophagus? This can be determined easily by checking to see if the reservoir bag expands and contracts as the animal breathes; if so, the endotracheal tube is probably in the trachea. Movement of the reservoir bag also tells the anesthetist that the endotracheal tube is connected to the Y piece and that the tube is not blocked. Other procedures used to determine the location and patency of the endotracheal tube include palpation of the neck and compression of the reservoir bag to see whether the chest rises.
- Is the endotracheal tube inserted past the thoracic inlet? If the tube enters one bronchus, exposure to the anesthetic is restricted to only one lung. Only one side of the chest will rise when the patient is bagged.
- Is air leaking around the endotracheal tube? If so, the patient is probably breathing room air, which dilutes the anesthetic gas entering the lungs. Air leakage can be detected by closing the pop-off valve, inflating the reservoir bag, and gently pressing on the bag while listening for the sound of air escaping from the animal's mouth. A soft hiss of escaping air is acceptable, but a large gush of exiting air should alert the anesthetist that either the endotracheal tube is too small or the cuff is not sufficiently inflated.
- Is the animal holding its breath? This is most commonly seen immediately after the intubated animal is connected to the machine. Prolonged breath-holding may

lead to arousal from anesthesia, since vaporized anesthetic is not entering the lungs or the bloodstream. If arousal appears imminent, it may be necessary to periodically bag the animal with a mixture of oxygen and anesthetic.

- Are the patient's respirations too shallow to draw sufficient anesthetic into the lungs? Rapid shallow respiration commonly seen in toy dogs and obese animals may be associated with insufficient anesthetic depth. The anesthetist should assist ventilation by bagging these patients (vaporizer on) every 5 seconds.
- Is the anesthetic machine assembled correctly? Occasionally, hoses become detached from the machine or the endotracheal tube, in which case the patient obviously does not receive any anesthetic from the machine.
- Is the oxygen flow rate adequate to vaporize anesthetic? For most precision vaporizers, a minimum flow rate of 500 ml/minute is necessary for accurate delivery of anesthetic.
- Is the exaggerated respiratory movement actually an agonal (near death) phenomenon, indicating dangerous anesthetic depth rather than a light plane?
- Is the anesthetic machine functioning adequately? Repeated episodes of awakening during anesthesia may indicate poor vaporizer function. If a halothane or isoflurane vaporizer setting of 3% to 4% seems necessary to maintain anesthesia in many patients, cleaning and recalibration of the vaporizer are probably necessary.

If the answers to the questions listed above do not explain the patient's arousal, the anesthetist should consult with the veterinarian. It may be necessary to increase the vaporizer setting or switch to a different anesthetic in order to achieve the desired anesthetic depth. If possible, the anesthetist should avoid abrupt increases in vaporizer concentration, because reflex apnea and even cardiac arrest may result.

Animal too deeply anesthetized

An animal that is too deeply anesthetized will usually show the following signs:
- Respiration rate is 8 breaths per minute or less; respirations may be very shallow or may be "rocking boat" in character
- Mucous membranes are pale, may be cyanotic
- Capillary refill is greater than 2 seconds
- Bradycardia is present (less than 60 to 70 bpm in a dog or 100 bpm in a cat)
- Pulse is weak; systolic blood pressure is less than 80 mm Hg (indirect measurement)
- Cardiac dysrhythmias may be present; QRS complexes are irregular on the ECG, or abnormal complexes may be present
- The animal's extremities and ears are cold, body temperature is often less than 35° C
- Reflexes are completely absent, including palpebral and corneal reflexes

- Muscle tone is flaccid
- Pupils may be dilated and pupillary light reflex is absent

The anesthetist should evaluate carefully his or her interpretation of the signs listed above. The presence of one or two signs may not indicate excessive depth, provided the other signs are absent. Vital signs also vary depending on the preanesthetic and general anesthetics used (e.g., atropine may affect heart rate and pupil dilation). The anesthetist should observe as many parameters as possible before making an assessment of patient depth.

There are several reasons why anesthetic depth may be excessive. In most cases, the vaporizer setting is too high for the patient being anesthetized, or in the case of injectable agents, too high a dose has been given. Occasionally, the animal may have a preexisting problem such as shock or anemia, increasing its susceptibility to anesthetic overdose. Excessive depth may also result from inadequate ventilation.

After concluding that the anesthetic depth is excessive, the anesthetist should immediately decrease the vaporizer setting (to zero, if necessary) and inform the veterinarian. If the veterinarian decides that the animal's condition has deteriorated such that resuscitation efforts are warranted, the anesthetist should begin to bag the animal with pure oxygen. (This discussion assumes that the patient is intubated and undergoing gas anesthesia. If an injectable agent has been used, intubation and oxygen delivery by means of an anesthetic machine should be initiated immediately.)

Bagging is achieved by closing the pop-off valve part way, filling the reservoir bag with oxygen, and gently squeezing the bag until the animal's chest rises slightly. This procedure should be repeated every 5 seconds until the animal shows signs of recovery, including increased heart rate, stronger pulse, and improved mucous membrane color and refill. The use of intravenous fluids, external heat, and drugs such as doxapram and specific reversing agents (yohimbine, naloxone) may also expedite recovery.

Occasionally the anesthetist may be unsure of whether a patient's depth is excessive. If the veterinarian is not immediately available to advise on the patient's condition, it is safest to assume that the animal is too deep and to decrease the vaporizer setting, while observing the animal carefully for signs of arousal.

Pale mucous membranes

Pale mucous membranes may arise from several causes. Patients are sometimes presented with preexisting anemia resulting from diseases such as feline leukemia, bleeding disorders, neoplasia, or chronic hepatic or renal disease. In other cases blood loss may have occurred during surgery. Some anesthetic agents, particularly inhalation agents and acetylpromazine, cause vasodilation and decrease blood pressure, resulting in poor perfusion of capillary beds and pale mucous membranes in some animals. Hypothermia, pain, and use of xylazine can also reduce blood supply to the tissues, causing pale mucous membranes.

If pale mucous membranes are observed during surgery, the anesthetist should ascertain the animal's anesthetic depth and monitor vital signs including heart rate, respiration, pulse strength, and capillary refill time. The veterinarian should be consulted, as it may be necessary to initiate intravenous fluid therapy or a blood transfusion to stabilize the patient's condition.

Prolonged capillary refill

The observation of a prolonged capillary refill (greater than 2 seconds) suggests that blood pressure is inadequate to perfuse superficial tissues. The presence of hypotension (or its life-threatening sequela, shock) should be suspected in any animal with a slow capillary refill time. Hypotension may have been present before the induction of anesthesia, as in the case of animals undergoing emergency surgery following trauma. Hypotension or shock also may arise as a result of blood loss during surgery or may occur in patients that are at a very deep plane of anesthesia. Some anesthetics, including acetylpromazine and the inhalation agents, also may cause severe hypotension in susceptible patients.

The anesthetist who observes a prolonged capillary refill time should immediately check the animal's blood pressure reading if available. In a dog or cat, an indirect systolic blood pressure under 80 mm Hg suggests that significant hypotension is present. If blood pressure readings are not available, the anesthetist can roughly estimate the systolic pressure by palpating a peripheral pulse. As a general rule, the absence of a palpable pulse at the metatarsal artery indicates a systolic pressure under 80 mm Hg, and the absence of a palpable pulse at the femoral artery indicates a systolic pressure under 60 mm Hg.

If pulse pressure is reduced, the anesthetist should closely observe the animal for other signs of shock, including hypothermia and tachycardia. In the hypothermic animal, circulation to the extremities deteriorates, and the surface temperature of the ears and paws is reduced. Tachycardia is seen because the heart responds to the fall in blood pressure by increased rate and force of contraction, although this effect may not be present in deep anesthesia.

The treatment for shock in the anesthetized patient is similar to that in the conscious patient and should be done under the supervision of a veterinarian. Intravenous fluids should be administered at a rapid rate. Over the first 15 minutes, 20 ml/kg should be given, and the animal should be observed closely for a response. The maximum fluid administration rate is 90 ml/kg for the first hour in the dog and 50–70 ml/kg in the cat. The use of colloid therapy or blood transfusions may be appropriate in some situations. Anesthetic depth should be reduced if possible, and 100% oxygen should be administered. The patient must be kept warm through the use of supplemental heat in the form of warm towels, circulating warm water heating pads, hot water bottles, or similar devices. Various drugs are recommended for the treatment of shock, including corticosteroids (prednisone sodium succinate, dexamethasone), cardiac ionotropes such as dopamine or dobutamine, and sodium bicarbonate.

Dyspnea and/or cyanosis

Any patient showing cyanosis or dyspnea during the administration of an anesthetic should be immediately brought to the veterinarian's attention. The presence of *dyspnea* (respiratory difficulty) indicates that the animal is unable to obtain sufficient oxygen or remove adequate CO_2 using normal respiratory movements. *Cyanosis* (a bluish discoloration of the mucous membranes) indicates that tissue oxygenation is inadequate. Dyspnea and cyanosis often are seen together and may be followed by respiratory arrest, in which respiratory efforts cease and oxygen is no longer delivered to the tissues.

The chief sources of respiratory distress during anesthesia are:
- The animal is unable to obtain oxygen from the anesthetic machine because the oxygen supply has run out, the flowmeter has been turned off, or the anesthetic circuit or endotracheal tube is blocked.
- The animal is unable to breathe normally because of airway obstruction or respiratory pathology. Causes of airway obstruction include endotracheal tube blockage, excessive flexion of the head and neck, laryngospasm, aspiration of stomach contents after vomiting or regurgitation, and brachycephalic conformation. Respiration is likely to be compromised in animals with pneumothorax, pulmonary edema, diaphragmatic hernia, and pleural effusion. Use of heavy surgical drapings or constricting bandages also may impair normal respiration.
- The animal is too deeply anesthetized, such that respiration and other vital functions are adversely affected.

Respiratory problems are life-threatening and should be addressed as follows:
1. The anesthetist must first ensure that oxygen is being delivered to the patient. If the oxygen tank has run out, the patient must be disconnected from the machine until another oxygen source can be secured. If the endotracheal tube is blocked, it must be removed and replaced.
2. Once oxygen flow has been established, the vaporizer should be turned off, and the animal should be bagged with 100% oxygen. If the anesthetic machine is unavailable, an Ambu bag (Fig. 6-1) can be used to deliver room air to the patient. While initiating bagging, the anesthetist should observe the chest for movement. If the chest does not rise when the animal is bagged, the endotracheal tube or airway may be blocked, and the blockage must be relieved. If the chest does rise when the reservoir bag is squeezed, oxygen is being delivered to the lungs and bagging should be continued until the mucous membrane color improves.

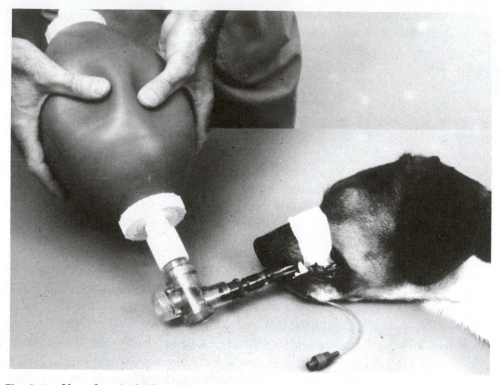

Fig. 6-1. Use of an Ambu bag to deliver room air to an intubated patient. (From Muir WW III, Hubbell JAE: *Handbook of veterinary anesthesia,* St Louis, 1989, Mosby.)

3. On rare occasions, dyspnea and cyanosis may be caused by complete airway obstruction. If intubation is not possible under these circumstances, the veterinarian may elect to perform an emergency tracheostomy, a surgical opening of the trachea to allow the insertion of a breathing tube. Alternatively, a 14-gauge intravenous catheter can be placed through the cricothyroid membrane and into the trachea. The catheter is connected to the barrel of a 3-cc syringe, which is in turn attached to the Y piece of an anesthetic machine.

4. Administration of intravenous fluids or emergency drugs such as doxapram may be helpful in reviving patients suffering from respiratory depression or arrest.

5. It is important that the anesthetist closely observes the patient during resuscitative efforts to ensure that cardiac arrest does not occur. If a pulse or heart beat cannot be detected, cardiac compressions should be initiated in conjunction with continued bagging.

6. If necessary, supplemental oxygen should be continued into the recovery period, using a mask, oxygen cage, or intranasal insufflation.

Tachypnea

Tachypnea, which is a rapid respiratory rate, must be differentiated from dyspnea, in which respiratory distress is present. Tachypnea may arise at any time during anesthesia and may be disconcerting to the anesthetist. It is particularly common during procedures in which neuroleptanalgesics, such as Innovar-Vet, are used. Tachypnea also may be seen if anesthetic depth is inadequate, in which case it is often accompanied by tachycardia and spontaneous movement. Paradoxically, tachypnea also may occur in deep anesthesia, as a response to low blood oxygen and high blood carbon dioxide.

If tachypnea is seen, the anesthetist should assess the anesthetic depth and check the CO_2 absorber crystals to ensure that hypercarbia is not present. If anesthetic depth, body temperature, and vital signs appear to be within acceptable limits, the anesthetist should refrain from changing the vaporizer setting, as the condition will usually correct itself within 1 to 2 minutes. Occasionally, injection of an analgesic, such as butorphanol, may be required.

Obese patients are prone to tachypnea, which may result in inefficient ventilation. It may be necessary to assist or control ventilation in these patients.

Abnormalities in cardiac rate and rhythm

Abnormalities in cardiac rate and rhythm include tachycardia, bradycardia, and cardiac dysrhythmias, all of which may be seen in anesthetized patients.

Tachycardia is present if the heart rate during stage III anesthesia is greater than 120 bpm for a large dog or greater than 160 bpm for a small dog or cat. It may result from the administration of drugs such as atropine, ketamine, or epinephrine. Tachycardia may be a preexisting condition in animals suffering from hyperthyroidism, shock, congestive heart failure, and other conditions. An elevation in heart rate is also a common response to surgical stimulation, although it does not necessarily indicate insufficient anesthetic depth unless accompanied by rapid respiration, spontaneous movement, or active reflexes.

Not all cases of tachycardia require treatment, particularly in patients with otherwise normal cardiac function, but the anesthetist should notify the surgeon before assuming that tachycardia is not significant. It is also important to check the vaporizer setting and anesthetic depth and adjust them if necessary.

Bradycardia is usually defined as a heart rate less than 60 bpm in a medium sized or large dog, less than 70 bpm in a small dog, and less than 100 bpm in a cat. Bradycardia may be caused by the administration of xylazine or opioid agents, particularly if preanesthesia with an anticholinergic was omitted from the anesthetic protocol. As discussed in Chapter 1, bradycardia also may result from increased activity of the parasympathetic system. This may occur in response to endotracheal intubation, ocular surgery (which may stimulate the vagus nerve), or handling of the viscera by the surgeon. Bradycardia may also occur if the animal is very deeply anesthetized, and when seen in this context is a warning that respiratory and cardiac arrest may be imminent. Other causes of bradycardia include hyperkalemia, hypothermia, and hypoxia.

Treatment of bradycardia depends on the cause of the condition. If anesthetic depth is excessive, the vaporizer setting should be adjusted and bagging with oxygen may be helpful. Bradycardia caused by the administration of drugs or excessive vagal stimulation is best treated with intravenous administration of atropine or glycopyrrolate. These drugs, however, are more effective when given as premedication agents rather than during the course of anesthesia. It should be noted that not all cases of bradycardia require treatment: if capillary refill and pulse strength appear normal, tissue perfusion is probably adequate and treatment may be unnecessary. The veterinarian should be consulted for direction.

The term *cardiac arrhythmia* (or more correctly, cardiac dysrhythmia) refers to any one of a number of abnormalities, including "dropped beats," premature ventricular contractions (PVCs) arising spontaneously from individual heart muscle cells, and sustained episodes of tachycardia. These abnormalities are most easily detected through the use of an ECG. The alert technician also may note that a pulse deficit is present in animals with some types of dysrhythmias.

Cardiac dysrhythmias commonly arise in animals given dysrhythmogenic drugs such as barbiturates, xylazine, and halothane. Such dysrhythmias may be of short duration and well tolerated in young healthy patients, but may be a significant problem in animals with preexisting heart disease and in geriatric patients. Dysrhythmias are particularly common during induction and light anesthesia and in some cases may be due to respiratory depression and subsequent hypoxia. Other causes of cardiac dysrhythmias include preexisting heart disease, gastric volvulus, thoracic surgery, and endotracheal intubation if an anticholinergic has not been given. Electrolyte imbalances and hypercarbia also may cause dysrhythmias. These conditions may arise from poor anesthetic technique including exhaustion of the CO_2 absorber crystals or inadequate oxygen flow rates.

Treatment of cardiac dysrhythmias should be done in consultation with the veterinarian. The anesthetist should rule out carbon dioxide accumulation within the circuit or inadequate oxygen flow. Ventilation should be increased by periodic bagging or use of a ventilator. In some cases, antidysrhythmic drugs such as atropine, procainamide, or lidocaine (without epinephrine) may be administered on the veterinarian's orders.

Respiratory arrest

Respiratory arrest is the cessation of respiratory efforts by the patient. It may lead to cardiac arrest and is therefore a potentially fatal condition.

Not all cases in which respiration stops require immediate action by the anesthetist. Respiratory efforts may temporarily cease after the intravenous injection of ketamine, barbiturates, and other respiratory depressants. Minimal or no respiratory efforts also may be present following a period of prolonged bagging with oxygen and, in such a case, would reflect low blood carbon dioxide and high blood oxygen levels. In both types of ventilatory arrest (that caused by drug administration or bagging with oxygen), the anesthetist must be sure that although respiration has ceased, other vital signs, particularly heart rate and mucous membrane color, are normal. If the heart beat is regular, the heart rate is greater than 80 bpm, the pulse is strong, and mucous membranes are pink, the patient does not usually require immediate treatment for respiratory arrest. Occasional "breaths" of oxygen (one every 30 seconds) can be delivered to the patient during this period to prevent hypoxia. However, excessive bagging with oxygen may extend the period of apnea by removing carbon dioxide from the blood, which is a stimulus for the patient to resume breathing. The anesthetist who suspects that respiratory efforts have temporarily ceased because of administration of drugs or ventilation with oxygen should closely monitor the patient's heart rate and mucous membrane color for 1 to 2 minutes before assuming that a serious condition exists. If spontaneous respiration does not resume within this time, the veterinarian should be consulted, and it may be advisable to begin regular bagging of the patient with oxygen.

True respiratory arrest is much more serious and requires immediate attention. This condition may arise because of anesthetic overdose, cessation of oxygen flow, or preexisting respiratory disease such as pneumothorax or diaphragmatic hernia. Affected animals may show warning signs such as dyspnea and/or cyanosis before respiratory arrest occurs. Other vital signs, such as heart rate, capillary refill, pulse strength, and pupil dilation, are often abnormal.

Treatment of respiratory arrest involves the following steps:

1. Inform the veterinarian. If the patient is not intubated, an endotracheal tube should be immediately inserted and the patient connected to an anesthetic machine delivering 100% oxygen.
2. Check the heart rate to ensure that cardiac arrest has not occurred.
3. Turn off the anesthetic vaporizer and nitrous oxide flow.
4. Ensure oxygen flow is adequate by checking the tank pressure gauge and flowmeter.
5. Ensure the airway is not obstructed by bagging the patient and observing that the chest rises on "inspiration."
6. Bag with oxygen at a rate of once every 3 to 5 seconds. Continue bagging until vital signs improve, particularly mucous membrane color and heart rate.
7. If an intravenous catheter is present, administer IV fluids at a rate suitable for treatment of shock.
8. The veterinarian may advise that doxapram or other drugs be given.
9. Ensure that the patient is kept warm.

Bagging should continue until heart rate and mucous membrane color have been restored to normal. Once this is achieved, the anesthetist should discontinue bagging for 15 to 30 seconds and closely observe the patient for respiratory efforts. If none are seen, bagging should resume.

On occasion, the anesthetist may be faced with a patient in respiratory arrest in the absence of an anesthetic machine. It is possible to substitute an Ambu bag (Fig. 6-1) or even mouth to endotracheal tube or mouth to muzzle resuscitation in these cases.

Cardiac arrest

Cardiac arrest may occur at any time during anesthesia. In most cases the anesthetist receives some warning that arrest is imminent, in the form of a short period in which cyanosis, dyspnea or respiratory arrest, and prolonged capillary refill are evident. If cardiac arrest appears imminent, the anesthetist should immediately alert the veterinarian and the hospital staff, while continuously monitoring the heart by auscultation, by palpation of the chest, or through the use of an ECG. A patient suffering from cardiac arrest shows the following signs:

• No heartbeat can be auscultated, palpated, or seen on an ECG
• No palpable arterial pulse is present, and blood pressure readings (if available) are 25 mm Hg or less
• Mucous membranes are gray or cyanotic, capillary refill may be prolonged
• Pupils are widely dilated with no response to light
• Respiration is absent, except for abrupt gasps

Coordinated action by all hospital staff members is essential to reverse cardiac arrest. Once arrest occurs, permanent brain damage may result if oxygen delivery to the brain is not reestablished within 4 minutes, either by cardiopulmonary resuscitation or restoration of cardiac function. Ideally, at least five staff members should participate in the resuscitative efforts as follows: one performs chest compressions, one bags the animal, one assesses pulse during compressions and when compressions are temporarily suspended, one draws up and administers drugs on the veterinarian's orders, and one maintains a record of patient status and resuscitative treatments.

The essential steps in responding to a cardiac arrest may be summarized with the mnemonic: ABCD (establish a patent *a*irway, *b*ag the patient with 100% oxygen, initiate internal or external *c*ardiac massage, and administer epinephrine and other *d*rugs).

1. If the animal is intubated and connected to an anesthetic machine, one staff member should immediately initiate respiratory support by turning off the vaporizer and nitrous oxide flow and bagging the animal with 100% oxygen at the rate of one breath every 3 to 5 seconds. Mask administration of oxygen is inadequate: if an endotracheal tube is not present, it is essential

that the animal be intubated immediately. Additionally, the anesthetist must ensure that the patient's chest rises slightly during bagging, indicating that the airway is not blocked.

2. Cardiac compressions should be initiated. The animal should be turned on its right side with its feet toward the person doing compressions and the head tilted down if possible. For a large dog, a firm object such as a book, sandbag, or rolled up towel should be placed under the dog's chest just behind the elbow. The heel of the compressor's hand should compress the chest against this object, with the pressure applied at the point where the chest is widest. For a large dog, both hands should be used to compress the chest. In the case of a medium-size dog, the person should place one hand under the dog's chest and the other hand at the fifth intercostal space, just over the dog's heart (Fig. 6-2). The chest is then compressed between the two hands. For a cat or small dog, compression may be done by using the thumb to compress the chest against the fingers of the same hand. Regardless of the size of the animal, rate of compressions should be 1 to 2 times per second (80 times per minute for a large dog and up to 120 times per minute for a small dog or cat), and the chest should be compressed approximately one third the diameter of the chest wall. The aim of the compressions is to manually force blood through the heart and, ultimately, to the tissues. It is believed that compressions also may assist circulation by increasing pressure in the chest, indirectly inducing blood flow. Each compression should result in a palpable femoral pulse, which should be periodically monitored by another staff member, if possible. If a pulse is not detected and the mucous membrane color does not improve, the method of compression should be adjusted by changing the rate or intensity, repositioning the patient, or assigning the compression task to another staff member.

Bagging and compressions should be delivered simultaneously. In the case of a technician working alone, 10 compressions should be given alternately with 2 breaths. Once CPR is initiated, it should not be discontinued for longer than 20 to 30 seconds at a time.

3. If external cardiac compressions are not effective, as shown by failure to achieve a palpable pulse or pink mucous membranes within 2 minutes, internal compressions may be attempted. In the case of dogs weighing over 20 kg, some authorities suggest that internal compressions should be initiated immediately after cardiac arrest is identified. There is understandable reluctance on the part of many veterinarians and technicians to enter the chest in order to perform internal massage; however, controlled studies have demonstrated that the success rate for resuscitation of large dogs is much greater if internal cardiac massage is performed. Investigators have shown that external chest compression in dogs weighing more than 20 kg results in less

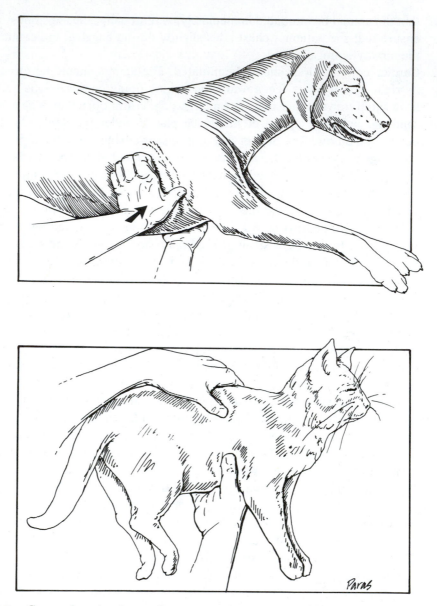

Fig. 6-2. Correct location for cardiac compressions for a medium size dog or a cat. (From Muir WW III, Hubbell JAE: *Handbook of veterinary anesthesia,* St Louis, 1989, Mosby.)

than 17% of normal cardiac output, whereas internal massage results in outputs up to 70% of normal. In the case of dogs undergoing a laparotomy at the time of arrest, the surgeon may immediately initiate internal compressions by opening the diaphragm, entering the thorax, and compressing the heart.

To perform internal compressions, the lateral thorax is quickly shaved and sprayed with alcohol, a self-adhering sterile drape is applied to the prepared area, and a skin incision is made between the seventh and eighth ribs, using a scalpel. The incision is extended through the muscle until the chest cavity is encountered. Care should be taken to avoid incising lung tissue, which lies immediately below the pleura. The operator's hand is inserted between the ribs (use of a retractor may be necessary to separate the ribs adequately). The heart is grasped, and gentle but firm pressure is applied to the ventricles at a rate of 80 times per minute. If resuscitation efforts are successful, a palpable heartbeat may return within seconds to minutes. Surgical closure and antibiotic therapy are essential after reestablishment of cardiac function by internal compression.

4. When doing compressions, it is necessary to stop periodically to determine whether the heart has resumed spontaneous contractions. This is relatively easy to ascertain by palpation when doing internal compressions but more difficult with external compression methods. Spontaneous contractions can be detected by discontinuing external compression and either palpating for a spontaneous pulse or observing an ECG for QRS complexes. Auscultation may also be useful.

   If spontaneous contractions are not observed, external or internal compressions can be resumed, although after 15 minutes they are unlikely to be successful in establishing a heart beat. Use of a defibrillator is helpful in some situations, but should be authorized and directly supervised by a veterinarian.

5. If spontaneous contractions are observed, cardiac compressions should be discontinued, although bagging must be maintained until spontaneous breathing is established, which may require up to several hours. The anesthetist should periodically check the capillary refill, mucous membrane color, and heart rate and should discontinue bagging only if these vital signs appear normal. If mucous membrane color deteriorates or if spontaneous respiration does not occur within 1 minute after bagging is discontinued, bagging should be resumed.

6. Drugs are commonly administered to aid recovery. In all cases, the veterinarian, if present, should authorize the type of drugs to be administered, the route, and the dosages.

If an intravenous catheter is present, the drugs are normally given through it, followed by intravenous fluids at a dosage of 20 ml/kg (cats) or 40 ml/kg (dogs) as rapidly as possible. Caution should be used when administering fluids to patients in cardiac arrest, as overhydration and pulmonary edema are common sequela.

If intravenous access is difficult, drugs may be given by injection into the base of the tongue or by intratracheal administration. Intratracheal administration may involve injection of the drug directly into the tracheal lumen, or the drug may be administered by means of a urinary catheter passed through the endotracheal tube. For intratracheal administration, the dose of emergency drug given should be twice the recommended intravenous dose.

Intracardiac injections should be avoided if possible, since injections by this route require the interruption of cardiac compressions and have some potential to damage the myocardium.

Commonly administered agents include epinephrine, prednisolone sodium succinate, dopamine, dobutamine, doxapram, atropine, lidocaine, and sodium bicarbonate. The current recommended dosage of emergency drugs is given in Tables 6-2 and 6-3.

Epinephrine is the drug most commonly recommended for initial treatment of cardiac arrest. The currently recommended dose is 0.5 ml for cats, 1 ml for small dogs, 2 ml for medium-size dogs, and 3 ml for large dogs, all drawn up from a 1 : 1000 solution. If halothane has been given to the patient, the same volume of a 1 : 10,000 solution should be used, because of an increased chance of ventricular fibrillation if the higher dose rate is used.

Dopamine or dobutamine infusions are also advised by many authorities, because these drugs increase the force and rate of cardiac contractions. Bicarbonate administration is no longer recommended unless the animal is hyperkalemic or cardiac arrest has been present more than 10 minutes. Calcium injections are also no longer advocated, except in hyperkalemic animals.

7. Successful cardiac resuscitation is often dependent on the quality of nursing care given to the patient. As with many recovering patients, restoration of body temperature is important. Other procedures, such as the installation of ophthalmic lubricant and regular repositioning of the patient, are similar to those outlined in Chapter 2 under anesthetic recovery.

Unfortunately, many patients suffering from cardiac arrest cannot be revived. In the case of those patients in which cardiac function is reestablished, conditions such as pulmonary edema and cerebral edema may occur. Cerebral edema is manifested by seizures, failure to return to consciousness, and temporary or permanent neurologic damage.

Repeated cardiac arrests are also common. This type and severity of complications partially depend on the length of time required to reestablish cardiac function.

Potential problems in the recovery period

Regurgitation during anesthesia and postanesthesia vomiting

Regurgitation is a passive phenomenon that occurs even during deep anesthesia. In a regurgitating animal, stomach contents exit through the cardiac sphincter, move up the esophagus, and enter the pharynx, nasopharynx, and oral cavity. Once in the pharynx, stomach contents may be aspirated into the respiratory tract. Regurgitation is most common in animals placed in a head-down position during surgery, because this causes increased pressure on the stomach. Unlike vomiting, regurgitation is not accompanied by retching or other outward signs, and in fact, the only sign apparent to the anesthetist may be a small amount of fluid draining from the animal's mouth or nose. Treatment of regurgitation involves immediate intubation (if a cuffed endotracheal tube is not already present) and removal of as much regurgitated material as possible through suction.

Vomiting during anesthesia is a relatively common phenomenon, particularly in brachycephalic dogs. Unlike regurgitation, vomiting is an active phenomenon, often accompanied by retching. Vomiting usually occurs as the animal is losing consciousness during induction or returning to consciousness during anesthetic recovery. It is potentially most dangerous if the animal is unconscious and the airway is not protected with an endotracheal tube. In this situation, the vomitus may be easily aspirated into the trachea. Aspiration of vomitus may cause immediate signs of dyspnea and cyanosis as a result of airway obstruction and bronchospasm. If the patient survives this episode, signs of aspiration pneumonia, including fever, increased respiratory rate, and increased lung sounds, may appear over the next 24 to 48 hours. It is imperative, therefore, that the anesthetist prevent the accumulation of vomitus within the oral cavity of the unconscious patient and the subsequent aspiration of the material into the air passages. To do this, an endotracheal tube should be immediately inserted if time allows. If this cannot be achieved, the animal's head should be placed at a lower level than the rest of its body (e.g., over the edge of the surgery table), which helps prevent passive flow of liquid material into the trachea. When the vomiting stops, it may be necessary to manually clean the oral cavity, using suction if available. If respiratory arrest occurs because of airway blockage, the animal should be intubated and bagged with oxygen.

Unconscious animals have a low risk of aspiration if a cuffed endotracheal tube is in place during the vomiting episode. It is for this reason that the endotracheal tube is customarily left in place until the patient regains the swallowing reflex and is close to consciousness. If vomiting is seen in an unconscious animal that has a cuffed endotracheal tube in place, the anesthetist should ensure that the cuff of the tube is inflated and should position the animal's head lower than the rest of its body to prevent accumulation of vomitus within the oral cavity.

Fortunately, most vomiting episodes occur after the animal has regained consciousness and the ability to swallow. It is not usually necessary to intubate conscious animals during a vomiting episode; however, the anesthetist should ensure that the head is kept extended and as low as possible.

Occasionally the technician may be called on to anesthetize an animal that has not been fasted before induction. These patients are at greatly increased risk of vomiting and/or regurgitation during induction, maintenance, and recovery. The anesthetist can help avoid problems by ensuring that rapid induction and intubation techniques are used. For this reason, an injectable agent is preferred over masking in these patients. A cuffed endotracheal tube with adequate diameter is essential. If possible, head-down positions should be avoided during surgery to prevent excessive pressure on the stomach. The anesthetist should also ensure that suction is readily available in case of regurgitation or vomiting. Use of antiemetic drugs, such as metaclopramide, may be helpful in some cases.

Postanesthesia seizures

Seizures are occasionally seen in animals recovering from anesthesia. Seizures may be caused by the administration of ketamine, diagnostic procedures such as myelography, or patient disorders such as epilepsy or hypoglycemia.

It is important that the anesthetist differentiate seizures from excitement during recovery. Excitement usually occurs following barbiturate anesthesia, particularly after the use of pentobarbital, and most often appears as spontaneous paddling of the limbs and occasionally as vocalization. Usually, treatment is unnecessary other than calm reassurance of the patient, although sedatives can be helpful (one of the reasons for the use of preanesthetic tranquilizers). In contrast, seizures appear as violent uncontrolled movements of the head, neck, and limbs and are often triggered by a stimulus such as sound or touch.

The anesthetist may occasionally observe signs of excitement in animals that have been given opioids for postoperative pain. Seizure-like activity may result after the administration of opioids to animals that have not been tranquilized, particularly cats.

Animals undergoing postoperative excitement or seizures should be brought to the veterinarian's attention. Elimination of stimuli such as light, sound, and touch may be adequate to resolve the seizure episode. Adequate postoperative analgesia should be provided. Many animals respond well to administration of intravenous or intramuscular diazepam at a dosage rate of 0.2 mg/kg. If diazepam is not effective or is unavailable, the animal may be masked with halothane or isoflurane, or pentobarbital may be administered in sufficient quantity to induce anesthesia.

Animals undergoing seizures or excitement during recovery require surveillance and nursing care to prevent self-injury. In the case of cats recovering from ketamine anesthesia, it may be necessary to trim the front claws or bandage the paws to prevent the animal from scratching its face.

All animals undergoing seizures should be monitored for hyperthermia and cyanosis. Hyperthermia can be treated by the application of cool wet towels. Cyanosis should be treated by the administration of oxygen by face mask.

Dyspnea in the anesthetic recovery period

Dyspnea resulting from upper airway obstruction is the most common cause of death in the postanesthetic period. Dyspnea in cats is usually caused by laryngospasm, whereas dyspnea in dogs is most commonly associated with breed-related (brachycephalic) obstruction of the entrance to the trachea.

Laryngospasm is a condition in which the cartilages in the laryngeal area become so tightly closed that air is unable to enter the trachea. This condition commonly arises in cats because of their extremely active laryngeal reflex. In some recovering cats, the removal of the endotracheal tube initiates reflex closure of the airway. This reflex is normally useful to the cat in that it prevents the aspiration of food or water into the larynx in the conscious animal; however, in the unconscious animal it may well result in complete airway blockage.

Cats undergoing laryngospasm may breathe with an audible stertor or wheeze and typically show exaggerated thoracic movements, gasping, and upward movement of the head during inspiration. If conscious, the animal usually appears anxious or excited. Laryngospasm must be differentiated from growling, which is common in cats recovering from anesthesia. In the case of growling, the noises are particularly evident on *expiration,* whereas in laryngospasm the respiration is labored and the noise is most evident during *inspiration.*

If a cat shows signs of laryngospasm during recovery from anesthesia, the anesthetist should check the mucous membrane color. If the cat's mucous membranes appear pink, the situation may resolve without treatment, although administration of oxygen by face mask may be helpful provided it does not stress the cat. If cyanosis is present and is not alleviated by the administration of oxygen by face mask, the animal must be intubated. To intubate the cat, it may be necessary to reinduce anesthesia by administration of intravenous ketamine or thiobarbiturates. If intubation is impossible, the veterinarian may elect to perform a tracheotomy to reestablish air flow. Once the animal is stabilized, the veterinarian may administer corticosteroids to reduce edema and swelling around the laryngeal area, in an attempt to prevent reoccurrence of the laryngospasm when the endotracheal tube is subsequently removed.

Laryngospasm is easier to prevent than to treat. Gentle intubation technique is essential when anesthetizing cats, to avoid unnecessary laryngeal trauma. Use of lidocaine spray and/or gel is also helpful during intubation. Early extubation is recommended in cats, in order to remove the tube before the laryngeal reflex returns.

Dyspnea in brachycephalic breeds of dogs usually occurs because the airway is obstructed by the soft palate or other redundant tissue in the pharynx. However, there are many other potential causes of obstruction, including foreign objects such as blood clots, gauze sponges, or loose teeth. Animals that have undergone surgery of the pharynx or larynx often undergo postoperative tissue swelling that may lead to airway obstruction.

However it arises, airway obstruction will usually not become evident until after the endotracheal tube is removed. Strategies to prevent and treat postoperative dyspnea in brachycephalic dogs are outlined on p. 247.

Prolonged recovery from anesthesia

Animals experiencing prolonged recovery from anesthesia should be examined by the veterinarian. There are many possible reasons that a patient may be slow to recover, including impaired renal or hepatic function, hypothermia, individual susceptibility to a particular anesthetic, breed variation (particularly sighthounds), or the presence of a disorder such as hypothyroidism, shock, or hemorrhage. Excessive anesthetic depth or prolonged anesthesia may also result in delayed recovery. Use of certain agents, including methoxyflurane, intramuscular ketamine, or repeated injections of barbiturates, may be associated with prolonged recovery even in healthy animals.

Recovery may be hastened in several ways:

- The patient should be placed in a location in which frequent observation is possible. If possible, emergency and monitoring equipment and oxygen should be available in the immediate area.
- It is often helpful to administer intravenous fluids, which hasten renal elimination of anesthetics and support circulation. The recommended rate of fluid administration for most intensive care patients is 3 to 5 ml/kg/hr.
- Oxygen may be administered by face mask at a rate of 1 to 4 L/minute, particularly if the patient is cyanotic or the respirations are shallow. Alternatively, oxygen can also be directed through a bottle of distilled water (for humidification) and delivered to the patient by means of a nasal catheter.
- Good nursing care is important, and the patient should be turned frequently and kept warm. If the patient's temperature is less than 37° C, active warming procedures should be instituted, including the use of fan heaters, reflective blankets, circulating warm water pads, chemical warmers, or towels warmed in a dryer.

• The animal should be periodically monitored for vital signs and reflexes. Urine production also should be monitored and should be at least 2 ml/kg/hr.

Reversing agents and analeptics are used occasionally to hasten anesthetic recovery. However, the anesthetist whose patients consistently demonstrate slow recoveries should not rely on pharmacologic solutions to solve what may be a problem of technique. The anesthetist should reexamine the anesthetic protocol and consult with the veterinarian to determine whether more appropriate agents or means of administration should be used. It is important to ensure that animals are not maintained at excessively deep levels of anesthesia for routine procedures. Finally, the anesthetist should ensure that every effort is made to avoid hypothermia in the anesthetized patient, since a subnormal body temperature will often result in prolonged anesthetic recovery.

KEY POINTS

1. Although anesthetic complications are uncommon, the technician must be able to anticipate and respond to emergencies in an efficient and knowledgeable fashion.

2. Human error may result in anesthetic problems: such error may arise from failure to obtain an adequate history or physical examination, lack of familiarity with the anesthetic machine or drugs used, incorrect administration of drugs, fatigue, inattentiveness, or distraction.

3. Equipment failure or operator carelessness may result in carbon dioxide absorber exhaustion, failure to deliver sufficient oxygen to the patient, misassembly of the anesthetic machine, failure of the vaporizer or pop-off valve, or endotracheal tube problems.

4. Anesthetic agents may cause problems during anesthesia, and the anesthetic protocol must be chosen to reflect the special needs of each patient. The anesthetist must be familiar with the adverse side effects associated with the use of each agent in the anesthetic protocol.

5. Some patients are at increased risk of anesthetic complications, due to preexisting factors such as old age, organ failure, recent trauma, or breed-related conformation.

6. Geriatric patients have less reserve than younger patients and have reduced anesthetic requirements. Neonatal patients also require reduced dosages of injectable agents and are prone to hypothermia and hypoglycemia.

7. Brachycephalic dogs suffer from anatomic characteristics that make respiration difficult, particularly during the recovery period. Preoxygenation before induc-

tion, rapid induction and intubation, and close monitoring during recovery are essential.

8. Thiobarbiturate drugs should be used with extreme care in sighthounds.

9. Obese animals should receive anesthetic dosages according to their ideal body weight.

10. Pregnant animals presented for cesarean section are at increased anesthetic risk. Various anesthetic techniques including epidural anesthesia, balanced anesthesia, and neuroleptanalgesia are sometimes used as alternatives to inhalation anesthesia in these patients. Almost all anesthetic agents may cause depression of fetal respiration and/or circulation, and the use of reversing agents may be advisable.

11. If possible, patients that have undergone recent trauma should be stabilized and thoroughly evaluated before anesthesia.

12. Animals suffering from cardiovascular or respiratory disease may require special anesthetic techniques such as preoxygenation and manual control of ventilation.

13. Hepatic or renal disease may cause delayed excretion of injectable agents, and prolonged recovery times may be seen. Inhalation anesthesia is often preferred to the use of injectable agents in these patients.

14. Emergency care is ideally a team effort involving all hospital personnel. It is helpful to have preauthorized emergency protocols and periodic "dress rehearsals."

15. It may be difficult to maintain adequate anesthetic depth in some patients: incorrect placement of the endotracheal tube, incorrect vaporizer setting, inadequate endotracheal tube size, and many other factors may contribute to this problem.

16. Excessive anesthetic depth may result from excessive administration of anesthetic agents or from preexisting patient problems. It may be necessary to bag the patient with 100% oxygen to achieve a lighter plane of anesthesia.

17. Pale mucous membranes may arise as a result of anemia, hemorrhage, or poor perfusion. Prolonged capillary refill suggests that hypotension (or, if severe, shock) is present.

18. Cyanosis is a critical emergency and arises because of insufficient delivery of oxygen to the tissues. It may result from a machine problem, airway or endotracheal tube blockage, or respiratory difficulties resulting from excessive depth, pneumothorax, or respiratory disease. Oxygen delivery to the patient must be reestablished through masking, intubation, or tracheostomy.

19. Abnormalities in cardiac rate and rhythm may result from the administration of

anesthetic agents, electrolyte abnormalities, hypercarbia, hypoxia, and many other factors.

20. Respiratory arrest that is accompanied by cyanosis and/or bradycardia is an emergency and must be treated by ventilation with 100% oxygen.

21. Cardiac arrest should be treated according to the principles of ABCD (establish a patent *a*irway, *b*ag the patient with 100% oxygen, initiate internal or external *c*ardiac massage, and administer epinephrine and other *d*rugs).

22. Regurgitation and/or vomiting may be dangerous in the anesthetized animal because of the danger of airway obstruction and aspiration pneumonia.

23. Postanesthesia seizures may be treated by eliminating external stimuli and administering diazepam.

24. Dyspnea caused by laryngospasm or brachycephalic airway obstruction may be treated by administration of oxygen by mask, reintubation of the patient, or tracheostomy.

25. Animals experiencing prolonged recovery from anesthesia require close observation and nursing care. An effort should be made to determine the reason for delayed arousal of each patient.

REVIEW QUESTIONS

1. When an animal scheduled for a surgical procedure is brought in by a neighbor who is in a hurry, the best thing to do is:
   a. Instruct the receptionist to have the neighbor sign the consent form
   b. Ask the neighbor to take the animal back home
   c. Ask the neighbor some quick questions about the animal
   d. Have the neighbor sign the consent form and then ensure that the owner is called before the procedure is initiated so a more thorough history can be obtained

2. In preparation for an anesthetic procedure, you have drawn up a syringe of barbiturate and an identical syringe of saline. You are then called to the front office to assist the veterinarian. About 10 minutes later you return to prepare the animal for induction. With the IV catheter in place, you are just about to inject some saline into the animal when you realize that you are not sure if the syringe contains saline. The best thing to do would be to:
   a. Inject a small amount of the solution and see what effect it has
   b. Discard both syringes and start over
   c. Ask the person who was holding the animal which syringe had saline in it
   d. Discard both syringes, label some new syringes, and start over

3. You have just begun working at a new veterinary practice, and one of your duties will be to oversee all anesthetic procedures. You notice that there is an anesthetic machine in the corner, but there is no date or information to indicate when the CO_2 absorber was last changed. The best thing to do would be to:

    a. Use the machine first and see if any of the granules change color during the procedure

    b. Ask the other staff members if they know how old the chemical in the absorber canister is

    c. Discard the contents of the canister and put in fresh granules

    d. Discard half of the contents and fill the remainder of the canister with fresh chemical

4. You are about to use the anesthetic machine and notice that although the flowmeter is working, the pressure gauge on the oxygen tank is reading close to zero. The best thing to do would be to:

    a. Assume that the pressure gauge may be faulty and wait and see if the flowmeter stops working

    b. Assume that the pressure gauge may be faulty and have another tank available for use

    c. Call the repair person to have the pressure gauge checked

    d. Change the oxygen tank for a fresh tank

5. While monitoring a patient on an anesthetic machine, you realize that the oxygen tank has become empty. The best thing to do would be to:

    a. Leave the patient and get another oxygen tank

    b. Remove the circuit from the patient to allow him to breathe room air

    c. After disconnecting the patient from the circuit, put on a new oxygen tank and then reconnect the patient to the circuit

6. A precision vaporizer is designed to have any of the three commonly used volatile anesthetics put into it.

    True   False

7. If the pop-off valve is inadvertently left shut, it will:

    a. Stop the oxygen flow from entering the circuit

    b. Cause a significant rise of pressure within the circuit

    c. Cause the flutter valves to malfunction

8. You look at the oxygen tank and note that 1000 psi of pressure is left in the tank, but the flowmeter now reads 0 and you cannot obtain a flow by twisting the knobs. The best thing to do would be to assume:

    a. The oxygen tank pressure gauge is malfunctioning and recheck the flowmeter

    b. The oxygen is okay and the flowmeter just is not registering the flow

    c. That the animal is not getting oxygen, and remove the animal from the circuit until a new machine is found or the problem is corrected

9. A geriatric patient is considered to be one that:

    a. Is greater than 10 years old

    b. Is greater than 15 years old

    c. Has reached 50% of its life expectancy

    d. Has reached 75% of its life expectancy

10. An obese dog about to receive an injectable anesthetic should receive:

    a. The dose prescribed on a mg/kg basis

    b. A reduced dosage

    c. A dosage based on ideal weight

    d. An inhalation anesthetic only

11. Brain damage may occur when there is inadequate oxygenation of the tissues for longer than _____ minutes.

   a. 2
   b. 4
   c. 6
   d. 8
   e. 10

12. When a technician is performing CPR alone, the ratio of cardiac compressions to ventilation should be:
   a. 5:1
   b. 10:1
   c. 5:2
   d. 10:2

13. To ensure that the benefit an animal obtains from CPR is not lost, one should not discontinue the CPR for longer than:
   a. 30 seconds
   b. 60 seconds
   c. 90 seconds
   d. 120 seconds

14. Respiratory arrest is always fatal.
   True   False

15. A systolic blood pressure below _____ mm Hg suggests that the animal is hypotensive.
   a. 60
   b. 80
   c. 100
   d. 120

The following questions may have one or more correct answers.

16. Endotracheal tubes may malfunction because of:
   a. Blockage from blood or mucus
   b. Improper positioning of the endotracheal tube
   c. Kinking of the tube from poor positioning

17. One may suspect that the endotracheal tube is malfunctioning even if it is in the trachea because:
   a. Compression of the reservoir bag does not result in the raising of the chest
   b. The animal is severely dyspneic
   c. The animal cannot be kept at an adequate plane of anesthesia
   d. The reservoir bag is not moving or is moving very little

18. One may suspect that the pop-off valve has been closed or that it is malfunctioning if the:
   a. Reservoir bag is distended with air
   b. Patient has difficulty exhaling
   c. Patient wakes up
   d. Flow rate starts to drop

19. Recovery from anesthesia in a geriatric animal may be slower because of:
   a. Decreased renal function
   b. Decreased hepatic function
   c. Hypothermia
   d. Tachycardia

20. Administration of the normal rate of fluids (10 ml/kg/hr) during an anesthetic procedure is more likely to result in overhydration in the:
   a. Neonate
   b. Geriatric
   c. Feline patient
   d. Brachycephalic

21. Brachycephalic dogs may be an increased anesthetic risk because of their:
   a. Physical size
   b. Excess tissue around the oropharynx
   c. Increased vagal tone
   d. Small trachea in comparison to their physical body size
   e. Increased susceptibility to barbiturates

22. To decrease the anesthetic risk associated with a brachycephalic dog, the anesthetist may elect to:
   a. Use atropine as part of the anesthetic protocol
   b. Preoxygenate the animal before giving any anesthetic
   c. Use an injectable anesthetic to hasten induction rather than masking
   d. Ensure intubation is done quickly after induction

23. The thiobarbiturates are well suited to induction of:
   a. Sighthounds
   b. Retrievers
   c. Spaniels
   d. Afghan hounds

24. The animal about to undergo cesarian section is at increased risk for anesthesia because of:
   a. Decreased respiratory function
   b. Increased chance of aspiration vomitus
   c. Increased chance of hemorrhage
   d. Increased work load of the heart

25. The traumatized patient may be an increased anesthetic risk within the first few hours after the trauma because of:
   a. Hypovolemia
   b. Cardiac dysrhythmias
   c. Decreased respiratory function
   d. Resistance to the effects of atropine

26. Anesthetic agents or drugs that one may want to avoid in the animal with cardiovascular disease include:
   a. Halothane
   b. Isoflurane
   c. Xylazine
   d. Opioids

27. An animal that has liver dysfunction may be hypoproteinemic and therefore requires _____ for induction compared to that needed for a normal dog.
   a. More barbiturate
   b. Less barbiturate
   c. The same amount of barbiturate

28. Too light a plane of anesthesia may be the result of:

    a. A flow rate that is too low
    b. Incorrect vaporizer setting
    c. Incorrect placement of the endotracheal tube
    d. Use of an anesthetic with a low solubility coefficient

29. An animal that is too deeply anesthetized may show which of the following?
    a. Weak pulse
    b. Pale mucous membranes
    c. Bradycardia
    d. Hypoventilation

30. Which of the following would you want to undertake if an animal was showing excessive depth of anesthesia?
    a. Turn off the vaporizer
    b. Administer 100% oxygen
    c. Establish an IV line and administer IV fluids
    d. Intubate and bag the animal
    e. Immediately transfuse with whole blood

31. Clinical signs that one may observe in a patient in the initial stages of circulatory shock include:
    a. Tachycardia
    b. Weak pulse
    c. Pale mucous membranes
    d. Hypothermia
    e. Slow capillary refill

32. Tachypnea may result from:
    a. Increased levels of arterial oxygen
    b. Increased levels of arterial CO_2
    c. The use of ketamine
    d. Too light a plane of anesthesia

33. Causes of bradycardia may include:
    a. Hyperkalemia
    b. Hypoxia
    c. Hyperthermia
    d. Increased vagal tone

34. Drugs that may induce cardiac dysrhythmias may include:
    a. Xylazine
    b. Barbiturates
    c. Isoflurane
    d. Halothane

35. Cardiac dysrhythmias may be seen as a result of:
    a. Nitrous oxide administration (with oxygen)
    b. Hypoxia
    c. Hypercarbia
    d. Light stages of anesthesia

36. Temporary cessation of respirations may occur due to:
    a. Use of acetylpromazine as a premedication
    b. Too deep a plane of anesthesia
    c. Bagging the animal with oxygen
    d. Barbiturate induction

37. If a patient has stopped breathing, things that the technician may consider doing include checking:
 a. The level of anesthesia
 b. To see that the heart rate is adequate
 c. To be sure the pulse is strong
 d. The capillary refill time and color of mucous membranes
 e. The packed cell volume
38. Prolonged recovery from anesthesia may be the result of:
 a. Hypothermia
 b. Hepatic dysfunction
 c. Renal dysfunction
 d. Repeated administration of thiobarbiturate

ANSWERS FOR CHAPTER 6

1. d **2.** d **3.** c **4.** d **5.** c **6.** False **7.** b **8.** c **9.** d **10.** c
11. b **12.** d **13.** a **14.** False **15.** b **16.** a, b, c **17.** a, b, c, d **18.** a, b
19. a, b, c **20.** a, b **21.** b, c, d **22.** a, b, c, d **23.** b, c **24.** a, b, c, d **25.** a, b, c
26. a, c **27.** b **28.** a, b, c **29.** a, b, c, d **30.** a, b, c, d **31.** a, b, c, d, e
32. b, d **33.** a, b, d **34.** a, b, d **35.** b, c, d **36.** b, c, d **37.** a, b, c, d
38. a, b, c, d

SELECTED READINGS

Clarke KW, Hall LW: A survey of anaesthesia in small animal practice: AVA/BSAVA report, *J Assoc Vet Anaesth* 17:4-10, 1990.

Dodman NH: Aging changes in the geriatric dog and their impact on anesthesia, *Compendium* 6(12):1106-1112, 1984.

Dyson DH, Mathews K: Recommendations for intensive care management in small animals following anaesthesia, *VCOT* 5:66-70, 1992.

Harvey RC: *Cardiopulmonary resuscitation in small animal practice,* Knoxville, 1991, University of Tennessee (unpublished).

Harvey RC, Paddleford RR: Management of anesthetic emergencies and complications, *Vet Tech* 12(3):237-242, 1991.

Haskins SC: *Opinions in small animal anesthesia,* Vet Clin North Am (Small Anim Pract) 22(2), Philadelphia, 1992, WB Saunders.

Holland, M: Anesthesia for feline cesarean section, *Vet Tech* 12(5):397-402, 1991.

Marcella KL, Short CE: Anesthetic management of the pregnant animal, *Compendium* 6(10):942-948, 1984.

Paddleford RR: *Manual of small animal anesthesia,* New York, 1988, Churchill Livingstone.

Raffe MR, Hardy RC: Anesthetic management of the hepatic patient, *Compendium* 4(10):842-848, 1982.

Robinson EP: Anesthesia of pediatric patients, *Compendium* 5(12):1004-1011, 1983.

Sawyer DC: Anesthesia for problem and high-risk patients, *Vet Tech* 15(2):61-69, 1994.

Wittnich C, Belanger MP, Salerno TA, Slutsky AS, Trudel JL: Canine cardiopulmonary resuscitation: External versus internal cardiac massage, *Compendium* 13(1):50-56, 1991.

Special techniques

7

PERFORMANCE OBJECTIVES
After completion of this chapter, the reader will be able to:

Define or explain the terms local analgesia, line block, nerve block, epidural anesthesia, controlled ventilation, assisted ventilation, manual ventilation, and mechanical ventilation.

Understand the advantages and disadvantages associated with the use of local analgesic agents.

Understand the various ways in which analgesic agents may be administered, including topical, infiltration, regional, epidural, and intravenous routes.

Describe the technique for performing an epidural block, and list the clinical situations in which this block could be used.

Understand the risks involved and the adverse side effects that may be manifested with the use of local analgesic agents.

Explain the difference between assisted and controlled ventilation.

Understand the techniques of assisted and controlled ventilation and their application to canine and feline anesthesia.

Describe the indications for the use of neuromuscular blocking agents and the hazards associated with their use.

Define the terms tidal volume, respiratory minute volume, atelectasis, and sigh.

State the difference between the two major types of neuromuscular blocking agents.

Explain the concept of "reversing" neuromuscular blocking agents.

The anesthetic agents and techniques used for routine procedures on most patients have been described in previous chapters. Occasionally, however, a patient is presented in which a specialized technique such as local analgesia, mechanical ventilation, and/or the use of neuromuscular blocking agents may be indicated. This chapter describes these techniques and indicates the circumstances in which they may be useful.

LOCAL ANALGESIA

The term *local analgesia* refers to the use of a chemical agent on sensory and motor neurons to produce a temporary loss of pain sensation and movement. Although less commonly used than general anesthetics, local analgesics are an effective and practical alternative in many situations involving canine and feline patients. The choice of local analgesia or general anesthesia is made by the veterinarian based on such factors as the temperament, age, and physical status of the patient, cost, time available, the nature of the surgery to be performed, and the anesthetist's skill in performing the local analgesia procedure. Local analgesia offers the advantages of low patient toxicity, low cost, and minimal patient recovery time. There are several disadvantages, however, including the following:

* There is some risk of overdose, particularly in smaller patients (see Toxicity on p. 294).
* Local analgesics may not provide sufficient patient restraint when used alone.
* Effective use of local analgesics often requires precise placement of the drug immediately adjacent to the target nerve. The veterinarian and/or technician performing the procedure must be familiar with the technique involved for each type of nerve block. For example, it is possible to block the sensory nerves of a dog's canine tooth in a manner similar to that employed by a dentist for humans, but few veterinarians or technicians have the patience or expertise to perform these blocks in small animals, given the convenience, safety, and effectiveness of general anesthetics.
* Local analgesics are relatively ineffective in areas composed of fat, bone, cartilage, fascia, tendon, and other connective tissues.

Agents used in veterinary anesthesia

Many local analgesic agents are available; they vary in strength, duration of effect, and method of use (see Table 7-1). Lidocaine (Xylocaine), bupivacaine (Marcaine), mepivacaine (Carbocaine), and procaine (Novocaine) are the agents most commonly used for skin infiltration and application to mucous membranes. Tetracaine (Pontocaine) and proparacaine (Ophthaine) are reserved chiefly for ophthalmic use.

Characteristics of local analgesia

Local analgesia differs from general anesthesia in several important respects:
* Local analgesics are not anesthetics, and the term *local anesthetic* is a misnomer. The term *anesthetic* is reserved for those drugs, such as barbiturates, ketamine, or inhalation anesthetics, that primarily affect neurons in the brain. Local analgesics also exert their effect on neurons, but *only* on those neurons in the peripheral nervous system and spinal cord.

TABLE 7-1
Local analgesics

Agent (generic name)	Trade name	Potency (Procaine = 1)	Dosage	Onset and duration of action
Lidocaine	Xylocaine	2	0.5%-2% for injection 2%-4% for topical use	Immediate onset; 2 hour duration with epinephrine
Mepivacaine	Carbocaine	2.5	1%-2% for injection	Immediate onset; duration 90-180 minutes
Tetracaine	Pontocaine	12	0.1% for injection 0.2% for topical use	Onset 5-10 minutes; duration 2 hours
Bupivacaine	Marcaine	8	0.25%-0.5% for injection 0.75% for epidural	Immediate onset; duration 4-6 hours

From Skardo RT: Local and regional analgesia. In Short CE: *Principles and practices of veterinary anesthesia,* Baltimore, 1987, Williams & Williams.

- Because local analgesics normally do not affect the brain, they have little sedating effect. The patient remains fully conscious unless other agents such as tranquilizers or neuroleptanalgesics are used. This is in contrast to general anesthetics, which produce complete unconsciousness.
- When properly used, local analgesics have relatively few effects on the cardiovascular or respiratory systems. In contrast, general anesthetics may cause significant cardiovascular and respiratory depression. For this reason, local analgesia may be preferable to general anesthesia for use in certain high-risk patients.
- Whereas general anesthetics are widely distributed throughout the body, local analgesics primarily exert their effects in the area closest to the site of injection. Unlike general anesthetics, local analgesics are not normally transferred across the placenta to the fetus. For this reason, local analgesia is sometimes used for cesarean sections and obstetric manipulations.

Mechanism of action

The peripheral nervous system and spinal cord are composed of many types of neurons. From the standpoint of the anesthetist, the most important of these are the neurons that convey sensations (pain, heat, cold, and pressure) from the skin, muscles, and other peripheral tissues to the brain. These neurons are termed *sensory neurons* and are affected by even small amounts of local analgesics, provided the drug is deposited in close proximity to the neuron. Another type of neuron, called *motor neurons,* conveys impulses from the brain to muscle fibers and is responsible for initiating and controlling voluntary movements. Motor neurons are also sensitive to the effect of local analgesics, resulting in temporary paresis (weakness) or paralysis (loss of movement) in the area served by the affected motor neurons after infiltration with a local analgesic.

Loss of sensation and loss of motor ability are seen concurrently. For example, use of a local analgesic near the terminal end of the spinal cord (called an epidural block) will result in loss of sensation and voluntary movement to all areas innervated by the affected sensory and motor neurons. The patient sensations that are lost include (in order of loss) pain, cold, warmth, touch, joint sensation, and deep pressure in the caudal abdomen and pelvic limbs. The patient also will be unable to move the pelvic limbs, and the muscles will appear relaxed.

A third type of neuron, those of the autonomic nervous system, is also affected by local analgesics. These neurons convey impulses from the brain to the blood vessels and internal organs (including the heart). If these neurons are exposed to local analgesics, their function is lost, resulting in a *sympathetic blockade.* The main effect in the peripheral tissues is vasodilation, resulting in flushing and increased skin temperature of the affected area. Vasodilation may lead to hypotension in some patients. A sympathetic blockade is commonly seen after epidural blocks, because sympathetic ganglia adjacent to the vertebrae are affected by the local analgesic. If a sympathetic blockade occurs within the proximal spinal cord (as may occur if local analgesic is allowed to infuse into the thoracic spinal canal), sympathetic innervation to the heart may be blocked, resulting in bradycardia and decreased ventricular contractions.

The mechanism of action of local analgesics is not fully understood, but appears to involve a blockage of transmission of electrical impulses along the nerve fiber. The local analgesic appears to block the membrane channels through which sodium flows into the neuron. A local analgesic drug therefore acts as a membrane stabilizer, stopping the process of nerve depolarization. The result is a loss of nerve conduction. Reversal of this effect occurs when the drug is absorbed into the local circulation. Local analgesics are then redistributed to the liver, where they are inactivated.

Route of administration

Topical use

Local analgesics are usually ineffective when applied directly to intact skin, since the drug molecules are unable to penetrate the epidermis and reach the dermis, where the peripheral nerves are located. However, local analgesics can be absorbed by mucous membranes, including the conjunctiva and respiratory epithelium. These drugs therefore can be used in the form of topical sprays or drops applied to these areas. One common topical use of local analgesics is administration of lidocaine spray to the larynx of a cat before intubation. Another local analgesic, cetacaine, was commonly used for this purpose in the past, but at present it is seldom used because it has the potential to induce methemoglobinemia in this species. Another common situation in which local analgesics are topically administered is the application of proparacaine or tetracaine to the surface of the eye. This is done to desensitize the cornea and conjunctiva before performing procedures such as conjunctival scrapings or tonometry. Local analgesics also may be used in the form of a gel, which can, for example, be applied to a urinary catheter to ease the catheterization process. In each case, analgesia of the mucous membrane results within 60 to 90 seconds, allowing procedures to be performed with less discomfort to the patient.

Infiltration

Local analgesics may be infiltrated (injected) into tissues, preferably in close proximity to the nerve that is to be affected. The local analgesic can be given intradermally, subcutaneously, or between muscles, depending on the area to be treated. Infiltration techniques are used most commonly to provide analgesia for surgery involving superficial tissues, including skin biopsies, removal of small skin tumors, and repair of minor lacerations.

The procedure used for local analgesia infusion is relatively simple. Before infiltration of local analgesic, the area must be clipped and a skin antiseptic applied in a manner similar to that used for a surgical prep. This prevents inadvertent contamination of the tissues with skin bacteria when the local analgesic is injected. A small gauge needle (23- or 25-gauge) is often used because these needles create little tissue damage and allow for more precise placement of the drug. The amount of the drug to be injected varies with the location and procedure used, but is typically between 0.5 and 1 ml per site.

The two types of procedures used for local analgesia infusion are nerve blocks and line blocks (Fig. 7-1).

Nerve blocks. A nerve block is achieved by injecting local analgesic in close proximity to a nerve, in order to desensitize a particular site. Reference texts contain illustrations that indicate the exact location of nerve blocks for different species and particular areas of the body. Nerve blocks are used very commonly in large animal anesthesia and also may be employed in small animals provided the location of the nerve is known exactly. Before placing a nerve block, it is helpful to palpate the nerve to determine its location, although this may not always be possible. A small amount of local analgesic is injected immediately adjacent to the nerve. The drug diffuses through the tissues to reach the target nerve. Caution should be

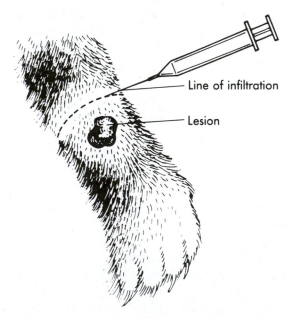

Fig. 7-1. Procedure for performing a line block.

used to avoid injecting directly into a nerve because temporary or permanent loss of nerve function can occur. It is also important to avoid intravenous injection of the drug, which not only is ineffective in producing local analgesia, but also may cause unwanted central nervous system and cardiovascular effects. For this reason, it is advisable to aspirate before injecting a local analgesic, and if blood appears in the syringe, the location of the injection should be changed.

Line blocks. Often the veterinarian will do surgery on an area of tissue that is served by numerous small neurons. In this situation, a *line block* consisting of a continuous line of local analgesic can be placed in the subcutaneous or subcuticular tissues immediately proximal to the target area (see Fig. 7-1). It is important to place the line block between the target area and the spinal cord, because this will block the sensory neurons most effectively. Placement of a line block can be easily accomplished by inserting the needle along the proposed line of infiltration and gradually withdrawing the needle while simultaneously injecting a small amount of local analgesic.

Regardless of whether the veterinarian prefers to use a nerve block or a line block, the onset of analgesia is usually 3 to 5 minutes after the injection of lidocaine. It is advisable to test the effectiveness of the block before surgery commences, by gently pricking the skin with a 22-gauge needle. If sensation appears to be present, the anesthetist should wait several minutes longer and consider repeating the infusion or using another anesthetic protocol if the block does not take effect.

The infusion of local analgesics is not universally effective. Deep tissues such as muscles are unlikely to be affected when only superficial neurons are blocked. Additionally, diffusion of local analgesic is impeded by obstacles such as scar tissue or fibrous tissue, fat, edema, and hemorrhage, and the procedure is often ineffective in these areas. Local analgesia is also relatively ineffective when injected into inflamed areas. In areas of active inflammation, tissue pH is acidic, which results in rapid inactivation of the drug.

Once the local analgesic reaches the neuron, the duration of effect depends on the type of drug being used (Table 7-1) and the rate of absorption by local blood vessels. This, in turn, depends on whether epinephrine is used with the local analgesic. Lidocaine, the drug most commonly used for local infusion, may be purchased with or without epinephrine. The concentration of epinephrine used is 5 micrograms per ml (1:200,000 solution).

Epinephrine is added to local analgesics for two reasons:
1. Epinephrine causes blood vessels in the area of the injection to constrict. This decreases the rate of drug absorption and thereby prolongs the effect of the local analgesic.
2. By causing vasoconstriction, epinephrine reduces the concentration of local analgesic that enters the circulation at any given time, thereby reducing toxicity of the drug.

Lidocaine *without* epinephrine may be preferred to lidocaine *with* epinephrine in some situations. A solution containing epinephrine should not be used at an incision site because it may impair tissue perfusion and healing. Epinephrine also increases the risk of ventricular dysrhythmias and should be used with caution in animals with known cardiac disease.

Regional analgesia

Regional analgesia is a technique whereby a local analgesic is injected into a major nerve plexus or in close proximity to the spinal cord. This results in the blockage of nervous impulses from a relatively large area, such as an entire limb or the entire caudal portion of the body.

Several procedures are commonly used for regional analgesia in veterinary and human anesthesia. These include epidural, spinal (intrathecal), and brachial plexus analgesia. When used in animals, these techniques often are combined with the use of neuroleptanalgesics or other injectable medications. This helps to assure adequate restraint, allowing accurate and safe injection of the local analgesic and preventing patient movement during the surgical procedure.

Epidural analgesia. Epidural analgesia is a regional analgesia technique that is used very commonly in large animal anesthesia and, to a lesser extent, in small animal anesthesia. The procedure is not difficult (see the box below) and once mastered allows the anesthetist to reliably block sensation and motor control of the rear abdomen, pelvis, tail, pelvic limbs, and perineum. The technique therefore can be used for tail amputation, anal sac removal, perianal surgery, urethrostomies, obstetric manipulations, cesarean sections, and surgery to the rear limb.

Epidural anesthesia is particularly valuable in two classes of patients: (1) debilitated patients that are deemed to be at high risk for general anesthesia and (2) patients requiring profound analgesia of the limbs, pelvis, or caudal abdomen.

Anatomic considerations for epidural analgesia. To understand the technique used for epidural analgesia, the anesthetist must be familiar with the anatomy of the terminal spinal cord region (Fig. 7-2). The spinal cord (containing the sensory,

---

Procedure for epidural analgesia in the dog and cat

Gather the necessary equipment. This includes a short-bevelled spinal needle with a stylet (18- to 20-gauge, 1.5 inches for small or thin dogs, and 2 to 3 inches for large overweight dogs), and several sterile 3-ml or 5-ml syringes. If a catheter is to be placed, a thin-walled, 18-gauge, 3-inch needle is required.

Sedate the patient to achieve adequate restraint, and place in sternal or lateral recumbency. The head is sometimes positioned higher than the spinal cord for at least the first 10 minutes of analgesia.

Identify the right and left cranial dorsal wings of the ilium, the spinous process of L7, and the sacral crest. Shave and surgically prepare the area surrounding the injection site (between L7 and the sacral crest). Wear surgical gloves for the procedure.

The anesthetist palpates the lumbosacral space (between L7 and the sacrum), halfway between the dorsal iliac wings and just caudal to the dorsal spinous process of L7 (see Fig. 7-3). Place the spinal needle in the area of greatest depression, perpendicular to the skin surface and exactly on the midline. Advance the needle in a slight cranial or caudal angle, as needed. Resistance may be encountered, and a distinct *pop* often can be felt as the needle is advanced through the ligamentum flavum (see Fig. 7-2). Immediately after penetrating the ligamentum flavum, the needle enters the epidural space. This usually occurs at a needle depth of 1 to 3 cm, depending on the size of the animal.

Remove the stylet, and examine the needle hub for blood or cerebrospinal fluid. If cerebrospinal fluid is encountered, the needle is in the subarachnoid space. (If this is the case, the procedure may be abandoned or the anesthetist may choose to administer 50% of the original dose, inducing spinal analgesia.) If blood and cerebrospinal fluid are not observed, the needle should be aspirated to ensure that neither is present. To further check for proper needle placement, 1 to 2 ml of air can be injected: no resistance to air passage should be felt.

The dosage of 2% lidocaine (with or without epinephrine) or 0.75% bupivacaine with epinephrine will vary with the extent of analgesia required. The anesthetist often will elect to produce anesthesia as far cranial as L2 (which is sufficient for most caudal abdominal procedures and all pelvic and rear limb procedures). To achieve this, inject a dose of 1 ml lidocaine or bupivacaine for each 5 kg of body weight. If analgesia is required to the level of T5, increase the dose to 1 ml of local analgesic for each 3 kg of body weight.

Inject the calculated dose of lidocaine or bupivacaine over 1 minute. More rapid injection may result in local analgesic infiltrating too far forward along the spinal canal (see p. 295). Injection will be resistance-free if the needle is positioned correctly. If continuous epidural analgesia is required, a polyethylene catheter may be advanced through the needle and the needle subsequently withdrawn, leaving the catheter in place. Advance the catheter only 1 cm into the epidural space.

Onset of analgesia is approximately 5 minutes after lidocaine infusion or 20 minutes after bupivacaine infusion. The block normally affects the most distal body parts (toes and tail) first. If a bilateral effect is desired, position the patient in dorsal recumbency for 20 minutes after the injection. If unilateral analgesia is required, place the patient in lateral recumbency, with the desired side positioned ventrally, allowing for gravitation of the local analgesic within the epidural space to the targeted side of the spinal canal.

It has been reported that 12% of correctly performed epidural blocks are ineffective, perhaps because of individual variations in anatomy. Failure of the block may be determined by testing with a needle prick or may become evident during patient preparation or application of towel clamps.

Duration of analgesia is 4 to 6 hours for bupivacaine with epinephrine and 1.5 hours for lidocaine with epinephrine.

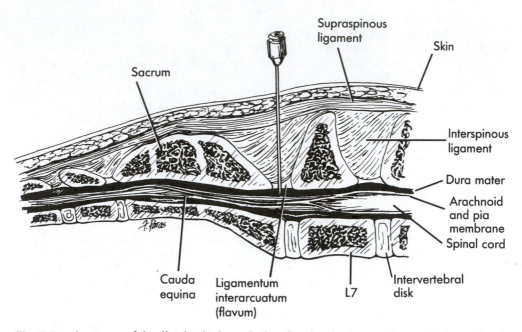

Fig. 7-2. Anatomy of the distal spinal canal, showing the placement of a needle for epidural analgesia. (From Muir WW, III, Hubbell JAE: *Handbook of veterinary anesthesia,* St Louis, 1989, Mosby.)

motor, and sympathetic neurons) is surrounded by three membrane layers: the pia, arachnoid, and dura mater. The subarachnoid space, which is the area between the arachnoid and the pia, is filled with cerebrospinal fluid. This fluid surrounds the entire spinal cord and communicates with the cerebrospinal fluid in the ventricles of the brain. The spinal cord and its membrane layers are encased within the spinal canal, consisting of bony vertebrae (cervical, thoracic, lumbar, sacral, and coccygeal), which protect the spinal cord from injury. In addition to the vertebrae, the vertebral canal is protected by several ligaments, including the supraspinous ligament (directly under the skin, see Fig. 7-2), the ligamentum flavum (also called the ligamentum interarcuatum), and the interspinous ligament. Neurons that supply the tissues exit from the spinal cord at regular intervals, emerging between the vertebrae and ultimately terminating in the skin and other tissues. The spinal cord itself terminates in a group of neurons collectively called the cauda equina.

In performing epidural analgesia, local analgesic is deposited in the epidural space, between the dura and the vertebrae. In dogs the location of the block is between the last lumbar vertebra (L7) and sacrum (Fig. 7-3). When properly performed, injection of local analgesic into this area is unlikely to damage the spinal cord, since the cord normally ends at the sixth or seventh lumbar vertebra (L6 or

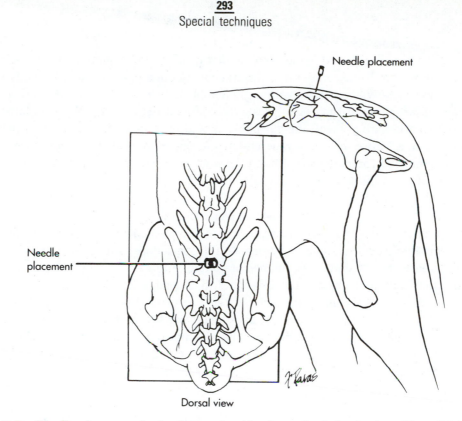

Needle placement

Needle
placement

Dorsal view

Fig. 7-3. Needle placement for lumbosacral epidural anesthesia in the dog. (From Muir WW, III, Hubbell JAE: *Handbook of veterinary anesthesia,* St Louis, 1989, Mosby.)

L7). In cats the spinal cord extends further caudally (as far as S1), and there is a slightly increased risk of spinal cord damage when performing an epidural. Inadvertent injection of local analgesic into the subarachnoid space also is more common in the cat than in the dog.

Epidural analgesia must be differentiated from spinal analgesia, which is commonly performed in human patients. In spinal analgesia, the local analgesic is infiltrated into the subarachnoid space, where it mixes with the cerebrospinal fluid.

Use of epidural analgesia to treat postoperative pain. Recently considerable interest has focused on the use of epidural blocks to provide prolonged and effective analgesia to patients suffering from severe injuries or postoperative pain affecting the caudal abdomen, pelvis, or rear limbs. Several drugs have been used for this purpose, including local analgesics (lidocaine, mepivacaine, bupivacaine) and opiates (morphine). The advantage of this technique is that relatively small amounts of drug are used and systemic effects are minimized. Duration of effect appears to be long, particularly if opiates are used. A single injection of 0.1 mg/kg of morphine may provide up to 24 hours of analgesia.

The procedure used is the same as that described for epidural analgesia in the box on p. 290. Either epidural or intrathecal injection may be used. It is advisable that single-use vials of drug without epinephrine or preservatives be used. In the case of morphine, 0.1 mg/kg of preservative-free drug (Duramorph) is preferred. If preservatives are present, the morphine should be diluted in 0.13 ml/kg of physiologic saline before injection. Side effects are uncommon, but the procedure is not recommended for patients suffering from septicemia, coagulation defects, or inflammation of the lumbosacral spinal area.

Intravenous infusion

Intravenous infusion of local analgesics is not performed commonly in dogs or cats, but may be useful in some situations. In this procedure, a tourniquet is applied to the area to be affected (e.g., immediately above the elbow if the foreleg is to be anesthetized), and a calculated amount of local analgesic is injected into a superficial vein using a 22-gauge, 1.5-inch needle. The usual dose used is 2 to 3 ml of 1% lidocaine without epinephrine, not to exceed 4 mg/kg. Within 3 to 5 minutes, there is total desensitization of the limb distal to the tourniquet, allowing 25 to 30 minutes of analgesia. An additional advantage of this technique is the relatively blood-free surgery site that it affords. As with other local analgesic procedures, however, patient restraint may be a problem unless concurrent sedation or neuroleptanalgesia is provided.

Sensation returns to the affected area within a few minutes of release of the tourniquet. It is very important to remove the tourniquet soon after the procedure is completed. If the tourniquet is in place more than 2 hours, prolonged hypoxia of the tissues of the limb may result, leading to tissue necrosis. In all patients removal of the tourniquet should be gradual (over a 5-minute period), since this helps prevent an excessive concentration quantities of the local analgesic from reaching the heart and brain.

Toxicity

The use of local analgesics is not without risk, and several adverse side effects have been recorded:

1. If local analgesic is injected into a nerve fiber, temporary or permanent loss of function may result.
2. Tissue irritation may occur with the use of some local analgesics. Mepivacaine (Carbocaine) is preferred over other local analgesics by some veterinarians because it appears to have little local toxicity.
3. Paresthesia, an abnormal sensation of tingling, pain, or irritation, may be present in an anesthetized area during recovery from local analgesia. Humans also experience this sensation; it occurs during recovery from ''freezing'' of the

oral cavity with Novocaine. Animals should be monitored during recovery because they may occasionally chew or otherwise traumatize affected areas.

4. Humans and animals may exhibit allergic reactions to local analgesics, usually in the form of a skin rash or hives. Anaphylaxis is also occasionally seen. Local analgesics should not be used in patients in which a previous allergic reaction to these drugs has been observed.

5. Systemic toxicity may occur, particularly if a local analgesic is inadvertently given intravenously without the use of a tourniquet.* Systemic toxicity may be seen even if the drug is placed in the subcutaneous tissues, particularly if a large amount of local analgesic is injected.

   The most common signs of systemic toxicity originate in the central nervous system and include muscle twitching, sedation or hyperexcitability, convulsions, and respiratory depression. Treatment of CNS signs may include injection of diazepam and administration of oxygen through an endotracheal tube.

   Cardiovascular effects may be observed because of the direct effect of local analgesics on the heart. In particular, intravenous injection of lidocaine has a profound effect on conduction of electrical impulses within the heart muscle. This characteristic is undesirable when performing local analgesia, but makes this drug of use in treating certain types of ventricular dysrhythmias.

6. Epidural anesthesia and spinal anesthesia may be hazardous if incorrectly performed. It is possible to traumatize the spinal cord or cauda equina, particularly if the animal is struggling during placement of the needle. Inflammation and fibrosis have been reported after epidural infiltration of local analgesics containing preservatives. Additionally, myelitis (spinal cord inflammation) and meningitis (inflammation of the pia, arachnoid, or dura mater) may occur if asepsis is not maintained.

7. If local analgesics are permitted to infiltrate into the cranial portion of the spinal cord, serious toxicity and even death may occur. If the local analgesic reaches the midthoracic vertebrae, innervation of the intercostal muscles may be blocked, interfering with normal respiration. If local analgesic diffuses as far forward as the cervical spinal cord, the phrenic nerve may be blocked. This nerve innervates the diaphragm, and loss of function may result in respiratory paralysis. Diffusion of local analgesic into the cervical and thoracic spinal cord also may affect sympathetic nerves supplying the heart and blood vessels, resulting in a sympathetic blockade and symptoms of bradycardia, decreased cardiac output, and hypotension.

8. Hypotension resulting from blockade of sympathetic neurons may occur after epidural infusion and other local analgesia techniques. Careful monitoring of

---

*It has been reported that up to 2 mg/kg of lidocaine may be injected intravenously without significant adverse side effects.

capillary refill time and pulse rate will alert the anesthetist to a fall in blood pressure. Treatment consists of intravenous fluid administration at a rate of 20 ml/kg over a 15- to 20-minute period.

In general, local analgesic toxicity can be minimized by following a few simple rules:

1. The dose of lidocaine given subcutaneously to any patient should not exceed 10 mg/kg. The smallest possible dose should be used.
2. Small, undamaged needles must be used for injection.
3. The injection site should be surgically prepared, and the injection should be given in an aseptic manner.
4. The anesthetist should always aspirate before injecting local analgesic, to ensure that inadvertent intravenous administration does not occur.
5. When performing epidural analgesia, care should be taken to keep the head elevated to avoid gravitational flow of the analgesic into the anterior spinal canal around the thoracic and cervical spinal cord. The anesthetist should be prepared to intubate and artificially ventilate any patient undergoing epidural analgesia, because this may be necessary if intercostal and phrenic nerve function is impaired.

CONTROLLED VENTILATION

The anesthetist commonly is called on to assist or control patient ventilation during anesthesia. In *assisted ventilation,* the anesthetist ensures that an increased volume of air is delivered to the patient, although the patient initiates each inspiration. In *controlled ventilation,* the anesthetist forcefully delivers all of the air that is required by the patient, and the patient does not make any spontaneous respiratory efforts. The anesthetist controls the volume of air, rate of respiration, and the pressure of air introduced into the animal.

Types of assisted or controlled ventilation

Ventilation assistance or control may take several forms, including the following:

- Squeezing the reservoir bag once every 5 to 10 minutes. The anesthetist thereby assists the patient's breathing on an intermittent basis.
- Continuous ventilation of the patient by bagging every 5 seconds. Usually, the anesthetist controls patient ventilation in this case.
- Continuous ventilation of the patient by means of a mechanical ventilator. The anesthetist adjusts the ventilator to completely control patient ventilation. Mechanical ventilators also can be used to assist, rather than control, patient ventilation.

Any procedure by which the anesthetist forcefully delivers oxygen and anesthetic gas to the patient's lungs may be termed *positive pressure ventilation (PPV)*. In positive pressure ventilation, the lungs are filled with air by the pressure of gas entering the airways, either from the reservoir bag or a mechanical ventilator. This differs from normal patient breathing, in which air is drawn into the lungs by the movement of the animal's diaphragm, intercostal, and abdominal muscles. Whether achieved by bagging the patient or by mechanical ventilation, PPV is intended to ensure that the animal receives adequate oxygen and is able to exhale adequate amounts of carbon dioxide. This is a concern in veterinary anesthesia because the patient's own ventilation efforts are often inadequate to achieve these objectives.

Ventilation in the awake animal

To understand the use of positive pressure ventilation in anesthesia, it is necessary to first review the mechanics of normal breathing and the reasons why these mechanics may be ineffective in the anesthetized animal. Ventilation is the physical movement of air and anesthetic gases into and out of the lungs and upper respiratory passageways. Ventilation has two parts: an active phase (inhalation) and a passive phase (exhalation). Inhalation is initiated by the respiratory center in the brain, which is triggered by an increased level of carbon dioxide in the arterial blood ($Paco_2$). As $Paco_2$ rises above a threshold level, the respiratory center initiates the active inspiratory phase by stimulating the intercostal muscles and diaphragm to move, expanding the thorax. This creates a negative pressure (partial vacuum) within the chest, which causes the lungs to expand. As the lungs expand, air moves through the air passages and into the alveoli. When the lungs reach an adequate volume, nerve impulses feed back to the respiratory center, signaling the brain to stop the active phase of respiration. The intercostal muscles and diaphragm then relax, and exhalation takes place as the thorax and lungs collapse. Exhalation is passive, which means that no active muscle movement occurs. During exhalation, the carbon dioxide level in the blood begins to rise again, and after a short pause the respiratory center responds by initiating another inspiration.

Normally, inspiration lasts approximately twice as long as exhalation. For example, in an animal breathing 20 times per minute, each inspiration will last approximately 2 seconds and each exhalation will last approximately 1 second.

The amount of air that passes in or out of the lungs in a single breath is the *tidal volume*. Animals that are breathing deeply have a relatively large tidal volume, whereas animals that have shallow breathing (or are panting) have a relatively small tidal volume.

The *respiratory rate* is the number of tidal volumes that occurs in 1 minute. The *respiratory minute volume* is the total amount of air that moves in and out of the lungs in 1 minute. This value can be found by multiplying the average tidal volume by the respiratory rate.

Ventilation in the anesthetized animal

Ventilation in the anesthetized animal differs significantly from normal ventilation described above. These differences include the following:

1. Tranquilizers and general anesthetics may decrease the responsiveness of the respiratory center in the brain to carbon dioxide. This means that inspiration does not occur as often in the anesthetized animal as in the normal awake animal, despite the fact that carbon dioxide may be significantly elevated. The respiratory rate of an anesthetized animal is therefore reduced compared to that of a normal awake animal. This explains the observation that a respiratory rate of 12 to 20 breaths per minute is very common in cats and dogs under inhalation anesthesia, whereas the same animal would normally have a respiratory rate between 20 and 30 breaths per minute when awake.

2. Tranquilizers and general anesthetics relax the intercostal muscles and diaphragm, causing them to expand less than normal during the inspiratory phase. Since the chest does not expand fully, the tidal volume is reduced compared to normal. Tidal volume in the normal animal at rest is approximately 10 to 15 ml/kg. In the anesthetized animal, tidal volume may be less than 8 ml/kg. The anesthetist may become aware of the reduced tidal volume by noting that the reservoir bag does not expand appreciably during expiration (i.e., the volume of gas exhaled is relatively small).

Because tidal volume and respiratory rate are decreased, respiratory minute volume is also decreased. The amount of air entering and leaving the lungs in the anesthetized animal is therefore considerably reduced compared to the normal awake animal. This has several consequences:

1. Pa_{CO_2} rises in the anesthetized animal (i.e., carbon dioxide produced by the body is not eliminated as rapidly as normal). As blood CO_2 rises, it joins with water molecules in the bloodstream to form bicarbonate ions (HCO_3^-) and hydrogen ions (H^+). The accumulation of hydrogen ions causes the pH of circulating blood to fall, leading to respiratory acidosis. Blood pH in the normal awake animal is between 7.38 and 7.42, whereas in the anesthetized animal, blood pH may be as low as 7.20.

2. If the anesthetized animal is breathing room air, Pa_{O_2} will fall below normal values, as a result of the decreased respiratory minute volume. This occurs because less oxygen is entering the lungs, and therefore less is available to be absorbed into the blood.

3. Because tidal volume is reduced, the alveoli do not expand as fully as normal on inspiration. In fact, some sections of the lung may partially collapse, and the alveoli may not expand at all. This condition is called *atelectasis*.

The anesthetist has several ways of compensating for these effects. The Pao_2 can be elevated to normal levels (and, in fact, often above normal levels) if the patient is supplied with adequate oxygen. This is easily achieved, since animals connected to anesthetic machines normally receive 100% oxygen (or a mixture of oxygen and nitrous oxide). The anesthetized patient connected to an anesthetic machine is unlikely to have a reduced Pao_2 unless a problem exists (e.g., the machine runs out of oxygen, oxygen flow rate is too low, or insufficient oxygen is provided with nitrous oxide).

It is more difficult to prevent atelectasis or an increase in $Paco_2$ and resulting respiratory acidosis. In animals anesthetized for prolonged periods or in patients with very depressed respiration, these problems may become significant. The anesthetist should take active steps to counter these changes in the anesthetized patient by assisting ventilation. This can be done in one of two ways:

1. Intermittent or continuous bagging of the patient using the reservoir bag (also called manual ventilation). For most patients, intermittent bagging (once every 5 minutes) is adequate.
2. Mechanical ventilation using a ventilator

Whichever method is chosen, the patient must be intubated and connected to an anesthetic machine before ventilation can be assisted. (Temporary ventilation assistance also can be given in the absence of an endotracheal tube, using an Ambu bag.) Air enters the respiratory passages under pressure and causes the alveoli to expand. Exhalation is passive and occurs when the positive pressure is discontinued, allowing the lungs to empty. This type of ventilation can be contrasted to normal ventilation, in which active expansion of the chest cavity causes a partial vacuum to form within the alveoli, which draws air into the lungs.

Manual ventilation

Manual ventilation can be used to assist or totally control the ventilation cycle, by means of pressure placed on the reservoir bag by the anesthetist's hand. The procedure is very similar to that used to treat respiratory arrest, described in Chapter 6. The pop-off valve is closed and the reservoir bag is compressed until the lungs are inflated. When pressure is released on the reservoir bag, exhalation can occur. The anesthetist must use caution to ensure that the pressure used is not excessive: the patient's chest should only rise to the same extent as with normal awake respiration, and the pressure manometer reading should not exceed 20 cm H_2O (14 mm Hg).

Manual ventilation can be performed on an occasional basis (once every 5 minutes) on any anesthetized patient. These periodic "sighs" help to expand collapsed alveoli and reverse atelectasis.

It is advisable to turn the vaporizer setting to zero before bagging the patient, if an in-circle, nonprecision vaporizer is in use. This helps prevent sudden vaporization of large amounts of anesthetic caused by increased flow of carrier gas through the vaporizer. If a precision vaporizer is in use, it is not necessary to turn the concentration setting to zero, as back flow compensation is usually present. (If continuous manual ventilation is used, however, it may be advisable to reduce the precision vaporizer setting, or the patient's level of anesthesia may become too deep because of increased delivery of anesthetic to the lungs. The anesthetist should closely monitor the patient and adjust the vaporizer setting based on the patient's depth.)

For some patients, respiratory depression is so severe that hypercarbia and respiratory acidosis develop despite intermittent bagging. The anesthetist may be able to identify these patients by their shallow breaths (small tidal volume) and infrequent respirations (respiratory rate is 8 breaths per minute or less). These patients require more aggressive ventilation, in the form of continuous manual or mechanical ventilation. In this procedure, ventilation is assisted starting immediately after induction, at which point the anesthetist should use the reservoir bag to superimpose positive pressure on the animal's own spontaneous breathing efforts. The assisted ventilation rate should be 12 to 16 respirations per minute, at a manometer pressure of 15 to 20 cm H_2O (11 to 14 mm Hg). After 3 to 5 minutes, the patient's spontaneous breathing efforts usually disappear, and the anesthetist has gained control over ventilation. If the patient resists the anesthetist's efforts to control ventilation, it may be necessary to use a neuromuscular blocking agent, which paralyzes the muscles of respiration.*

Once control is established, a ventilation rate of 8 to 12 "breaths" per minute is usually adequate. A pressure of 15 to 20 cm H_2O is recommended, unless the chest is open, in which case a pressure of 20 to 30 cm H_2O may be required. When squeezing the reservoir bag, the inspiratory time should be 1 to 1.5 seconds. Expiratory time should be twice as long as inspiratory time. The pop-off valve must be closed when the reservoir bag is squeezed; however, it should be opened briefly between every 2 to 3 breaths, to allow gas to escape from the circuit. The anesthetist should not hold on to the reservoir bag between breaths because this causes

---

*Not all patients require this amount of effort in order to gain control over ventilation. For many patients it is adequate to give a few large tidal volumes manually, then connect the patient to a ventilator. The initial large tidal volumes depress the animal's urge to breathe by lowering the blood carbon dioxide levels. Once connected to a ventilator or undergoing continuous manual ventilation, the patient usually stops spontaneous breathing efforts within 1 minute.

increased pressure in the lungs, which may cause alveolar rupture or increased intrathoracic pressure.

Continuous manual bagging can be performed using either a rebreathing or a nonrebreathing system. Nonrebreathing systems usually lack a manometer, and the anesthetist must use sight and touch to determine the optimal tidal volume.

When the surgical procedure is nearing completion, it is necessary for the anesthetist to "wean the animal off" the controlled ventilation procedure. This is done by turning off the anesthetic and nitrous oxide, while continuing to ventilate the patient with oxygen. If a neuromuscular blocking agent has been used, it should be reversed if possible. The anesthetist should gradually reduce the rate of inspirations to approximately 5 per minute, while observing the animal for evidence of spontaneous breathing. When this is seen, the patient's ventilation can continue to be assisted by squeezing a small amount of air from the reservoir bag with each inspiration. Eventually, the animal regains the ability to maintain a normal rate and tidal volume, and ventilation assistance can be discontinued. Occasionally this may take several minutes to reestablish, particularly in older and debilitated patients and patients in which ventilation has been controlled for a long time. Stimulation of the patient by pinching the toe pads or gently rubbing the thorax and abdomen may help the patient regain spontaneous respiratory movements.

Continuously assisted ventilation, as described above, has many advantages to the patient. It prevents hypoxia, efficiently eliminates carbon dioxide, and prevents respiratory acidosis. It is particularly useful in animals with compromised respiration, including obese patients, debilitated patients, animals undergoing thoracic surgery, and animals with diaphragmatic hernia, pneumonia, or head trauma. It is also useful in animals showing hypoventilation from any other cause, including prolonged anesthesia.

Mechanical ventilation

Mechanical ventilation is similar to continuous manual ventilation in many respects. However, patient breathing is controlled by a ventilator, which replaces continual compression of the reservoir bag. The ventilator automatically compresses a bellows, which forces oxygen and anesthetic gas into the patient's air passageways via an endotracheal tube. There are many types of ventilators that can be used with a veterinary anesthesia machine; they vary in the number and complexity of the controls (Fig. 7-4). Ventilators can be attached to a circle system by removing the reservoir bag and attaching the outlet of the ventilator to the anesthetic machine. The scavenger should be attached to the exhaust port of the ventilator.

Depending on the type of ventilator used, the anesthetist may choose to deliver gases on inspiration according to a pressure cycle, volume cycle, or time cycle. The

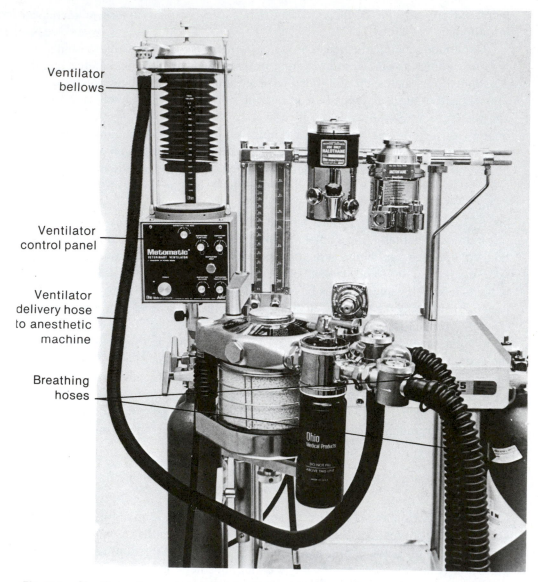

Ventilator
bellows

Ventilator
control panel

Ventilator
delivery hose
to anesthetic
machine

Breathing
hoses

Fig. 7-4. Ventilator for use in small animal anesthesia. Machine illustrated has two out-of-circuit vaporizers and one in-circuit vaporizer. Mechanical ventilation should not be attempted when in-circuit vaporizer is in use. (From Warren RG: *Small animal anesthesia,* St Louis, 1983, Mosby.)

pressure-cycled ventilator (such as the Bird Mark 7 Respirator) will supply air until the pressure reaches a preset level. A time cycle ventilator (Small Animal Ventilator, Drager) supplies air according to a set inspiratory time. A volume cycle type (such as the Ohio Meramatic) delivers a preset tidal volume regardless of the pressure required. In volume-cycled ventilators, the anesthetist must adjust the volume of gas to be delivered on inspiration (usually 15 to 20 ml/kg, less if respiration is to be assisted rather than controlled). The animal's chest should be observed to rise with each inspiration. Respiratory rate is usually 8 to 12 breaths per minute. Duration of inspiration is set at 1 to 2 seconds, and duration of expiration should be 2 to 4 seconds with an inspiratory:expiratory ratio of 1:2 to 1:3.

Like manual ventilation, mechanical ventilation is particularly indicated for patients with compromised respiration. It is not normally necessary in healthy anesthetized patients, in which intermittent manual bagging (once every 5 minutes) is usually sufficient. Mechanical ventilation is used most commonly in animals undergoing a thoracotomy or other lengthy surgery, in which continuous manual ventilation would be difficult for the anesthetist. Animals undergoing thoracic surgery often have preexisting cardiovascular and/or pulmonary disease and are at significant risk of cardiovascular collapse and/or respiratory arrest if conventional anesthesia with unassisted ventilation is pursued. In addition to mechanical ventilation, these patients benefit from preoxygenation and intravenous induction techniques (rather than mask or chamber induction). In these and other patients, mechanical ventilation may be combined with the use of neuromuscular blocking agents (see section below).

Risks of controlled ventilation

Controlled ventilation, whether by manual ventilation using a reservoir bag or by a ventilator, has the potential to damage the animal's lungs, if done incorrectly.

- Overventilation of the patient may rupture alveoli, resulting in pneumothorax or mediastinal emphysema.
- Cardiac output may be decreased if positive pressure is maintained throughout the respiratory cycle.
- If the ventilation rate is excessive, excessive amounts of carbon dioxide can be exhaled, leading to respiratory alkalosis.
- Controlled ventilation using an in-circle vaporizer is difficult and may be dangerous. Because of the lack of back pressure compensation in these vaporizers, the patient may receive excessive amounts of vaporized anesthetic.
- Mechanical ventilation is not intended to relieve the anesthetist of the necessity for patient monitoring. The anesthetist must closely monitor all animals in which ventilation is controlled or assisted, to ensure that patient depth and safety are maintained within acceptable limits.

NEUROMUSCULAR BLOCKING AGENTS

Neuromuscular blocking agents (also called muscle-paralyzing agents) are often used in human anesthesia, but have found only limited use in veterinary anesthesia. They are used most commonly in conjunction with mechanical ventilation, in order to paralyze the muscles of respiration. Use of neuromuscular blocking agents prevents spontaneous inspiratory efforts by the patient and allows more rapid and complete control of ventilation. These agents also are sometimes used in orthopedic surgery and other surgeries in which profound muscle relaxation is desired. They are used occasionally in conjunction with cesarean surgeries because they produce abdominal muscle relaxation but are not transferred through the placenta to the fetus. Neuromuscular blocking agents also may be useful in facilitating difficult intubation, including animals with laryngospasm. Occasionally muscle-paralyzing agents are used in conjunction with opioids, nitrous oxide, and other general anesthetic agents in "balanced anesthesia" techniques.

Neuromuscular blocking agents should be administered only after the patient has been anesthetized and respiration has been controlled by means of continuous manual or mechanical ventilation. These agents should be considered to be an adjunct to, rather than a replacement for, anesthesia with other agents. Use of neuromuscular blocking agents in a conscious animal is inhumane because these agents have no tranquilizing or analgesic properties. The patient given these drugs as the sole anesthetic agent will have normal sensitivity to pain, but will be unable to move or otherwise resist the surgeon's efforts. Control of respiration is also essential after the administration of these drugs, because the respiratory muscles will be paralyzed. As a result of this paralysis, it is difficult or impossible for the patient to breathe on its own.

Neuromuscular blocking agents act by interrupting normal transmission of impulses from the motor nerve to the muscle synapse. The site of action is the nerve-muscle junction where chemical transmitters such as acetylcholine are released by the nerve in close proximity to the muscle end plate. There are two ways in which muscle paralyzing agents may disrupt nervous transmission, and the agents used are classified as *depolarizing* or *nondepolarizing* according to which of the two mechanisms applies. Depolarizing agents, such as succinylcholine, act by causing a single surge of activity at the neuromuscular junction, which is followed by a period in which the muscle end plate is refractory to further stimulation. Animals given these agents may show spontaneous muscle movement, followed by paralysis. Nondepolarizing agents, such as gallamine, pancuronium, and atracurium besylate, act by blocking the receptors at the end plates. As their classification suggests, they do not cause an initial surge of activity at the neuromuscular junction.

Muscle-paralyzing agents are normally given by slow intravenous injection. The dose required varies between patients and the anesthetic protocol used. Most agents take effect within 2 minutes, and the duration of paralysis is approximately 10 to 30 minutes (although this varies considerably, depending on the agent used). If more prolonged paralysis is required, repeated doses can be given. Alternatively, some agents may be given by constant intravenous infusion.

Regardless of the agent used, only voluntary (skeletal) muscles are affected. Involuntary muscles, including cardiac muscle and the smooth muscle of the intestine and bladder, are unaffected by these agents. Skeletal muscles are affected in a predictable order: facial and neck paralysis is seen first, followed by paralysis of the tail, limbs, and abdominal muscles. The intercostal muscles and diaphragm are affected last.

Nondepolarizing agents may be reversed with an anticholinesterase agent, such as edrophonium or neostigmine. These reversing agents may have undesirable side effects, such as bradycardia and increased bronchial and salivary secretions, and should be given only after pretreatment with atropine. Neostigmine should not be given more than 2 to 3 times during the course of a single anesthesia, since cumulative effects may be seen.

The use of neuromuscular blocking agents is not without risk:

- Hypothermia is a common side effect, resulting from the decreased muscle tone seen in patients given these agents.
- Anesthetic depth may be difficult to assess because of the inhibition or absence of normal reflex responses and the absence of jaw tone.
- Muscle-paralyzing agents should not be used in animals with liver or kidney disease or in animals with glaucoma.
- Animals treated with aminoglycoside antibiotics, such as gentamicin, may show increased duration and intensity of muscle-paralyzing effects.
- Animals that have undergone recent treatments with organophosphate insecticides show an increased susceptibility to neuromuscular blocking agents. Other drugs, such as corticosteroids, furosemide and other diuretics, anticancer drugs, and epinephrine, have been shown to affect the potency of neuromuscular blocking agents. Concurrent use of isoflurane or halothane also increases the potency of these agents.

KEY POINTS

1. Local analgesia is the use of a chemical agent on sensory and motor neurons to produce a temporary loss of pain sensation and movement. Because of low patient toxicity, low cost, and minimal recovery time, local analgesia may be preferred to general anesthesia in some patients. Disadvantages include lack of patient restraint, risk of overdose in smaller patients, and technical difficulties.

2. If sufficient quantities of local analgesics reach the sympathetic ganglia, a *sympathetic blockade* may result. This causes flushing, increased skin temperature, and occasionally hypotension and bradycardia.

3. Local analgesics have many topical uses, including application to the conjunctiva or the epithelium of the respiratory or urogenital tracts.

4. Local analgesics may be injected in close proximity to a peripheral nerve, blocking sensation from the tissues served by the nerve. Surgical preparation of the area is necessary before local analgesia infusion. Epinephrine is commonly added to the local analgesic used for this procedure to delay absorption of the local analgesic agent from the site.

5. Epidural analgesia is achieved by injecting local analgesic in the epidural space, between the dura and the vertebrae. In dogs and cats, the injection is performed between the last lumbar vertebra and the sacrum. This technique is useful in debilitated patients and in patients requiring profound analgesia of the caudal abdomen, limbs, or pelvis.

6. Intravenous infusion of local analgesics may be useful for distal limb surgery, including amputation.

7. Local analgesics may be harmful if injected into a nerve fiber. They may also cause temporary *paresthesia,* which may result in self-mutilation.

8. Adverse systemic side effects of local analgesia include hyperexcitability, respiratory depression, and sympathetic blockade. Epidural analgesia may result in spinal cord trauma or paralysis of the muscles of respiration. Toxicity may be avoided by limiting the amount of lidocaine administered to the patient (maximum 10 mg/kg).

9. Controlled or assisted ventilation may be used to deliver oxygen and anesthetic to the patient. Either a mechanical ventilator or manual bagging may be used. These procedures are particularly useful in patients with poor respiratory function caused by the use of anesthetic agents or respiratory disease. Controlled or assisted ventilation helps prevent the development of respiratory acidosis and pulmonary atelectasis.

10. Manual ventilation can be achieved by gently squeezing the reservoir bag at a rate of 8 to 12 breaths per minute and a pressure of 15 to 20 cm H_2O. Inspiration time should be 1 to 1.5 seconds, and expiratory time should be 2 to 3 seconds. Manual ventilation is difficult if a nonprecision vaporizer is used.

11. Mechanical ventilators may be incorporated into either a rebreathing or nonrebreathing system. Depending on the type of ventilator used, the anesthetist may control the pressure or volume of gas to be delivered, the respiratory rate, and the length of inspiration and expiration.

12. If controlled ventilation is used, the anesthetist must use caution to avoid excessive expansion of the alveoli, continuous positive pressure, and excessive ventilation rates.

13. Neuromuscular blocking agents may be useful in some anesthetic procedures for allowing relaxation of voluntary muscles. They should never be used as the sole anesthetic agent.

14. Neuromuscular blocking agents may be depolarizing or nondepolarizing in their action. Nondepolarizing agents may be reversed by the administration of neostigmine.

15. Neuromuscular blocking agents may cause systemic effects, such as hypothermia, increased intraocular pressure, and respiratory failure. Mechanical or manual ventilation should be available when these agents are used.

16. Many drugs, including aminoglycoside antibiotics, organophosphates, and diuretics, may either potentiate or reduce the effectiveness of neuromuscular blocking agents.

REVIEW QUESTIONS

1. In the normal awake animal the main stimulus to breathe is the result of:
   a. Excess oxygen concentration in the blood
   b. Excess carbon dioxide concentration in the blood
   c. Insufficient oxygen in the blood
   d. Insufficient carbon dioxide in the blood
2. In the normal awake animal inhalation lasts _____ times as long as exhalation.
   a. $\frac{1}{2}$
   b. 2
   c. 3
   d. 4
3. The normal tidal volume in an awake animal is _____ ml/kg.
   a. 5-10
   b. 10-15
   c. 16-20
   d. 20-25
4. In the anesthetized animal that is breathing room air, the anesthetist may expect to see:
   a. An increase in the Pa_{CO_2} and a decrease in the Pa_{O_2}
   b. A decrease in the Pa_{CO_2} and an increase in the Pa_{O_2}

   c. A decrease in the Pa_{CO_2} and a decrease in the Pa_{O_2}

   d. An increase in the Pa_{CO_2} and an increase in the Pa_{O_2}

5. Local analgesic agents will have a direct effect on the:
   - **a.** Peripheral nervous system
   - **b.** Central nervous system
   - **c.** Peripheral and central nervous systems

6. Local analgesic agents may affect:
   - **a.** Sensory neurons
   - **b.** Motor neurons
   - **c.** Both sensory and motor neurons

7. Local analgesic agents work because:
   - **a.** They mechanically block nerve impulse transmission
   - **b.** They interfere with the movement of Na ions
   - **c.** They block the impulses at the spinal cord level

8. When an analgesic agent is infused around a major nerve, the procedure is referred to as a (an):
   - **a.** Line block
   - **b.** Epidural block
   - **c.** Local nerve block
   - **d.** Intravenous analgesia

9. Epinephrine may be mixed with a local analgesic agent to prolong the effects of the drug.

   True   False

10. When performing an epidural, one must be aware that the spinal cord in the _____ may extend as far caudally as S1.
    - **a.** Cat
    - **b.** Dog

11. The maximum subcutaneous dose of lidocaine for a patient is _____ mg/kg.
    - **a.** 1
    - **b.** 5
    - **c.** 10
    - **d.** 15

12. The blood pH of an anesthetized animal tends to be:
    - **a.** Acidotic
    - **b.** Alkalotic
    - **c.** Normal

13. The term *atelectasis* refers to:
    - **a.** Excess fluid in the respiratory system
    - **b.** A lack of breathing
    - **c.** Collapsing of the alveoli
    - **d.** Constriction of the bronchi

14. In the anesthetized patient we would expect to have a state of:
    - **a.** Respiratory alkalosis
    - **b.** Metabolic alkalosis
    - **c.** Respiratory acidosis
    - **d.** Metabolic acidosis

15. The term *to sigh* refers to giving:
    a. Oxygen to the patient
    b. An increased volume to the patient
    c. Only room air to the patient
    d. A decreased volume to the patient
16. If you are ventilating the patient, it may be necessary to:
    a. Increase the vaporizer setting
    b. Decrease the vaporizer setting
    c. Change the carbon dioxide absorber granules every hour
17. When you wish to stop ventilating a patient, it may take up to 5 minutes before the patient starts to breathe totally on its own again. This occurs because there is:
    a. A decreased oxygen concentration in the blood
    b. A decreased carbon dioxide concentration in the blood
    c. An increased carbon dioxide concentration in the blood
    d. An increase in anesthetic concentration in the blood
18. While a patient's breathing is being assisted manually, the exhalation phase should be:
    a. As long as the inhalation phase
    b. Half as long as the inhalation phase
    c. Twice as long as the inhalation phase
    d. Three times as long as the inhalation phase
19. A neuromuscular blocking agent will not only paralyze skeletal muscle, but it will also give some analgesia.
    True   False
20. When an animal is given a _____ drug, an initial surge of muscle activity may be seen before there is paralysis of the muscles.
    a. Depolarizing
    b. Nondepolarizing
21. The muscle type that is most dramatically affected by muscle relaxant drugs includes:
    a. Cardiac
    b. Smooth muscle
    c. Skeletal muscle
22. Both depolarizing and nondepolarizing drugs can be reversed.
    True   False

For the following questions more than one answer may be correct.

23. Problems that may result from controlled ventilation may include:
    a. A decreased cardiac output
    b. Muscle twitching
    c. A state of respiratory alkalosis
    d. Ruptured alveoli
24. Local analgesic agents work well when applied:
    a. Topically on the epidermis
    b. Topically on mucous membranes
    c. Topically on the cornea
    d. Only by injection

25. Factors that may interfere with the action of local analgesic agents include:
   a. Fat
   b. Scar tissue
   c. Rapid heart rate
   d. Hemorrhage
   e. Large muscle mass
26. Clinical signs of systemic toxicity from a local analgesic agent may include:
   a. Sedation
   b. Convulsions
   c. Muscle twitching
   d. Respiratory depression
27. The effects that could result from an epidural if the drug reached the cervical spinal cord include:
   a. Sympathetic blockade
   b. Paralysis of intercostal muscles
   c. Paralysis of diaphragm
   d. Hypertension

ANSWERS FOR CHAPTER 7

1. b   **2.** b   **3.** b   **4.** a   **5.** a   **6.** c   **7.** b   **8.** c   **9.** True   **10.** a   **11.** c
12. a   **13.** c   **14.** c   **15.** b   **16.** b   **17.** b   **18.** c   **19.** False   **20.** a   **21.** c
22. False   **23.** a, c, d   **24.** b, c   **25.** a, b, d, e   **26.** a, b, c, d   **27.** a, b, c

SELECTED READINGS

Heath RB: Lumbosacral epidural management, *Vet Clin North Am (Small Anim Pract)* 22:417-419, 1992.

Hubbell JAE: Disadvantges of neuromuscular blocking agents, *Vet Clin North Am (Small Anim Pract)* 22:351-352, 1992.

Ilkiw JE: Advantages of and guidelines for using neuromuscular blocking agents, *Vet Clin North Am (Small Anim Pract)* 22:347-350, 1992.

Muir WW, III, Hubbell JAE: *A handbook of veterinary anesthesia,* St Louis, 1989, Mosby.

Pascoe PJ: Advantages and guidelines for using epidural drugs for analgesia, *Vet Clin North Am (Small Anim Pract)* 22:421-423, 1992.

Short CE: *Principles and practice of veterinary anesthesia,* Baltimore, 1987, Williams & Wilkins.

Valverde A, Dyson DH, McDonell WN, Pascoe PJ: Use of epidural morphine in the dog for pain relief, *Vet Comp Orthop Trauma* 2:55-58, 1989.

Warren RG: *Small animal anesthesia,* St Louis, 1983, Mosby.

APPENDIX A

Standard values and equivalents

STANDARD VALUES

Metric weights

1 gram (1 g) = Weight of 1 ml water at 4° C
1000 g = 1 kilogram (kg)
0.1 g = 1 decigram (dg)
0.01 g = 1 centigram (cg)
0.001 g = 1 milligram (mg)
0.001 mg = 1 microgram (μg)

Metric volumes

1 liter (L) = 1000 milliliters (ml) or 1000 cubic centimeters (cc)
0.001 L = 1 ml
1 deciliter (dl) = 100 ml

Solution equivalents

1 part in 10 = 10.00% (1 ml contains 100 mg)
1 part in 50 = 2.00% (1 ml contains 20 mg)
1 part in 100 = 1.00% (1 ml contains 10 mg)
1 part in 200 = 0.50% (1 ml contains 5 mg)
1 part in 500 = 0.20% (1 ml contains 2 mg)
1 part in 1000 = 0.10% (1 ml contains 1 mg) = 1000 μg per ml
1 part in 1500 = 0.066% (1 ml contains 0.66 mg)
1 part in 2600 = 0.038% (1 ml contains 0.38 mg)
1 part in 5000 = 0.02% (1 ml contains 0.20 mg)
1 part in 50,000 = 0.002% (1 ml contains 0.02 mg)
1 part in 200,000 = 0.0005% (1 ml contains 5 micrograms)

The number of milligrams in 1 ml of any solution of known percentage strength is obtained by moving the decimal one place to the right. For example, a 1% solution contains 10 mg/ml. By definition, a percent solution contains the specified weight (in grams) of the solute in 100 ml of total solution. For example, a 5% dextrose and water solution contains 5 g of dextrose dissolved in each 100 ml of water.

Approximate equivalents

Weights

1 kg = 2.2 avoirdupois or imperial pounds
1 kg = 2.6 apothecary or troy pounds
1 oz = 30 g
(Avoirdupois or imperial = 28.350 g)
(Apothecary or troy = 31.1035 g)
1 lb = 453.6 g = 0.4536 kg = 16 oz

Volumes

1 liter = 1.06 U.S. quarts = 33.8 fluid ounces
1 U.S. pint = 473.2 ml
1 quart = 946.4 ml

Length

1 meter (m) = 39.37 inches (in)
1 in = $\frac{1}{12}$ ft = 2.54 centimeters (cm)

Pressure

1 lb per sq in (psi) = 0.070 kg/sq cm
= 51.7 mm of mercury (Hg)
= 70.3 cm of water (H_2O)

$$1 \text{ mm Hg} = 1.36 \text{ cm } H_2O$$
$$1 \text{ cm } H_2O = 0.73 \text{ mm Hg}$$
$$1 \text{ atmosphere} = 760 \text{ mm Hg}$$
$$= 14.7 \text{ lb/sq in}$$
$$= 29.9 \text{ in Hg}$$
$$= 1.03 \text{ kg/sq cm}$$
$$= 33.9 \text{ ft } H_2O$$
$$= 760 \text{ torr}$$
$$= 1013.25 \text{ millibars}$$
$$= 100 \text{ kilopascals (kPa)}$$

EQUIVALENTS OF CENTIGRADE AND FAHRENHEIT THERMOMETRIC SCALES

Fahrenheit to centigrade: $^\circ C = (^\circ F - 32) \times \frac{5}{9}$

Centigrade to fahrenheit: $^\circ F = (^\circ C \times \frac{9}{5}) + 32$

Centigrade degree	Fahrenheit degree	Centigrade degree	Fahrenheit degree	Centigrade degree	Fahrenheit degree
−17	+ 1.4	5	41.0	27	80.6
−16	3.2	6	42.8	28	82.4
−15	5.0	7	44.6	29	84.2
−14	6.8	8	46.4	30	86.0
−13	8.6	9	48.2	31	87.8
−12	10.4	10	50.0	32	89.6
−11	12.2	11	51.8	33	91.4
−10	14.0	12	53.6	34	93.2
− 9	15.8	13	55.4	**35**	**95.0**
− 8	17.6	14	57.2	**36**	**96.8**
− 7	19.4	15	59.0	**37**	**98.6**
− 6	21.2	16	60.8	**38**	**100.4**
− 5	23.0	17	62.6	**39**	**102.2**
− 4	24.8	18	64.4	**40**	**104.0**
− 3	26.6	19	66.2	41	105.8
− 2	28.4	20	68.0	42	107.6
− 1	30.2	21	69.8	43	109.4
0	**32.0**	22	71.6	44	111.2
+ 1	33.8	23	73.4	45	113.0
2	35.6	24	75.2	⋮	
3	37.4	25	77.0	⋮	
4	39.2	26	78.8	100	212.0

Catheter comparison scale

(For comparison of endotracheal tube sizes)

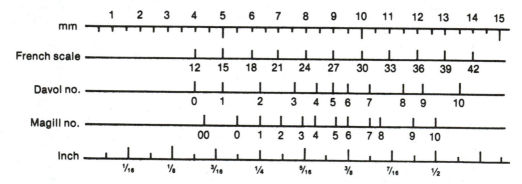

Modified from Lumb WV, Jones EW: *Veterinary anesthesia,* Philadelphia, 1973, Lea & Febiger.

APPENDIX C

Equipment and drugs for use in an emergency crash kit

The following list of equipment and supplies may be altered depending on the veterinarian's preference. Some supplies (i.e., laryngoscope, Ambu bag, sterile fluids) that are easily accessible within the clinical setting may be omitted from the kit.

EQUIPMENT AND SUPPLIES

a. Endotracheal tubes (various sizes)
b. Penlight
c. Adhesive tape (1-inch)
d. Gauze roll (1- or 2-inch)
e. Sterile gauze pads
f. IV fluid administration set
g. Burette for fluid administration
h. Intravenous catheters (18-, 20-, and 22-gauge)
i. Syringes (1-, 3-, 5-, 20-ml sizes)
j. Needles (18-, 20-, 22-gauge)
k. Alcohol swabs
l. Sterile surgery instruments, including scalpel handle and blades, hemostats, thumb forceps, scissors, needle holder

m. Sterile suture material (absorbable and nonabsorbable)
n. Sterile saline for injection
o. Sterile fluids (lactated Ringer's, saline, 5% dextrose)
p. Vacutainer needles and tubes (lavender and red top)
q. Stethoscope
r. Sterile gloves
s. Thermometer
t. Sterile lubricant and lidocaine gel
u. Ambu bag
v. Laryngoscope

DRUGS

a. Epinephrine (1 : 1000)—may be refrigerated
b. Dopamine
c. Sodium bicarbonate
d. Atropine
e. 10% calcium chloride or calcium gluconate
f. 2% lidocaine without epinephrine
g. Doxapram
h. Dexamethasone
i. Prednisolone sodium succinate
j. Diazepam
k. Naloxone
l. Yohimbine
m. Butorphanol
n. Heparin
o. Furosemide

NOTE: A list of emergency drug dosages should be posted or included in the kit.

Index